Neurosurgical Treatment of Persistent Pain

Pain and Headache

Vol. 11

Series Editor
Philip L. Gildenberg, Houston, Tex.

KARGER

Basel · München · Paris · London · New York · New Delhi · Singapore · Tokyo · Sydney

Neurosurgical Treatment of Persistent Pain

Physiological and Pathological Mechanisms of Human Pain

Jan M. Gybels, MD, PhD

Professor of Neurology and Neurosurgery, Chief of Clinic of the Department of Neurosurgery,
Director Laboratory Experimental Neurology, KUL University of Leuven, Leuven, Belgium

William H. Sweet, MD, DSc, DHC, FRCS Ed (Hon.)

Professor of Surgery Emeritus, Harvard Medical School,
Whilom Chief, Neurosurgical Service, Massachusetts General Hospital, Boston, Mass. USA

70 figures and 33 tables, 1989

KARGER

Basel · München · Paris · London · New York · New Delhi · Singapore · Tokyo · Sydney

Pain and Headache

Library of Congress Cataloging-in-Publication Data
Gybels, J.
Neurosurgical Treatment of persistent pain: physiological and pathological mechanisms of human pain / Jan M. Gybels, William H. Sweet.
(Pain and headache; vol. 11)
Includes bibliographies and index.
1. Intractable pain – Surgery. 2. Intractable pain – Pathophysiology. 3. Central nervous system – Surgery. I. Sweet, William Herbert, 1910– II. Title. III. Series.
[DNLM: 1. Nervous System – surgery. 2. Pain, Intractable – physiopathology. 3. Pain, Intractable – therapy. W1 PA293 vol. 11 / WL 368 G996n]
RD595.5.G83 1989 617′.48–dc 19
DNLM/DLC for Library of Congress 88–37194 CIP
ISBN 3–8055–4885–0

Bibliographic Indices
This publication is listed in bibliographic services, including Current Contents® and Index Medicus.

Drug Dosage

The authors and the publisher have exerted every effort to ensure that drug selection and dosage set forth in this text are in accord with current recommendations and practice at the time of publication. However, in view of ongoing research, changes in government regulations, and the constant flow of information relating to drug therapy and drug reactions, the reader is urged to check the package insert for each drug for any change in indications and dosage and for added warnings and precautions. This is particularly important when the recommended agent is a new and/or infrequently employed drug.

ISBN 3–8055–4885–0

Contents

To Hélène, Emmanuel, Marie,
Jan-Willem and Elisabeth
To Elizabeth, David,
Gwendolyn and Paula

Legend for the Cover Illustration

Munch described the motive of the painting appearing on the cover in the following words: "One evening I was walking along a path – on one side lay the city and below me the fjord. I was tired and ill – I stopped and looked out across the fjord – the sun was setting – the clouds were dyed red like blood.

I felt a scream pass through nature; it seemed to me that I could hear the scream. I painted this picture – painted the clouds as real blood. – The colors were screaming. – This became the picture *The Scream* from the *Frieze of Life*."

Preface

It is now almost two decades (1969) since White and Sweet wrote their second substantial treatise on pain entitled 'Pain and the Neurosurgeon'. Since that time, surgical techniques have changed. Previous open operations have been supplemented by the percutaneous introduction of electrodes under very brief general or local anesthesia with the opportunity of verifying by physiological means the nervous structures one aims to destroy. In addition the operating microscope may have disclosed subtle compressive lesions on cranial nerves which may give rise to paroxysmal neuralgias and possibly can be treated by removing the compression.

But perhaps more importantly, since that time the evidence that a complex system of pain suppressor mechanisms exists has presented a completely new vista of pain control by activation of these mechanisms. Included are both electrical stimulation at specific sites and introduction of chemicals to bind to either opiate or many nonopiate types of pain suppressor receptors. Clinical utilization of these new concepts is still in its early stages. Neurosurgeons have known since Foerster's comprehensive studies that pain often seems to 'run in front of the knife', i.e. the nervous system possesses a remarkable capacity, following destructive procedures on it, to return towards the status quo ante, and to develop little-used or new mechanisms either to cause recurrence of the original pain or to replace it by other types of pain. Although often appearing at a slower pace than the analogous development of tolerance to chemical analgesics, it is clear that both physician and surgeon are confronted by this major problem in pain control.

The new developments include awareness of both pain suppressor and pain inducer pathways, of a bewildering variety of normal chemical mediators at the synapses in these pathways, and the pharmacology of the less readily destroyed analogs of the pain suppressors and antagonists of the pain inducers. This knowledge, though increasing, is still in a state of flux very difficult for the clinician to analyze and apply.

This book is written primarily for neurosurgeons who seek but do not yet have a special expertise in the neurosurgical treatment of pain. Its second intention is to provide all students and therapists of pain with a survey of clinical observations re the effects on chronic pain of destroying, stimulating electrically, and applying drugs to specific parts of the human nervous system. Within the limits of the pages prescribed by the publisher this second objective can be met only incompletely.

For hundreds of hours spent in follow-up studies, collation of data, literature searches and typing of manuscripts, we thank our research assistants, Mrs. Monique Heeren, Deborah Wallace and Linda Berard.

May 1988 Jan Gybels and William Sweet

Introduction, Including Definitions and Generalizations

The interruption of pathways of the nervous system concerned with pain is a classical and indeed logical approach to the relief of intractable pain. Modern anatomical tracing techniques and functional analysis with the use of microelectrode recording have described the pathways subserving 'acute pain' often referred to as 'nociceptive pain' in great detail [for recent review, see Willis, 1985; Besson and Chaouch, 1987]. However, as stressed by Noordenbos [1959], there is every reason to postulate that chains of short neurons forming a multisynaptic afferent system (MAS) have an important function in the conduction of impulses which give rise to pain in man, and anatomy and physiology have largely failed to come to grips with this. Even more disturbing is the uncertainty as to how these nociceptive pathways are implicated in chronic pain. Because of ethical considerations and difficulties in evaluating chronic pain in animals, there are few experimental data in animal models of chronic pain [for review, see Gybels, 1984; Levitt, 1985; Coderre et al., 1986; Colpaert, 1987].

From a clinical point of view, two major categories of chronic pain have been recognized. One, often referred to as 'somatic pain', is hypothesized, in the absence of any actual data, to be due to prolonged activation of nociceptors responsible for acute pain. Guilbaud et al. [1985] have suggested that prolonged activation of nociceptors which are sensitized by the pathological process might produce changes in the central nervous system (CNS). The other category of pain, often referred to as 'central', or 'deafferentation', or 'dysesthetic' pain [Casssinari and Pagni, 1969; Tasker et al., 1983], results from injury to the nervous system. This pain does not depend on activation of peripheral nociceptors, but must be the result of changes in the signal elaborating machinery. Exactly where and how in the various subgroups of pain related to intrinsic neural abnormality the substrates of the pain sensation swing into action remains to be elucidated. It is also not clear how large a nerve trunk must be involved, e.g. by cancer, for the pain to become 'neurogenic' rather than 'somatic'.

The most popular designation for this group appears to be 'deafferentation pain'. One of the most inclusive definitions of deafferentation pain is that of Tasker et al. [1980]. They so classify, 'all painful states associated with neurological injury except the pain associated with neurological compression' and including specifically, 'the chronic pain of peripheral nerve injury, certain types of peripheral neuritis, arachnoiditis, avulsion of the brachial plexus, trauma to spinal cord or cauda equina, postcordotomy dysesthesia, postherpetic neuralgia, Wallenberg's syndrome, thalamic pain'. They include as well the pain 'after certain injuries and amputations and that associated with the destruction of neurological tissue by cancer'. Elimination from the definition of any requirement for clinical evidence of sensory loss permits them to include causalgia and other sympathetic dystrophies as well.

While many of the painful lesions primarily in the nervous system are accompanied by a greater or lesser degree of objective sensory loss, it is clearly not the feature of sensory loss which correlates with the presence of pain; it is the exact site and nature of the lesion which determines whether or not pain will be present. Three striking examples of this are: (1) Avulsion of roots of the brachial plexus from the spinal cord commonly causes continuing pain, e.g. in 90% of 122 patients of Wynn Parry with such proven lesions, whereas the same sort of sensory loss caused, he said, 'no significant pain' in any of his 290 patients in whom the injury was distal, causing stretching or rupture of the nerves without avulsion from the cord [Wynn Parry, 1980, 1983]. (2) Complete trigeminal posterior rhizotomy causes continuing severe pain in the well-known anesthesia dolorosa, in 2–15% of patients referred to the anesthetic zone [White and Sweet, 1969, pp. 212–213], whereas the same complete sensory loss almost never causes pain in the anesthetic zone following spinal posterior rhizotomy sufficiently extensive to produce such a zone [Sweet, 1981; White and Kjellberg, 1973]. (A further difference in pain between the lesions at the two sites is that a region or band of pain at the junction of the anesthetic trigeminal with the normesthetic upper cervical dermatomes does not occur, whereas such a painful region may develop in the boundary zone between anesthesia and normesthesia after spinal posterior rhizotomy.) (3) An attack of herpes zoster may be followed by a sustained sensory deficit which ranges from no loss to complete anesthesia. Severe continuing pain may occur in the presence of minimal to major objective sensory loss.

We think it remains to be established that as a unifying concept for a general type of pain, deafferentation is helpful in determining, e.g. the mode of therapy. However, we do agree that within any specific circumscribed pathologic process the degree or type of sensory loss may correlate with the severity of the pain. Thus, in Wynn Parry's patients the more roots avulsed the more severe was the pain [Sweet, 1984]. Moreover, when anesthesia follows trigeminal rhizotomy a constant pain is more likely than when analgesia without major loss of touch follows differential thermal rhizotomy. When the latter technique produces only hypalgesia a constant pain is still less likely to occur. So both the type and degree of sensory loss within a specific pathologic state may correlate positively with the presence of pain. However, this still leaves us far from explaining such facts as that total trigeminal anesthesia is accompanied by no dysesthesia or even paresthesia at all in many people, e.g. in 29% of Peet and Schneider's [1952] 382 patients. This is further striking evidence that our understanding of the mechanism of this type of pain is deficient.

Do all pains caused by neural injury have a central abnormal component and, hence, are they appropriately classed as 'central pain'? Further studies may reveal that this is always true, but for the present we shall designate as 'neurogenic' the pains associated with primary injury of neural tissues — peripheral or central — reserving the term 'central pains' for those in which the primary lesion is in brain or spinal cord and, for neural pains peripheral thereto, the designation peripheral neurogenic will be used. Since 'dysesthesia' has now been defined as 'an unpleasant abnormal sensation' we shall not be using it as indicative of or synonymous with either 'neurogenic' or 'central pain' [Merskey, 1979, 1982].

Long before the different mechanisms of these two categories of chronic pain began to be formulated, neurosurgeons in reporting their results of operative procedures in chronic pain management have made a distinction between chronic pain due to cancer and chronic pain of nonlethal etiology. In many neurosurgical cases this latter type of pain is due to involvement of the nervous system and concerns a very restricted group of the chronic pain patients [Gildenberg and De Vaul, 1985]. The cancer process will indeed usually activate nociceptors by distension, pressure, chemical substances, etc. and therefore usually gives rise to somatic pain, but not infrequently the cancer process will also destroy nervous tissue by invading nerves and plexuses and will then produce features of neurogenic pain as well. The same is true with respect to spinal operations, especially in those patients with previous unsuccessful surgery in the area.

In describing the different operative procedures designed to interrupt nociceptive pathways, we shall follow an anatomical order from the periphery to the cortex. Only those points of technique which present a specific interest will be described. With regard to older procedures, now no longer used, only those data will be mentioned which are of interest for the understanding of pain mechanisms.

To help decide on the relative frequency of the different procedures, use has been made of a simple questionnaire given to colleagues as occasions presented themselves. They were asked to indicate if since 1980 they never, occasionally, or often performed a certain type of operation and what the exact number was for the year 1984 or 1985. These colleagues belonged to five continents; some of them devoted a substantial part of their activity to functional neurosurgery, while others were rarely solicited to care for intractable pain patients.

A major difficulty arises when reporting results of interventions. This is of course not only the case in the neurosurgical literature, but can be observed in the whole field of pain therapy. Reports of results range from anecdotal accounts, through series giving percentages of categories of verbal reports, to evaluations also taking into account, on a semiquantitative basis, consumption of analgesics and activity levels and making a distinction between short-term results and long-term results as well [Cowie and Hitchcock, 1982]. Our subjective judgment as to how to report the results in the literature has been guided by the degree of critical assessment of the original authors, the number of their cases, the availability of thoughtful reviews, the reputation of the authors and our own experience. The criteria for 'success' and 'good' results are often inadequately specified. Possibly a committee of the International Association for the Study of Pain (IASP), which has already performed a great service in defining terms and syndromes relevant to pain, could nudge us all in the direction of more useful reports with a series of suggestions as to how this may be achieved. Current differences of opinion will be more likely to be resolved when we have firmer facts.

We who are seeking to allay persistent pain must all be as certain as possible that the cause is not amenable to direct attack. Then, having established that status as well as we are able, we as therapists of the pain confront a trichotomy of modes of management. On a background of sympathetic understanding of the patient's personality and general problems we have three major avenues of approach. The time-honored method relies largely on drugs. Broad analgesic effects are now known to be a component of the action of an enormous variety of agents such as, for example, steroidal and nonsteroidal anti-inflammatory, antihistaminic, psychotropic and anticonvulsant drugs. The conscientious psycho- or neuropharmacologist, like the neurosurgeon, has an understandable tendency to cling tenaciously to his patient and explore other regimes with which he is familiar even when the likelihood of success is small or the degree of relief inadequate. Likewise, the anesthesiologist may retain his hold on the patient, exploring diagnostic or therapeutic blocks with little hope of fruitful results.

As summarized by Portenoy and Foley [1986], opioids have for many physicians become 'the mainstay of therapy for patients with pain due to cancer'. These and other authors are also exploring their use for chronic noncancer pain. Taub [1982a] was one of the first to report a substantial series of such patients; 313 of 737 on analgesic medication were maintained on opioids and followed for up to 6 years. Although only 4.2% of those on opioids presented problems of tolerance or substance abuse, the effectiveness of the treatment was not reported. In a much smaller series of 38 well-studied patients treated with opiates (half of the 38 for 4–7 years), there were similarly only 5% of 'management problems' and no toxicity related to the drugs [Portenoy and Foley, 1986]. A major feature of the care of each of these patients was that a single physician took primary responsibility for the overall management of the patient's medical problems as well as therapies. It is likely that the general competence and personality of that physician played a major role in the outcome — a variable in all our appraisals which we cannot ethically eliminate. These authors frankly report that 37% of the 38 patients achieved 'inadequate relief' and for the whole group 'few substantial gains in employment or social function could be attributed to the opioid therapy'. The authors' frankness includes the statement that they are providing the inchoate (incomplete) evidence on which tentative conclusions can be based. When they state that this 'therapy can be a safe, salutary and more humane alternative to the option of surgery or no treatment', we assume they are referring only to the 63% whose relief was described as 'partial but acceptable or fully adequate'. Maruta et al. [1979] and recently Bouckoms [1989] have presented realistic and similar appraisals of the problems and benefits. The former's 144 reported patients at the Mayo Clinic, a major tertiary referral center, had chronic pain of nonmalignant cause. Drug dependency was already present in 24%, and 49% were drug abusers — a biased population, which does, however, point to a problem of consequential magnitude. The bias was eliminated in Bouckoms's series of 59 patients with nonmalignant pain who were carefully selected for and followed on narcotics for up to 108 months and an average of 36 months. Although no patient with a history of significant abuse or addiction was so treated, 27% developed new or unexpected serious abuse, i.e. consistently took much more opiate than prescribed, and 24% became addicted in the sense of drug-seeking behavior as defined by the WHO. Tolerance, sufficiently marked to be a treatment-limiting condition, developed in another 22%. On the other cheerful side of the ledger are the 34% who had satisfactory relief — complete or almost complete. The successes were largely confined to the 74% with somatic (nociceptive) pain; the results were poor in the 26% with primarily central pain. It is, however, becoming apparent that these two broad rubrics include many subcategories of different mechanisms of pain, each of which requires special analysis. That a variety of pains are not relieved at all by systemic morphine is well established [Arner and Arnér, 1985]. Portenoy and Foley [1986] also say: 'Opioid maintenance therapy should be considered only after all reasonable attempts at pain control have failed'. Since they do not mention neurosurgical treatment as a possibility one might infer that they do not regard this as reasonable.

The complexity of the problem is illuminated by the fact that in a number of centers for treatment of chronic pain an important component of the therapy is to get the patient with pain of nonlethal cause off of his narcotics. Thus, of Aronoff's [1987] circa 8,000 such patients approximately 50% arrived taking narcotics, elimination of which from the regimes of the great majority was followed by a significant component of improvement in their whole life-style. However, Aronoff does manage a few carefully selected patients on rigorously controlled narcotics.

The use of opioids via spinal or intraventricular catheters represents a minor invasive procedure via which anesthesiologists, neurologists and neurosurgeons are seeking by more precise placement of the opiate or other agent to achieve better control at lower risk.

Waiting in the wings are the two other groups of the triad: those with cognitive-behavioral multidisciplinary treatment programs and the anesthesiologist-neurosurgeon category each with more expensive and riskier alternatives to offer. The primary objectives of behaviorally oriented programs are 'treatment for excess disability instead of treatment for pain'. This concept 'highlights the major problem of people with chronic pain, namely that they are more functionally disabled than is necessary'. These therapists seek to diminish pain behaviors and 'increase activity levels without recourse to methods directed specifically at the source of nociception'. Society and patient both profit if he becomes more productive, and often an associated dividend is 'impressive reduction in the pain'. [Quotes from Fordyce et al. 1985].

The world literature is replete with deprecatory, even vitriolic appraisals of the publications of those from the other two groups, another symptom of the difficulties we all face. One critic of the paper of Portenoy and Foley even took to task the editor of Pain for publishing the paper at all, finding that 'the conclusions of the authors cannot be said to rest upon any data of significance', and that they 'make only a slighting and distorted reference to the outcome studies of cognitive behavioral treatment programs' [Sternbach, 1987]. In fact, Portenoy and Foley say that during opioid maintenance therapy concurrent use of ancillary cognitive-behavioral and physical therapies should always be pursued.

With respect to the third and invasive components of the trichotomy, anesthesiology and neurosurgery, this role is being aggressively down-played by the nonsurgeons, both because of better nonsurgical therapies, and as well unwarranted operations, especially in the spinal canal by neuro- and orthopedic surgeons. These have produced such hordes of failures in the USA that patients in this category there outnumber all others with chronic pain of nonlethal cause, leading some distinguished physicians to regard one of their main roles to be protection of the patient from the surgeon. We fear that some physicians have lost sight of the fact that a fully successful neurosurgical destructive procedure enables the patient to forget about his pain and that electrical stimulation for suppression of pain has no systemic side effects. Indeed, these are such alluring prospects to both patient and surgeon that the latter may fail to properly emphasize the risks of major adverse sequelae of some of the destructive operations and of failure to secure adequate relief. However, we do not think these facts justify neglect of what neurosurgery has to offer. In his recent book 'Pain', Fields [1987] devoted only four pages to all forms of neurosurgical stimulation and ablation. He omits mention of sympathectomy, cordectomy and cingulotomy (which can all be dramatically successful) and is skeptical about many other relevant types of neurosurgery. We hope our book will present a balanced survey of the neurosurgical menus and be of help to nonneurosurgeons as well.

Especially regarding many neurosurgical procedures for pain, the operator would do well to collaborate closely with appropriate medical colleagues for all phases of patient selection and long postoperative follow-up. A dramatic example of the wisdom of such association is the cooperation between the Department of Psychology at the Massachusetts Institute of Technology and the psychiatric and neurosurgical services at the Massachusetts General Hospital in the recognition of the valuable place of cingulotomy in the management of affective psychoses and pain (chapter 19). This has led to continuation of the operation by this group despite its abandonment in many places. In the more controversial areas it is beneficial to have a part of the appraisal performed by persons with no responsibility for any part of patient care, as occurred in the case of MIT's Department of Psychology. We do agree with Field's thought that the neurosurgical management of severe chronic pain remains in general in an experimental phase, in which respect we say it resembles closely the nonneurosurgical management of such pain. Continuing careful documentation of what we are doing and why is essential to further progress in this often unsatisfactory field.

It is our impression that all of the disciplines able to make a significant contribution to some cases of chronic pain should be capably represented in each treatment complex and should report their complications, failures and successes to the whole staff. The more cordial the intergroup relationship the greater is the likelihood that the right program of treatments will be matched with the proper patients. It is peculiarly important that neuroscientists work with the neurosurgeons since each operation is an experiment which may yield new concepts about the human nervous system obtainable in no other way.

Part I. Surgical Interruption of Nociceptive Pathways

Section I. Operations on the Cranial Nerves

Chapter 1.A. The Trigeminal Nerve

Trigeminal Neuralgia

Historical Note

Operations on the trigeminal nerve are frequently performed for this disorder, also called tic douloureux, which is possibly one of the most painful of all human afflictions. As can be seen from many of the entries in table 1/I tic douloureux has been surgically treated for many years by denervating that part of the territory of the trigeminal nerve from which the pain is triggered or provoked. Accounts of the evaluation of our knowledge include among others those of Horsley et al. [1891], Rose [1892], Stookey and Ransohoff [1959] and Sweet [1985]. All of the procedures in table 1/I down to and including No. 11, compression of the trigeminal root, have, with the exception of partial section of the sensory root at the pons, become almost obsolete. The results, however, of the open operations in the middle fossa do play a major role in our current thinking as will be discussed in the next section.

Physiopathology of Essential Trigeminal Neuralgia

Many hypotheses have been formulated concerning the pathophysiology of tic douloureux but generally they can be divided into the groups of those favoring a peripheral and those describing a central mechanism for the origin of the paroxysmal pain.

Peripheral Causes

The arguments for a peripheral extrinsic origin include pathological features often seen at the level of the posterior root and occasionally at the level of the Gasserian ganglion: (1) Unequivocal space-taking lesions, such as tumors, arteriovenous malformations or aneurysms against trigeminal structures in the posterior fossa and less frequently in the middle fossa. (2) An

Table 1/I. Landmarks in the surgical treatment of tic douloureux

1	First complete publication of a case	Wepfer [1727]
2	Unsuccessful peripheral section of a branch of the trigeminal nerve	Schlichting [according to Rose 1892]
3	Description of the disorder, coining of term tic douloureux, chemical destruction of peripheral branch	André [1756]
4	Gasserian ganglion resection	Krause [1896]
5	Retrogasserian rhizotomy	Horsley et al. [1891] Spiller and Frazier [1901]
6	Alcohol injection in a branch of the trigeminal nerve	Schloesser [1907]
7	Alcohol injection in Gasserian ganglion	Harris [1912]
8	Report of 298 consecutive Gasserian ganglionectomies without mortality	Cushing [1920]
9	Partial section of V root at the pons	Dandy [1929]
10	Electrocoagulation of Gasserian ganglion	Kirschner [1931]
11	Decompression of the trigeminal root	Taarnhøj [1952]
12	Compression of the trigeminal root	Shelden et al. [1955]
13	Vascular decompression	Gardner and Miklos [1959]
14	Temperature-controlled coagulation of Gasserian ganglion and rootlets	Sweet [1968]
15	Microvascular decompression	Jannetta [1976]
16	Retrogasserian glycerol injection	Håkanson [1981]
17	Percutaneous compression of Gasserian ganglion	Mullan and Lichtor [1983]

upward tilt of the petrous pyramid in aging persons due to demineralization of the base of the skull or associated with basilar impression [Gardner, 1953, 1968]. (3) A pulsation of the intrapetrous carotid artery against the ventral surface of the Gasserian ganglion [Kerr, 1967b]. (4) Combined dural and osseous constriction at the porus trigemini [Lee, 1937]. (5) Compression of rootlets by their dural roof in the middle cranial fossa [Taarnhøj, 1952]. (6) Compression at the foramen rotundum or ovale [Shelden et al., 1955]. (7) Vascular pressure in the posterior fossa [Dandy, 1934; Jannetta, 1967b], etc. None of these mechanical etiologies explains the great rarity of primary neuralgias confined to the first division in 1–2%, the presence in many autopsy cases of some of these mechanical compressive factors without the affliction during life of tic douloureux [Hardy and Rhoton, 1978], and the extraordinary variability in vulnerability to provocation of attacks with remissions lasting for hours to years.

The long-held concept that there are no associated histopathological changes in the Gasserian ganglion or root has been effectively challenged.

Electron microscopy [Beaver, 1967; Kerr, 1967a] of operative specimens has shown, in patients with trigeminal neuralgia, pathology characterized by vacuolated but intact ganglion cells, degenerative hypermyelination, segmental demyelination with denudation of axis cylinders and microneuroma formation in the rootlets. Kunc et al. [1978] have described similar lesions in his biopsies from the spinal trigeminal tract in such patients. Multiple sclerosis occurs in over 2% of the patients with trigeminal neuralgia in a literature summary of White and Sweet [1969]. The fundamental features of intact axons associated with patchy extensive demyelination also characterize the CNS lesions of multiple sclerosis in general, as emphasized by Adams and Kubik [1952]. (However, specific mention of preservation of axis cylinders in the plaques of the trigeminal lesions was lacking in the descriptions of the postmortem materials in many articles as noted by White and Sweet [1969, p. 145].) There are at least 5 patients in whom plaques also occurred in the contralateral spinal trigeminal tract or root entry zone without causing pain [Parker, 1928; Daum et al., 1960; Van Gehuchten and Brucher, 1962 (case 2); Olafson et al., 1966; Jensen et al., 1982]. Hence one infers that some other conjoined causative factor is required unless the axons had also degenerated in the painless lesions in these 5 patients.

The last decades have given experimental evidence of pathophysiological processes via which damaged nerves can contribute actively to pain syndromes. Of particular importance in trigeminal neuralgia seems to be the ectopic electrogenesis in trigeminal nerve root fibers demyelinated by trauma [Calvin et al., 1982; Burchiel, 1980], the high sensitivity of dorsal root ganglion neurons to mechanical distortion [Howe et al., 1977] and cross-talk between low and high threshold sensory channels [Granit et al., 1944; Seltzer and Devor, 1979]. Besides ephaptic conduction at demyelinated and/or traumatized regions, a mechanism frequently invoked is the dorsal root reflex. This is a prolonged centrifugal discharge of dorsal root fibers evoked with a latency of some milliseconds after the same or other dorsal root fibers carry a volley centripetally. Its origin is to be found in excessive presynaptic depolarization associated with presynaptic inhibition which may trigger an impulse that propagates backwards [Turnbull et al., 1961]. Moreover, it has been shown that presynaptic depolarization of A delta fibers is produced by activity in myelinated fibers. It has been hypothesized [Calvin et al., 1977] that excessive presynaptic depolarization of small 'pain' fibers from excess large fiber activity establishes a reverberatory circuit that causes the painful paroxysms. Too much inhibition can turn into excitation. Some drugs, such as phenytoin and carbamazepine which are effective in the treatment of trigeminal neuralgia, do indeed also depress the dorsal root reflex [Storrs and King, 1971]. Conversely, this reflex is increased in amplitude in the chronic animals with alumina gel in nucleus caudalis showing marked overreaction to light touch in the trigeminal domain [King, 1967].

Central Causes

Much of the evidence for a central origin of tic douloureux is speculative but the following clinical arguments have been advanced [King, 1967]: the clear association of tic douloureux and multiple sclerosis; the high incidence of herpes simplex and vascular stress in patients with tic douloureux; and the comparable paroxysmal clinical manifestations of tic douloureux and sensory epileptiform discharges. From the clinical neurophysiological point of view the latent period between the onset of the triggering tactile stimulus and the onset of the pain, the self-sustaining tendency of the attack once started; the at times refractory period, relative or absolute of up to minutes following an attack before another full-blown attack can be provoked, and the efficacy of anticonvulsant drugs all suggest that the mechanism responsible for the paroxysm of pain is situated centrally and may well be in structures related to the spinal fifth nucleus [Kugelberg and Lindblom, 1959]. Finally in experimental animals the application of substances such as strychnine, picrotoxin, penicillin or alumina gel into the trigeminal subnucleus caudalis produces hypersensitivity to tactile stimulation of the face resembling that of the trigger zone in trigeminal neuralgia [King et al., 1956; King and Barnett, 1957; Black, 1974; Sakai et al., 1979; Håkanson and Pearson, 1982]. This does not happen when these substances are applied to the Gasserian ganglion [Burchiel et al., 1978] or in the main sensory trigeminal nucleus [King et al., 1956].

The hypothesis of 'a peripheral cause and central pathogenesis' [Fromm et al., 1984] proposes that chronic irritation of the trigeminal nerve produces a failure of the normal segmental inhibition which follows each volley into the trigeminal nucleus, as well as an increased activity in the trigeminal nerve due to ectopic-spike irritation. The proposition that failure of segmental inhibition occurs is based on several arguments. For instance, pharmacological data show that carbamazepine, phenytoin, and baclofen, all of which often relieve trigeminal neuralgia, facilitate inhibitory mechanisms and depress excitatory mechanisms in the spinal trigeminal nucleus [Fromm et al., 1981]. In crushed sensory nerves a decrease of primary afferent depolarization can be observed [Horch and Lisney, 1981], indicating the existence of a failure of segmental inhibition in different conditions in which there is a partial denervation of the trigeminal nucleus. A combination then of increased activity in the primary afferent fibers with an impairment of inhibitory mechanisms in the trigeminal nucleus would lead to paroxysmal discharges of interneurons in the trigeminal nucleus in response to tactile stimulation. An attack of trigeminal neuralgia would occur when these bursts reached the threshold to activate nociceptive neurons in that nucleus. This hypothesis would explain why even peripheral lesions of the branches of the trigeminal nerve subserving the painful paroxysms can relieve trigeminal neuralgia since they would decrease the amount of afferent activity in the affected fibers, thereby decreasing the likelihood of paroxysmal discharges in the trigeminal nucleus. Painful paroxysms would cease and the refractory period that may follow the attacks of trigeminal neuralgia would point to a recovery of inhibition.

Thus, trigeminal neuralgia would have a peripheral cause and a central pathogenesis: trigeminal neuralgia would occur when disease of the nerve caused increased firing in it as well as impaired efficiency of the inhibitory mechanisms that normally control afferent activity in the trigeminal nucleus. When the ensuing paroxysmal bursts of neuronal activity in the trigeminal nucleus involved nociceptive trigeminothalamic relay neurons, the afflicted person would experience the excruciating paroxysms of trigeminal neuralgia. A recent hypothesis favors structural and functional changes in the trigeminal system following partial deafferentation and resulting in an alteration in the receptive field of wide-dynamic-range neurons (WDR, chapter 7); touch stimuli would then produce this activity in WDR neurons which in normal conditions is only produced by noxious stimuli [Dubner et al., 1987].

The complexity of the connections of nucleus caudalis which include an ascending trigeminal intranuclear pathway terminating on the rostral components of the trigeminal sensory nuclear complex plus afferents to n. caudalis from many nontrigeminal sources as well as efferents from this nucleus far and wide point to the likelihood of multiple mechanisms which may go awry as pointed out in many publications from King's group [Stewart et al., 1964].

None of the current hypotheses explains the curious phenomenon of relief of the pain for protracted intervals of months to years following modest manipulations in the vicinity of the trigeminal ganglion and/or rootlets. These observations became convincing when the 'decompression' operations were first introduced: (1) by Taarnhøj [1952] to open the dural roof of Meckel's cave, and (2) by the Pudenz-Shelden [1952] group to drill away bone at the foramina rotunda or ovale. When these two operations at different sites proved equally effective, Shelden et al. [1955] decided that mild trauma to the trigeminal pathways was the feature common to both types of operation. They accordingly advocated 'rubbing' of the ganglion and nearby rootlets after opening the overlying dura. By 1964 they had carried out 200 such compressions with immediate complete relief and only 50 recurrences. Loss of sensation was minimal and no severe dysesthesias were provoked. Many variations involving different types of minor manipulations were introduced, all with roughly similar success. By 1969 White and Sweet [pp. 200–205] had assembled 28 publications from 24 services reporting 1,790 such operations whose common denominator was some maneuver involving the trigeminal ganglion and root in the middle cranial fossa. All reports described a high percentage of initial relief, the highest failure rate being 25% of 12 cases [Schwartz, 1955]. Severe recurrences of pain requiring reoperation were reported in only 8–28% of the patients in six series of 90–200 cases each — most with multiyear follow-ups. The usual sensory loss was only subjective with fewer patients demonstrating any objective loss. Some noted that the more clear-cut the sensory loss, the less was the likelihood of severe recurrence [Svien and Love, 1959; White and Sweet, 1969]; no such correlation was seen by Gardner and Miklos [1959].

In the small series of White and Sweet [1969] of 18 cases with a Shelden-type compression operation from 1957 to 1964, follow-ups in 1987 revealed 9 recurrences in from 14 months to 11 years, averaging 5.5 years, and freedom from pain until death at 9–23 years in 6, averaging 16 years. Only 3 continuing with freedom from pain had short follow-ups of 2–7 years, averaging 4 years. All reports describe durations of relief vastly exceeding those occurring with spontaneous remissions. Under microvascular decompression we discuss the similar convincing evidence that minor manipulations in the posterior fossa to keep vessels from compressing the rootlets are also remarkably successful. That it is not necessarily the movement of the vessel but some modest derangement of the nerve that is the key to success is intimated by the reports of Varma and Frazer [1984]. They wrapped with muscle the rootlets in the posterior fossa in 19 patients, relieving them of their trigeminal neuralgia in all but the 2 with multiple sclerosis. There had been arterial contact in 9, venous contact in 3 and no vascular contact in 5. Follow-up was from 4 to 30 months. Sweet records 2 protracted remissions with minimal trigeminal manipulation in the first patient and none in the second. In case 1 a plastic cuff containing two platinum electrodes was passed around the second trigeminal division just behind the foramen rotundum with a view to controlling second-division neuralgia by electrical stimulation. The surgical gesture alone resulted in cessation of the pain for 8 years; when it recurred electrical stimulation was of no value. In the second patient after 6 years of trigeminal neuralgia the trigeminal rootlets in the posterior fossa were exposed in the hope of relieving first-division pain by displacing a vessel. An unusually easy exposure with almost no retraction disclosed the 2 superior cerebellar arterial branches well anterior to the trigeminal rootlets. No instrument came within 1 cm of the rootlets and Sweet closed the wound with a view to achieving first-division hypalgesia more precisely by radiofrequency heating. This never became necessary; he remained pain-free for 8.5 years until death from a heart attack. In 11 patients no longer responding to medical treatment Sweet has either punctured an artery or in one patient produced a major hematoma below the base of the skull and stopped the projected RF lesion before entering the foramen ovale. In 6 of these patients a remission occurred lasting for one month to over one year. One continues relieved at 13 years.

We comment further on these puzzling phenomena under microvascular decompression.

Current Treatments

Since the advent of phenytoin and carbamazepine and more recently of baclofen and clonazepam, nearly all of the patients with trigeminal neuralgia are initially relieved by one or a combination of these agents. However, especially those in the older age group and those with multiple sclerosis are prone to develop tolerance and/or toxicity to the drugs. This is especially true of the most effective of the four agents, carbamazepine. An insidious onset of mental and physical lethargy as its dose is increased is often mistaken for unavoidable 'aging'. Many of our patients have found themselves 'years younger' in their capacities within a month or two of stopping carbamazepine after operative complete relief had been achieved. However, both patients and their physicians are often loath to consider any invasive procedure savoring of risk. Maximal reduction of risk can be achieved by the use of percutaneous approaches of: (1) differential thermal rhizotomy and the less-tried more recent (2) differential glycerol rhizotomy, and (3) compression of trigeminal ganglion and root by a balloon 'microcompression'. While in nonneurosurgical disciplines operations directed at peripheral branches including the newly utilized cryotherapy [Nally, 1984] have their recent proponents, the likelihood of regeneration of fibers and return of pain within months to a year or two makes these methods less attractive than those directed at the less recoverable root area.

Dandy [1934] questioned the need for destructive procedures; he thought that the etiology of tic douloureux was to be found in the compression usually exerted by blood vessels on the trigeminal sensory root in the posterior fossa. His opinion has led to open operations in which a 'decompression' of the ganglion or posterior rootlets has been pursued, the other current principal alternative to the percutaneous approaches.

Thermal Rhizotomy

Historical Note

The University of Heidelberg's Kirschner [1931] introduced electrocoagulation of the Gasserian ganglion devising an apparatus that permitted accurate aiming of the electrode through the foramen ovale. He had operated on 1,113 patients by 1942 [Kirschner, 1942] with the Bovie type of electrodestructive unit long used for hemostasis since its first use in neurosurgery by Cushing. The Heidelberg group including Klar [1960] and Penzholz et al. [1975] applied the method conservatively and obviously with great success to 2,570 patients by 1967. A very long follow-up averaging 12.7 years with a maximum of 33 years was achieved by them in 315 patients who were under 46 years of age at the time of operation. The mortality in this group was zero with only 5 cases of anesthesia dolorosa and none of neuroparalytic keratitis but an 80% recurrence rate [Menzel, 1986]. However, when older patients were included and on virtually all other services the serious complications were greater because of erratic control of the lesion made with the Bovie type unit. By reducing the intensity of the electrocoagulation Thiry [1962] allowed preservation of a certain degree of tactile sensibility while not jeopardizing the therapeutic results, although some serious extratrigeminal complications still occurred.

Controlled Thermocoagulation

Hypothesizing that lightly or unmyelinated fibers including those concerned with pain might be destroyed by increments of graded heating with relative sparing of the heavily myelinated fibers, including those for touch, Sweet [1968, White and Sweet 1969, pp. 607–609] developed a method in 1965 which usually permits attainment of this objective. The neurophysiological evidence largely supports the concept that severe loss of pain sensation with preservation of much touch is associated with destruction of A delta and C fibers and sparing of many A beta fibers in animals [Letcher and Goldring, 1968; Uematsu et al., 1974b; Frigyesi et al., 1975; Broggi and Siegfried, 1977] and by compound action potential measurements in man by Macon et al. [1981] and Sweet and Poletti [1982]. Klumpp and Zimmermann [1980] describe the reverse behavior in the cat's posterior tibial nerve with two thirds of the C fiber potential persisting when the A fiber potential was less than 1% of control. Histological evidence shows that thermocoagulation destroys indiscriminately both small C and A delta fibers and large A beta fibers [Smith et al., 1981; Uematsu, 1982; Kanpolat and Onol, 1980]. A similar tendency for phenol selectively to produce analgesia 30 years ago was described despite the fact that histologists found nerve fiber destruction by phenol to be 'nondifferential, all sizes and types of nerve fibers being equally affected'. For details of literature see White and Sweet [1969, pp. 660–663]. A single destroyed A beta fiber in a histologic section is more conspicuous than 10 destroyed C fibers. We submit that the correlation between compound action potentials and clinical examination of touch and pinprick permits rapid reliable interpretation of more data than a nonquantitative survey of histologic sections. Tactics for controlled thermocoagulation of the trigeminal ganglion and rootlets have been described in detail by several authors [Sweet and Wepsic, 1974b; Siegfried and Vosmansky, 1975; Nugent, 1985; Nugent and Berry, 1974; Tew et al., 1978, 1982; Sweet, 1976b].

Current Recommendations

(1a) Reliable radiofrequency (RF) signal generators of a precisely controllable heat source [Sweet et al., 1960]. (1b) Reliable thermistors for use within a 20-gauge insulated needle electrode or preferably thermocouples within a 22-gauge electrode. The smaller the gauge of the device the less the risk of serious hemorrhage. (All three devices are manufactured by the Radionics Instrument Company, Burlington, Mass.) (2a) Neurolept agents and analgesics such as droperidol 1.25 mg and fentanyl 50 μg repeated as needed to permit an intermittently awake, cooperative patient. (2b) Very short acting methohexital (Brevital) to produce brief unconsciousness during the actual electrode placement and heating. No such general anesthesia is used by Schürmann et al. [1972] and Nugent [1985]. Sindou et al. [1987] prefer propranidid as providing a faster, shorter anesthesia with a more complete awakening. The allergic risks of this agent have discouraged anesthesiologists in the USA. (3) Precise direction of the electrode guided by fluoroscopic control through the appropriate part of the foramen ovale on a trajectory which will carry it only a few millimeters above the superior surface of the petrous pyramid. Final placement among the fibers from the division of pain, preferably from the area of the trigger zones, is achieved roughly from fluoroscopy and radiographs and more precisely with two modalities: (1) electrical stimulation at circa 50-cycle 1-ms pulses of a square wave, and (2) continuous radiofrequency heating. Sindou prefers a 5/s frequency noting that this slower rate brings out clonic masticatory movements indicating undesirable proximity to the motor root and the need to shift the electrode away from these fibers. A careful sensory examination follows each increment of heating, and stimulation by both electrical modalities may dictate readjustment of electrode position since the developing sensory loss may not be in the expected area, or subsequent stimulation may reveal an unsatisfactory shift in the area of reference of sensation. (4) Episodes of heating increasing by 5–10 °C steps for 1 min or less. Note should also be made of the milliamperage and voltage required and if these are unusually high for the temperature recorded the lesion should be stopped and sensation checked. (5) Stop heating if the first-division skin flushes or algesia there changes to analgesia during the heating . After the first lesions less or no brevital may be used to permit sensory testing during the actual heating in the final phases of the operation. (6) Patience to await adequate awakening of the patient for reliable sensory testing, 2 h or more, may be needed for the procedure. (7) Prompt termination of the operation upon modest indication for so doing. It is too simple to come back another day to warrant any avoidable risk.

Details of Surgical Technique

There are now 11 series of 600–1,500 procedures with minimal extratrigeminal morbidity and only 1 death in over 10,000 procedures. These have soothed many of us into a state of complacency regarding the current modus operandi. However, the reports of a poll we conducted of distinguished neurosurgeons around the world have revealed an incidence of serious extratrigeminal complications we must reduce [Sweet and Poletti, 1988]. The percutaneous intracranial approaches will always have some degree of trigeminal morbidity, but we should all be able to maintain a permanent extratrigeminal morbidity of almost zero. Several neurosurgeons having described to us difficulty with the method, we are giving an account which may seem unnecessarily detailed.

Details of Electrode Introduction and Lesion Production

We place an adhesive strip in the Frankfurt plane from mid external auditory canal to the inferior border of the orbit. This is marked at 1-cm intervals from the anterior wall of the external auditory canal forward along the inferior border of the zygoma. This acts as a rough external guide to the anteroposterior direction of the electrode which, when through the medial half of foramen ovale, will usually lie 2.0–3.5 cm in front of the anterior wall of the external auditory canal as measured along the lower border of the zygoma. In the coronal plane the shaft points usually from 0 to 5 mm lateral to the medial border of the lacrimal caruncle. The skin is punctured 3 cm lateral to the labial commissure usually with an electrode with a 10-cm shaft. The index finger of the hand not holding the electrode is applied to the oral mucosa. It follows the advancing shaft to ensure that the point does not penetrate the oral mucosa and pick up bacteria on its way. We have had 3 patients with enough dolichocephaly to require a longer 11-cm shaft. According to the anthropologist Martin, the distance from glabella to opisthokranion — the most prominent point in the midline of the occiput — averages in Swiss and German male adults around 188–192 mm whereas it is at 192–195 mm in white American males [Martin, 1928]. This is measured with the standard anthropologist's calipers in those with suspiciously big heads, and the electrode with the 11-cm shaft used in those over 200 mm. We also note those who have small or brachycephalic skulls so as not to thrust the electrode too deeply. One woman with a small head had as much as 33 mm of a 10-cm shaft outside the skin for a third-division lesion among the rootlets. In order to prevent the electrode once placed from slipping in, the shaft is passed through a small plastic disc which is applied against the cheek once the proper depth is attained. This grips the metal tightly, preventing inward slippage and attracting attention if the electrode migrates outward. Uninsulated metal clips should not be used against the skin for this purpose since the RF heats the metal and may burn the skin. We have routinely placed the ground electrode in the upper temporal ipsilateral scalp.

The fluoroscopic technique of Whisler and Hill [1972] and Onofrio [1975] is used with the head hyperextended and rotated 15–20° away from the side of the pain. A fluoroscopic screen presenting a standing image and minimal radiation permits detailed study to spot the foramen ovale, and may be supplemented by films to confirm the identification of the foramen. New has added the helpful detail of placing intracutaneously the length of a 22-gauge needle just under the skin for 2–3 cm so that its tip lies at the electrode puncture wound in the skin 3 cm from the labial commissure. This modifica-

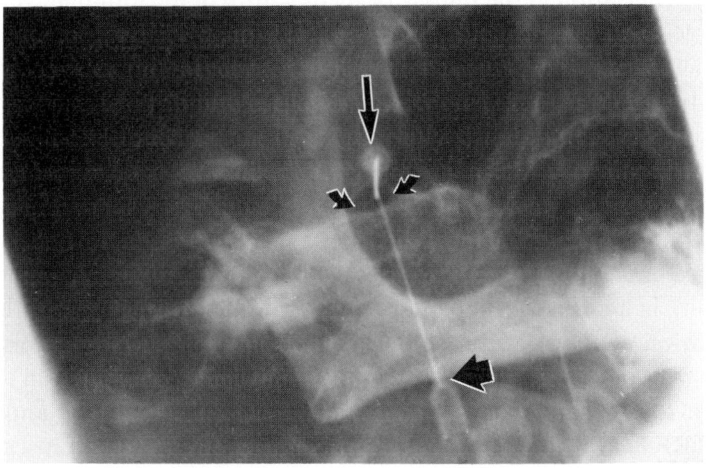

Fig. 1/1. Placement of needle-electrode in proper portion of foramen ovale guided by fluoroscopy and radiographs. Small arrows = medial and lateral boundaries of foramen ovale. Large arrowhead = small-gauge subcutaneously placed needle whose point lies at opening in skin 3.0 cm lateral to labial commissure via which the needle-electrode's point penetrates the skin. By fluoroscopy the point of the small needle is brought to overlie precisely the desired portion of the foramen ovale — in this case the medial part of the middle third of the foramen for V2/V3 neuralgia. During placement electrode shaft follows this trajectory. Long arrow = partially radiolucent hub of electrode with dense deep end of line of shaft indicating electrode point in proper part of foramen.

tion of the tactic of Apfelbaum [1978] enables one to fluoroscopically line up the skin puncture site with the foramen ovale so as to direct precisely the electrode to the desired portion of that opening (fig. 1/1).

Rarely the foramen proves elusive or the foraminal canal permits entry of the electrode but inadequate intracranial penetration. This has been attributed to a long pterygo-alar bar; a radiographic technique to show this has been described by Chouké and Hodes [1951]. Sweet failed to enter the foramen in 4 cases in the first 12 years. However, with the advent of high-resolution computerized tomographic (CT) scans difficult cases have been studied with the needle tip presumably near the foramen ovale and corrections applied. Failure to enter the foramen occurred in only 2 patients in the last 10 years; their foraminal area had been destroyed by middle fossa basal cancers. Siegfried [1983a] described no such failures in 1,000 neuralgia patients. In 8 other reports the failures ranged from 0.5 to 4% with an average of 2.7%.

If upon penetration of the middle or medial third of the foramen, venous blood emerges, the needle electrode is withdrawn a few millimeters, 0.5–1 ml saline is injected, and the stylet replaced. Sweet secured cerebrospinal fluid (CSF) in 846 or 73% of 1,147 procedures in which this was noted. It is not necessary to enter CSF to secure a satisfactory lesion.

Final placement of the electrode tip in the appropriate rootlets requires the aid of responses to electrical stimulation. The locus of sensation upon square wave stimulation is usually the same as that to RF heat, but if they are different one modality is not consistently more reliable than the other. Electrode site is modified in accordance with an inferolateral to superomedial disposition of the rootlets from IIIrd to Ist division. With increasing experience we, Sindou et al. [1987] and others have found it fruitful in those without previous lesions to try for threshold voltages of 0.05–0.2 and less than 50 °C RF heat. Lower effective temperatures and more circumscribed deficits are likely to ensue. Rovit [1985] seeks a threshold voltage of 0.15 or less. Full sensory testing to pin should be done after each lesion. Even if no hypalgesia to pin has developed the electrical threshold tends to increase. As stepwise increases in the lesion are made, the fibers near that electrode site may become unresponsive and sensation be referred to a neighboring division. Readjustment of electrode position into unaffected fibers of the target division is obviously required. In 9% of W.H.S.' patients the sensory loss appeared in a division to which electrical stimulus-evoked sensation was not referred — especially disappointing when this is the first division. Once significant hypalgesia is present it is often feasible to complete the lesion with little or no brevital so that one can test the patient during the lesion and stop it as soon as analgesia appears. This is hard enough to achieve consistently so that several neurosurgeons advocate settling for only hypalgesia — marked or even moderate [Kanpolat et al., 1982; Nugent and Berry, 1974].

Avoidance of Dysesthesia

The worst of the intratrigeminal sequelae is intolerable dysesthesia. We have concentrated on trying to eliminate this by seeking the patient's help in deciding how much numbness to produce. Many prefer dense numbness and may even like the reassurance given by this sensation that the pain is unlikely to recur. Others find the various symptoms associated with trigeminal denervation most distressing. As soon as clear-cut hypalgesia develops we wait for the patient to be really awake to concentrate on his facial sensations. If there is any question in his mind about their tolerability we urge termination of the procedure. Since 1983, having followed this tactic more rigorously, Sweet has had none of the patients develop such severe dysesthesias that they are not usefully helped by medication, i.e. anesthesia, analgesia or hypalgesia dolorosa.

Avoidance of Corneal Anesthesia

As one seeks to complete second-division analgesia or produce hypalgesia in a trigger zone in the first division, there is a disconcerting tendency for abrupt loss of both touch and pinprick sensation to appear in the first division. An earlier hope that facial flushing in this area would be a useful warning was especially encouraged by the study of Drummond et al. [1983] who used both pulse recording and thermography to document vasodilation and thought that in their 23 patients the division of the facial flush corresponded with subsequent analgesia. The hope that this would avoid corneal sensory loss has proven of minor value. Analgesia may develop despite no flushing and vice versa. In Kerr's [1975a] superb study of facial vasodilator mechanisms in the cat, vasodilator fibers from the greater superficial petrosal nerve were found to enter the Gasserian ganglion and pass peripherally in each branch. Electrical stimulation to one division caused vasodilation in that division's domain. Unfortunately, the first-division's vasodilator fibers were the least responsive. Stimulation of trigeminal rootlets caused no vasodilation and stimulation in the bulbar descending tract caused a little such response only in the area of the second division. Sindou et al. [1987] have confirmed the findings of Kerr during their RF lesions, noting a facial flush in 80% when the electrode was probably in the ganglion and in only 20% when it was in the root. However, Sweet saw an ipsilateral facial flush in many patients in whom the tip of the 5-mm bare electrode was 4 mm or more behind the profile of the clivus, almost certainly all in the rootlets. Broggi [1975] reports a single case of complete hemifacial pallor during the RF coagulation.

Testing the conscious patient during the lesion making is the most certain way to reduce the incidence of corneal anesthesia as already noted. Despite attempting to stop the lesion at hypalgesia in the first division for pain triggered in that division we have still had in 119 such patients an incidence of 18% corneal anesthesia. In the 10% of Tew and van Loveren's [1988] patients with first-division trigger zones, corneal sensation was lost in 28% in the course of obtaining full relief. Likewise Siegfried [1983a] produced corneal anesthesia in all 34 (21%) of his 135 patients with first-division pain. As described in the section on glycerol, this agent can be used so as to give a better chance of preventing such anesthesia yet achieve some V1 sensory loss.

We describe as anesthetic a cornea which does not feel the touch of a wisp of paper tissue. Such a state does not necessarily denote total anesthesia; many such patients wink lactose powder off the cornea. Another test suggested by Rovit [1985] is the response to dropping artificial tears in the eye. Especially if the patient can still feel touch on the eyebrow or eyelid he may have a useful warning sensation of a foreign body in the eye. The patient should wear a plastic unilateral 'trigeminal' eye shield when corneal sensation is much diminished or absent. This is attached unilaterally to the outer side of the lens to be worn constantly when awake. Patients should be instructed that if they 'get something in the eye' it will not hurt at all. If they think they may have a foreign body there, they should act as promptly to check this as they do when they have the usual pain in this state on the normal side. Artificial tears should be used 3 or more times a day in the eye. Any redness of the conjunctiva or blurring of vision should lead to an immediate visit to an ophthalmologist with prompt vigorous therapy of any corneal ulcer including tarsorrhaphy if recommended. A corneal erosion or ulcer developed in 3% of Sweet's patients. They have had this treated promptly. Temporary tarsorrhaphy was used in 1.6%.

Other Intraoperative Complications

Cardiac ischemia, bradycardia and brief cardiac arrest have all been spotted on the continuous ECG monitor by the anesthesiologist. Electrode placement, heating, glycerol injection and especially placement of the huge needle for microcompression [Belber and Rak, 1987] may provoke such changes which tend to return promptly to normal upon stopping the maneuver. Atropine i.v. provides prophylaxis against initial occurrence or recurrence of the drop in heart rate. Actual or potential cardiac ischemic episodes may be handled best by terminating the whole procedure. We have done this twice when the patient described substernal pain, and Sindou et al. [1987] have also stopped 2 of their 609 procedures because of the appearance of 'ischemic abnormalities'. The other 6 cardiac episodes of Sweet were more minor and none of the 8 has been followed by a myocardial infarct. One advantage of the procedure is the ease of stopping it at once upon any clue that this might be advisable. Rhoton [1985] reports one fatal myocardial infarct following over 1,500 procedures and Browne [1985] 2 fatal myocardial infarcts within 2 weeks of operation.

Convulsions have occurred infrequently. We have had 6 minor seizures without incident problems. There is a report of one patient fracturing the humerus in a convulsive seizure [Mittal and Thomas, 1986]. Sweet provoked a small intraorbital hemorrhage by entry into the inferior orbital fissure in one patient with transitory impairment of nerves II, III, IV and VI which cleared completely in 2 days. Such massive hematomas in the cheek developed 5 times that the procedure was terminated; 2 of these occurred in the same patient. The fascinating symptom of a transient global amnesia developed in 2 of Sweet's patients during the operation.

Results

We have classified the outcomes regarding pain as: (1) inadequate sensory loss — repeat lesion required in 4 weeks; (2) complete relief after one or 2 lesions; (3) mild, often brief, recurrences not requiring reoperation, and (4) recurrences requiring reoperation. Table 1/II reports results of 11 services with 600 to 1,500 procedures. In addition we have tabulated the results of other published articles. The following neurosurgeons with large series have also given us brief accounts including their numbers of procedures — all without lasting extratrigeminal morbidity or mortality — Burchiel more than 100, Churcher 150, Escobedo 202, Gardner 100, Norrell more than 100, Sujatanond 290, Taren more than 1,000, Turnbull 398, Vaernet 44, Wrenn more than 400 [all personal communications, 1985–1987].

Only 6 deaths have been reported in the publications to date. Their causes were: a 93-year-old whose RF lesion may have injured the cerebral peduncle [Apfelbaum, 1977], meningitis and temporal lobe abscess [Brandt and Wittkamp, 1983], pulmonary edema [Campos et al., to be published], intracerebral hemorrhage [Mittal and Thomas, 1986], pneumonia [Nugent, 1985], intracranial hemorrhage [Penzholz, 1986].

In a varying percentage of cases apparently satisfactory loss of algesia soon recovers. The percentages of patients requiring early reoperation vary from a low of 2% in Siegfried's [1981] experience to a high of 12% for Sweet. In the latter's series the percentages of both the early and later recurrences have risen in the last decade as the policy has been followed of stopping the procedure if the patient is at all uneasy about his tolerance of the new numbness. We cite the example of a prominent internist who, having seen 2 patients with anesthesia dolorosa, asked that the operation stop as soon as he had clear-cut hypalgesia in the trigger zones. This tactic resulted in 5 RF lesions between January 1966 and February 1969. However, he then remained free both of tic pain and any concern over other facial sensations until his death 171 months later.

Table 1/II. Trigeminal thermal rhizotomy: 11 services with 600 or more procedures

Author, year	Number of patients	Number of RF operations	Early complete relief[1], %	Follow-up period range, average	Recurrences not requiring reoperation, %	Recurrences requiring reoperation, %
Siegfried, 1983a	1,000		100	135 patients followed 5.5–8 years	4	21 at 5.5–8 years
Broggi et al., 1985	1,000		100	1–10 years		13
Maxwell, 1985		>600				
Nugent, 1985	643	~800		4.7 years		23
Rovit, 1985	550	600				19
Frank et al, 1985a[2]	939		100	6 months–5 years		21
Rhoton, 1985		~1,500				
Sindou et al., 1987	609		100	1–13 years		7
Thurel, 1987	890	1,150	96			23
Sweet, 1988a	702	1,119	99	1–21 years, 5.6 years	6	31
Tew and van Loveren, 1988	1,100		98	1–18 years	9	8

[1] Includes that after early reoperation.
[2] Three services.

Blessed with extraordinarily assiduous research assistants, we have follow-up data extending to patient death, to March 1987 or for more than 5 years in 766 patients with trigeminal neuralgia treated by RF lesions or glycerol.

Complete relief was achieved by one, 2 or rarely 3 operations in 96–100% of the patients in all of the large series of table 1/II recording these data. Sweet has had such failures to relieve the paroxysmal pains in 6 of 702 patients. In 14 of the 26 smaller series giving this information similar early success rates were obtained. Menzel et al. [1975] ultimately freed from pain 97% of their younger cases followed for an average of 12.7 years after the Kirschner type of electrocoagulation. Later recurrences requiring reoperation occurred in 7–31% of the cases in the 11 series of table 1/II.

Table 1/II. (cont.)

Anesthesia, analgesia, hypalgesia dolorosa, %	Dysesthesias controlled with drugs, %	Keratitis, %	Corneal anesthesia, %	Masticator paralysis, %	Masticator weakness, %	Oculomotor paresis temp.,%
3	24 at 5.5–8 years	0.8	2.8	15	25	4
7.9 'often unbearable'		tarsorr. 0.4	21	10		0.3
2		1				
1	5	0.5	2 last 600 ops		10	0.25
0.2	0.7		4			0.2
0.6	11.6		1	1		
			1 patient, loss of eye			
25 'painful'		20	35	lasting 2 temp. 25		6.5
0.6	7	2	6		25	0.7
2.1	6	3				
		tarsorr. 1.5	9	25	40	0.4
1	9	3			13 (curved electrode)	1.5

Note that there is no major advantage to carrying the lesion to analgesia as done by Sindou and Sweet in contrast to the lesser levels of hypalgesia as done by Nugent and Rovit.

As Sindou et al. [1987] point out, their lowest recurrence rate of 7% is accompanied by some higher complication rates, e.g. 23% corneal hypesthesia, 4% keratitis and 6.5% oculomotor paresis of which 0.3% were lasting. In general, few recurrences tend to be associated with more complications. Note that stopping of the procedure when hypalgesia has been achieved, recommended by Nugent and Rovit, resulted in 23 and 19%, respectively, of recurrences requiring reoperation — not significantly greater than in the series of most of us seeking analgesia as the end point. Moreover, these two surgeons have a gratifyingly small percentage of dysesthesias.

By far the most distressing sequela of the procedure is severe dysesthesias. We define pragmatically degrees of dysesthesia as: (1) severe or 'dolor-

Table 1/III. Trigeminal neuralgia (patients of W.H.S.): postoperative paresthesia and dysesthesia

	After 1,119 RF lesions		93 glycerol	
	number	%	number	%
Paresthesias	304	27	34	37
Of concern but no drugs needed	156	14	20	22
Of concern, controlled on medications	10	0.9	3	3
Dysesthesias				
Not requiring medication	27	2	5	5
Usefully helped by medication	64	6	19	20
Anesthesia dolorosa	13	1	2	2
Analgesia dolorosa	8	0.7	0	
Hypalgesia dolorosa	5	0.4	2	2

osa', not usefully relieved by any medical regime; (2) moderate — usefully relieved by medication; (3) mild — not requiring medication. Definitions in the literature vary, making comparisons difficult, but we have made an effort in table 1/II. Depending on the type of objective sensory loss, we classify the worst group as anesthesia, analgesia or hypalgesia dolorosa. Our occurrence rate was respectively 1, 0.7 and 0.4%; even the lesser loss of hypalgesia does not guarantee absence of the severely distressing state — hence our reliance on the patient's subjective appraisal during operation. The trigeminal zone was divided into 9 cutaneous and 9 internal areas for sensory examination. Touch was examined only in the 9 cutaneous zones, the nasal mucosa and tongue. Anesthesia to a wisp of tissue or to finger touch was recorded. The fact that anesthesia dolorosa occurred in 6.6% of those who had some anesthetic areas emphasizes again the desirability of avoiding this degree of loss. A more detailed breakdown of results regarding nonpainful and painful denervation sensations is given in table 1/III.

Postoperative Complications

Optic Nerve

These injuries related to needle placement can certainly be eliminated with routine properly interpreted radiographs which show the electrode much too far forward in the inferior orbital fissure via which it is possible to impale the optic foramen. Lateral films should always precede any lesion-making. Figure 5 of a 1976 publication of W.H.S. illustrates an unmistakable major misplacement into the orbital fissure corrected before a lesion was made [Sweet, 1976b]. Responses to electrical stimulation may be grossly misleading as revealed by our neurosurgical poll [Sweet and Poletti, 1988]. Three operators made the lesions without radiographic control at the site of reference of sensation to the second division. All were followed by lasting ipsilateral blindness. Three other operators report the same sequela without further details.

Sweet also made a small lesion in the inferior branch of an oculomotor nerve at the inferior orbital fissure as a consequence of the following sequence of events. The electrode had been inserted only into the canal of the foramen ovale as shown on film in order to make a peripheral lesion. This was done, but the ensuing basal view of the skull was unsatisfactory because of difficulty in positioning the 340-lb.(155-kg) patient. On renewed electrical stimulation the third-division reference of pain was again secured and two more lesions made. A dilated ipsilateral pupil was noted; we then saw that the last head manipulation had resulted not only in the electrode sliding out of the foramen ovale but in skidding along the skull base to enter the inferior orbital fissure! Full recovery from the IIIrd nerve palsy required 2 months. Marked extension of the head for a basal view may cause enough discomfort and may shift the electrode just enough, so that we now rely more on fluoroscopy which requires less extension of the head. W.H.S. has also placed an electrode tip in CSF at a site which yielded with both square wave and RF heating the desired sensation in the cheek. Radiographs showed the tip to be in the pars nervosa of the jugular foramen! — 2 more examples of the less than total reliance we should place on responses to electrical stimulation. There were 18 oculomotor palsies mentioned in the poll, all but one or 2 of which were temporary. The incidence on 11 services is given in table 1/II.

Cranial Nerves III–XII

One patient of Mittal and Thomas [1986] had involvement of VI, VII as well as V and another became deaf. Brandt and Wittkamp [1983] noted temporary involvement in 6 patients, 2 each of II, VII and XII and a permanent VIth and a recurrent laryngeal nerve. Thiry and Hotermans [1974] had 3 patients with affection of XII and Hitchcock et al. [1983] has had this temporarily in one.

Infections

In the poll and 42 other reports that we studied there were 10 intracerebral (usually temporal lobe) abscesses of whom 3 died and 1 was left with a lasting mental deficit. There were 32 bacterial meningitides with death in only one and no lasting sequela in the others. Symptoms may not appear until after the patient has gone home and he should be warned of their possible occurrence.

Rovit [1985] routinely uses a prophylactic oral dose of 1.5 g ampicillin every 6 h for 5 days. Our infectious disease consultants say that the risk of the antibiotic approximates the risk of infection and counsel against its use in the absence of special indication. The patient of Sweet with a brain abscess developed it after 3 sessions in 5 days to secure an adequate lesion. We now use prophylactic antibiotics if the procedure is repeated in 10 days or less. We use steam autoclaving for all but the thermistors and thermocouples which are gas sterilized. The few aseptic meningeal reactions have been short-lived.

Hemorrhages

These are the greatest hazard. A bleeding diathesis may be provoked by many of the drugs in current use. Hence complete blood counts including a platelet count, prothrombin and partial thromboplastin times plus the especially important bleeding time are valuable in the workup. In 14% of our recent studies of 219 patients the bleeding time was elevated at greater than 9.5 min. In this event 20 mg prednisone 3 times daily plus elimination of the offending drug may help restore this level to normal in a few days — provided the hematologist does not uncover some other cause for a hemorrhagic diathesis. Sharp rises in blood pressure incident to electrode placement and heating occur to varying degrees in most patients [Sweet et al., 1985]; these are best discerned by an intra-arterial monitoring of the pressure at every heartbeat. The initial resistance of Sweet to subjecting the patient to an intra-arterial line was overcome by the demonstration of systolic pressure rises of 100 mm Hg in a few seconds — too rapid to be spotted promptly by the automatic brachial cuff inflation systems. We do not shut off the heat until the brief blood pressure elevations move above the low 200 mm Hg range. Too much vasodilator drug was followed in one patient of a colleague by such protracted severe hypotension that a nonfatal myocardial infarct ensued. The neurosurgical poll revealed 15 major intracerebral hemorrhages unrelated to puncture of a vessel by the electrode; 8 patients died; 4 had major residual sequelae. One hopes the foregoing precautions will sharply reduce such sequelae. However, some of these aged patients are already on the verge of a stroke which, though most unusual, has to remain one of the unavoidable hazards of any operation in the older age group.

Intracerebral Hemorrhages Due to Needle Puncture via Foramen Ovale. It has become apparent that aspiration of venous blood intracranially in this procedure, usually from entry into the cavernous sinus, does not cause a significant hemorrhage with the 20- to 22-gauge needle. After proper replacement of the needle-electrode we have routinely made lesions at the same sitting without sequelae. The neurosurgical poll revealed 10 intracranial hemorrhages related to needle puncture — 4 intratemporal and one subtemporal hematoma and 5 more arterial subarachnoid hemorrhages. Death occurred in 5 of these with lasting disablement in one. Sweet has once aspirated arterial blood when the radiographs showed the needle tip to be in the usual proper locus for a lesion. Prompt withdrawal of the needle was followed by no symptoms and clear CSF upon lumbar puncture. Nugent and Berry [1974] describe a similar case. Sweet treated his patient at a later date by open operation. On another occasion initially clear CSF became very bloody and did not clear during the withdrawal of 13 ml. The procedure was terminated with no lesion and no sequela. The small or accessory middle meningeal artery enters the foramen ovale to supply trigeminal pathways in the middle fossa. Possibly such an enlarged artery was responsible for the bleeding in these 3 cases.

As pointed out by Håkanson [1981] the data from intracisternal lidocaine blocks and metrizamide injections show that clear CSF can come from just beneath the temporal lobe rather than the trigeminal cistern. Thus, when the needle was in the position of figure 1/2 it lay in the CSF above the trigeminal cistern as attested by the failure of 1.65 ml 2% lidocaine to achieve a trigeminal block, whereas with the minimal replacement of the needle tip into trigeminal cisternal CSF, as shown in figure 1/2 (right), 0.1 ml of the lidocaine provoked a complete trigeminal analgesia. If the electrode tip were 2–3 mm higher it would probably be in the temporal lobe.

On many occasions deep insertion of the electrode has yielded no CSF and no response to electrical stimulation at up to 0.5 V. Then on withdrawal of the needle (anteriorly and inferiorly) CSF was obtained along with a low-voltage sensory response, strongly suggesting that the tip had originally been in the inferior temporal lobe or the midbrain — to date always without sequela. Especially in brachycephalics, puncture through the canal of the foramen ovale can also conduct the electrode tip into dangerously high posterior territory as illustrated by a recent case (fig. 1/3a). The tip here lies

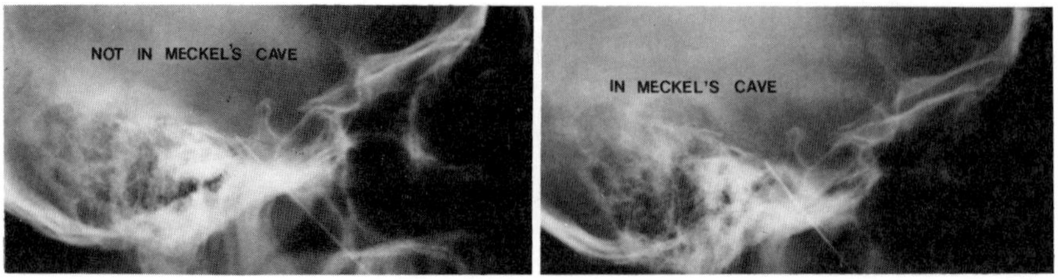

Fig. 1/2. Similarity of lateral views with electrode in trigeminal cistern or above it. On left, electrode tip slightly higher above petrous bone than after replacement on right. In position of left film tip was in CSF under temporal lobe; on right, tip in CSF of trigeminal cistern. See text for supporting evidence.

14 mm above the petrous bone, higher than we have seen in any other patient, 6 mm behind the top of the posterior clinoid process. From this site came clear, colorless CSF. Only after 9 mm further withdrawal of the electrode to the position of figure 1/3b did the threshold finally drop to 0.20 V for sensation in cheek and both lips. In view of the foregoing considerations we now recommend securing radiographic assurance that the electrode is not going to lie too far above the petrous pyramid as it is advanced.

An obvious way to reduce the hazard of bleeding is to use an electrode of smaller diameter — of 22-gauge with a cross-sectional area of 0.43 mm^2 (compared with 0.67 mm^2 for a 20-gauge, 0.92 for a 19-gauge and 1.32 mm^2 for an 18-gauge needle) and to guide the electrode by fluoroscopy and films. The smaller cross-section of the 22-gauge shaft may also decrease the likelihood of protracted pain referred to the mandibular division and related to the longitudinal penetration of this nerve at the foramen ovale. This however has never been a persistent problem with the 20-gauge electrode.

Another hazard may perhaps be related to the most unusual fact of previous radiation therapy. Mittal and Thomas [1986] describe a patient who 38 years earlier had had radiotherapy after removal of a right temporal astrocytoma. She did not awaken after her right trigeminal RF lesions and CT scan showed 'diffuse right intracranial hemorrhage with blood in the right lateral ventricle' leading to death in 19 days. The radiation-induced vascular and fibrotic changes may have increased the risks of bleeding from the needle. This was the only major complication in their series of 280 RF lesions.

Arterial Puncture below the Base of Skull or through a Wrong Foramen. There have been several reports in which the surgeon identified the foramen lacerum (anterior) with puncture of the internal carotid at this site. Another site for entry of the internal carotid is just below the opening in the petrous bone via which the artery enters this structure. Usually prompt withdrawal of the electrode has been followed by no sequela [Broggi, 1975; Graziussi et al., 1982; Hitchcock et al., 1983; Kanpolat et al., 1982; Nugent and Berry, 1974; Silverberg and Britt, 1978]. However, Rish [1976] reports a patient in whom the foramen lacerum was entered on 2 successive days with an 18-gauge electrode. Each day the needle was replaced into the foramen ovale and a second-division lesion made — inadequate the first day. Four hours after the second set of lesions a contralateral weakness appeared which by 12 h became a hemiplegia. The ipsilateral intrapetrous carotid artery showed on angiogram a mural irregularity. There was a gradual useful degree of recovery. Thiry and Hotermans [1974] had 2 patients whose arterial punctures were followed by a cerebral ictus. The hemiplegia of one recovered in a week, but a Sylvian softening without recovery persisted in the other. Although a carotid puncture heals with a thrombus, continued manipulations with their accompanying bursts of hypertension may convert enough of the thrombus to an embolus to lead to the stroke experienced by these patients. Although there are several reports of continuation of the procedure at the same session after an arterial puncture, we prefer to wait about a week before reoperation until the thrombus at the puncture site is covered with endothelium.

A third possibility is entry into the intrapetrous portion of the internal carotid artery through the occasional osseous deficiency in the inferior wall of its canal; and if the superior wall is also deficient one can continue on through into the brain. Sweet did this once in the postmortem room. We know of no reports of this misadventure in vivo.

The Foramina or Canals of Vesalius and of Arnold. On 9 occasions Sweet has placed the electrode through a small opening in the medial part of the floor of the middle cranial fossa which lies a variable distance anterior and/or medial to the foramen ovale. Anatomy texts and several skulls were studied after the first such misplacement without revealing any ancillary opening. No sequela was seen with the first 8 such errors (5 reported in 1976), but the 9th patient gradually developed a hemorrhage in the ipsilateral (dominant) temporal lobe, apparent only after an appropriate lesion had been made in the rootlets (fig. 1/4a, b). Happily her dysphasia cleared in 2 weeks. This episode led to further study of this opening, earlier erroneously described by

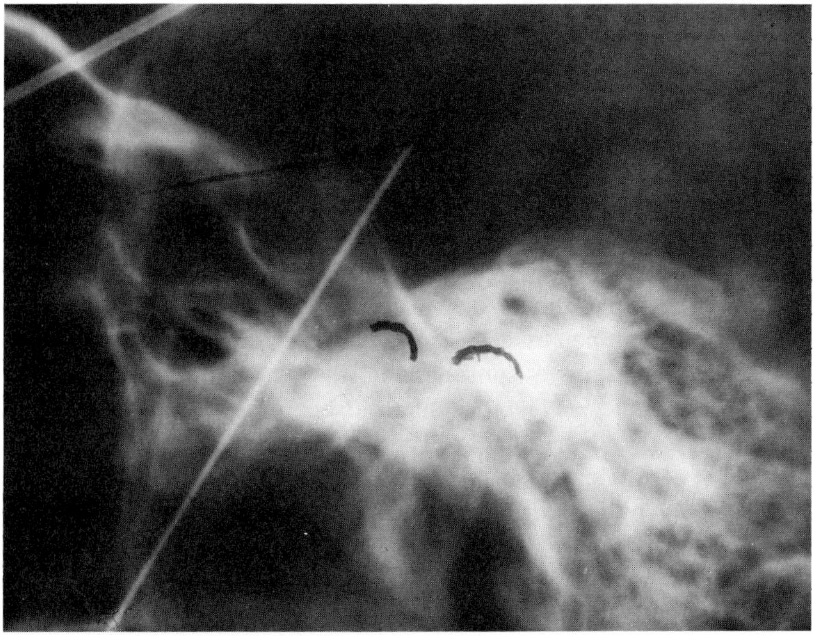

a

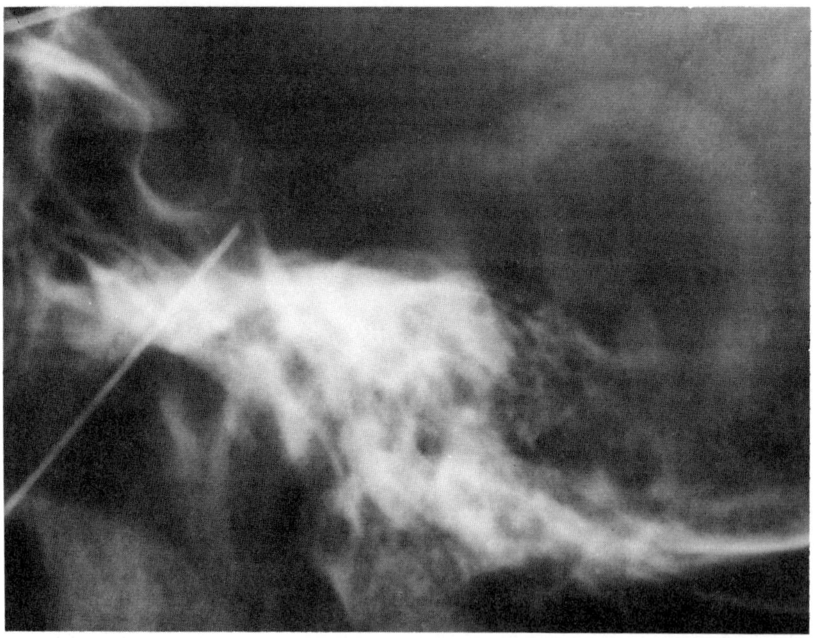

b

Sweet [1976b] as unnamed. It proves to have the ultra-distinguished name of the foramen or canal of Vesalius. It always lies behind the foramen rotundum and may be close enough to the foramen ovale so that the range of variation in the external landmarks for directing the needle shaft both from the lateral and sagittal directions includes entry into this opening as a major possibility. The anatomical texts of Testut [1896], Gray [1901] and Paturet [1957] all describe it (fig. 1/5). Gray's latest edition by Warwick estimates its incidence on at least one side as 40%. Lasjaunias and Berenstein [1987], in a text of neuroangiography, describe not only an emissary vein but also a branch of the accessory meningeal artery as utilizing this foramen. All five anatomists describe the foramen of Vesalius as varying in size, often absent and transmitting a small vein. Sweet has only once been able to identify it in a basal radiograph of the skull in these 9 cases even when the electrode passed through it. Paturet adds that its inferior opening is at the base of the pterygoid apophysis below and lateral to the opening for the Vidian canal.

We illustrate the foramen or canal of Vesalius on the left side only, in 2 dry skulls shown from above (fig. 1/6). The larger opening is easily traversed by an 18-gauge needle, the other only by one of 19 gauge. Figure 1/7, lateral radiographs with the needle shaft extending intracranially, shows the maximal difference between an anteriorly and posteriorly directed 20-gauge electrode. Sindou et al. [1987] in their first 200 procedures describe entering 'a false route' in 10 cases — 2 in the carotid canal, one in the jugular foramen and 7 in the pterygomaxillary fissure. If their electrode went on into the intracranial cavity it may have been in the foramen of Vesalius instead of the pterygomaxillary fissure.

Only Paturet of the five anatomists describes another opening, the innominate canal of Arnold for another emissary vein, lying posterior to the foramen ovale (fig. 1/5). One notes that this opening is in or lateral to the sagittal plane of the lateral third of the foramen ovale — so the needle here would be likely to pass lateral to the trigeminal pathways and go into the brain. DeRougemont [1973] tells us that he has once passed an electrode through this 'trou innomine'.

Fig. 1/3. Electrode trajectory much too high despite entry via foramen ovale. *a* with 14 mm shaft exposed, tip 14 mm above petrous bone and 6 mm behind top of posterior clinoid process in CSF. *b* 23 mm shaft exposed, tip 2 mm in front of profile clivus — probably in V ganglion.

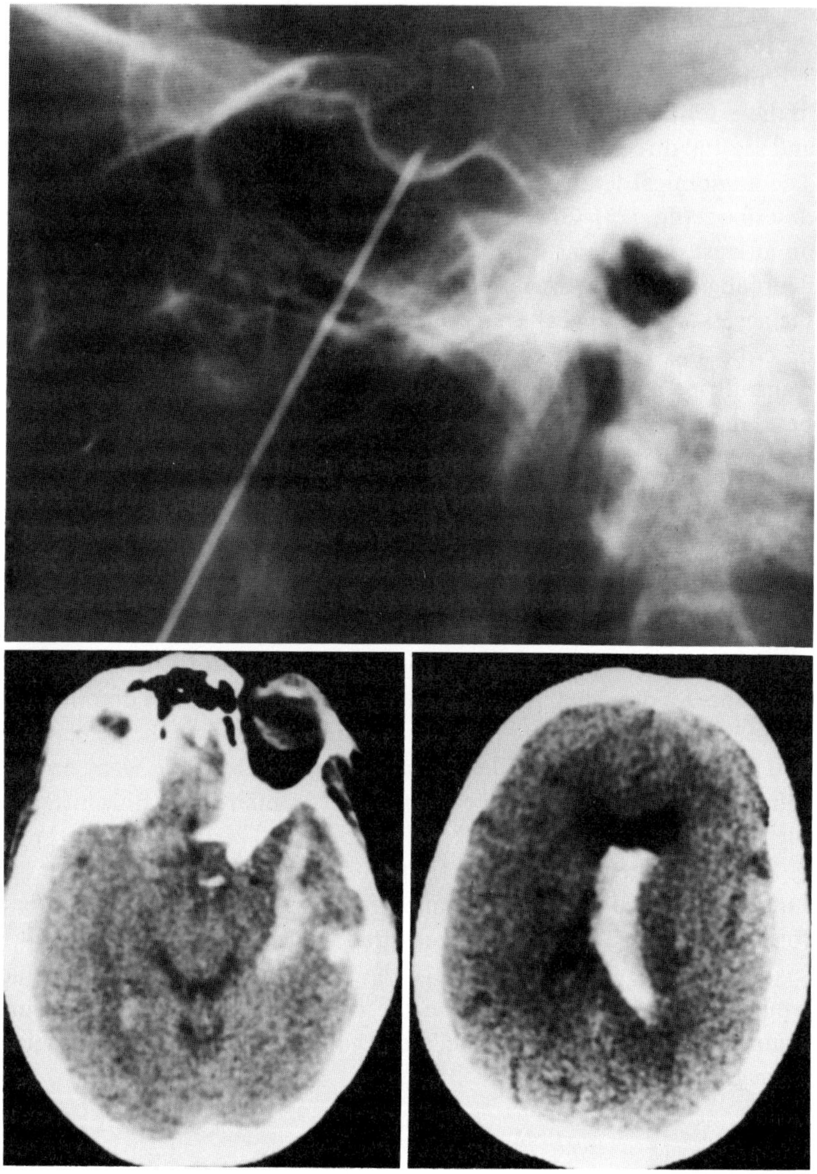

a

b

Fig. 1/4. a Electrode passes through foramen of Vesalius. Tip not in blood or CSF. Electrical stimulation: 0 response at 0.5 V. *b* CT scan later same day: on left image hemorrhage within left temporal lobe; on right image — blood also in left lateral ventricle. Fortunate complete resolution of symptoms (aphasia) in 2 weeks.

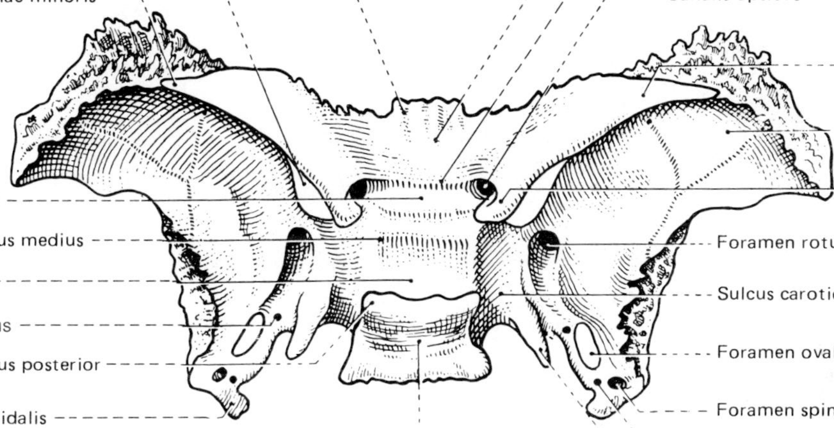

Fig. 1/5. Superior view of isolated sphenoid bone showing foramen of Vesalius (trou de Vésale, foramen venosum) and innominate canal of Arnold both sides. From Paturet [1957].

Now that it is clearly possible to provoke an intratemporal hemorrhage via the route of Vesalius, we are further convinced that one should establish, with fluoroscopy and radiographs as needed, that the medial half or two thirds of the foramen ovale is being entered. As Nugent points out, we should aim in the lateral projection for the junction of the profile of the clivus with the upper surface of the petrous bone. However, if this surface has less than the usual upward slope as it moves backward, one may need to enter the foramen ovale in a more horizontal direction in order to avoid too superior a trajectory. Figure 1/2 shows the usual upward slope; figure 1/3 shows a flatter upper petrous surface which led to too high an electrode entry. Piercing the skin 10 mm or more above the horizontal plane of the labial commissure may correct this problem.

Rarely, Sweet has placed the electrode tip as far back as 15–16 mm behind the clivus and still in CSF, in order to secure needed second- or first-division reference of sensation. The further back the electrode the more

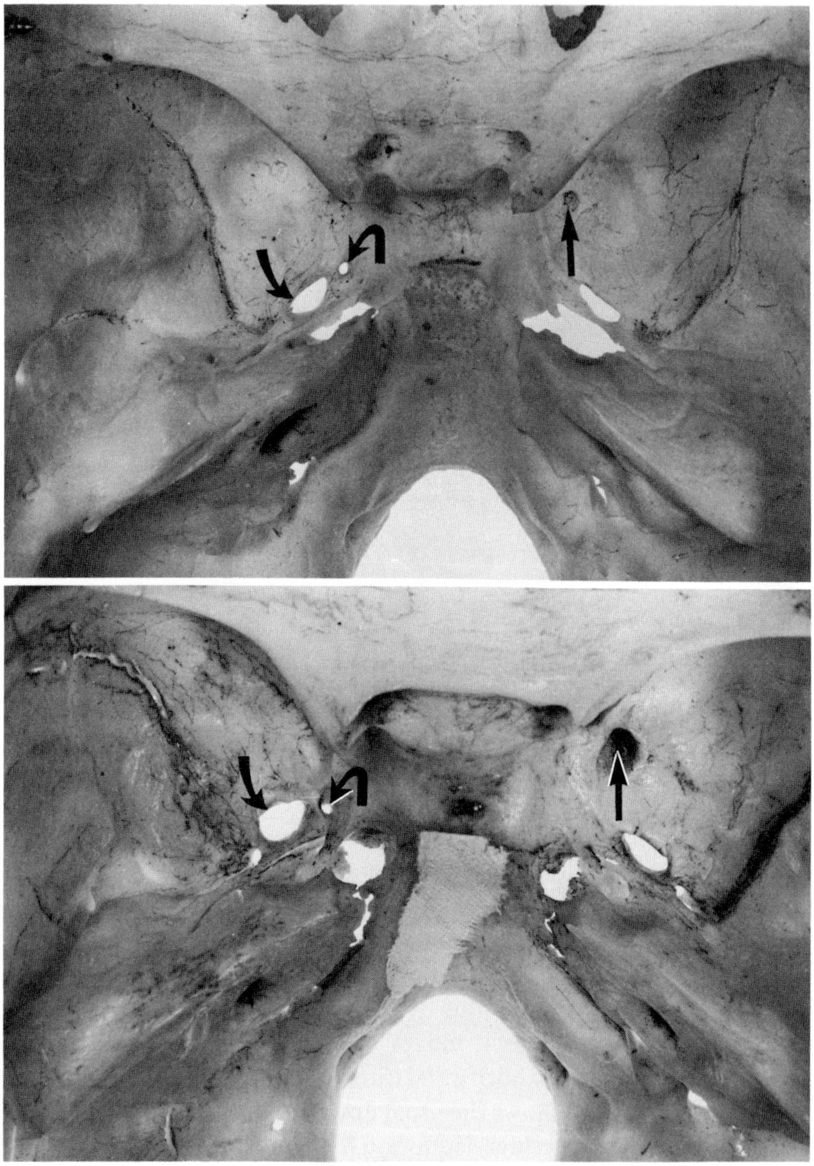

Fig. 1/6. Basal views from above of 2 dry skulls to show a foramen of Vesalius on left side only in each skull. In all views recurved arrow = foramen of Vesalius: curved arrow = foramen ovale; long straight arrow = foramen rotundum; jagged foramina without arrows and medial to ovale = foramen lacerum.

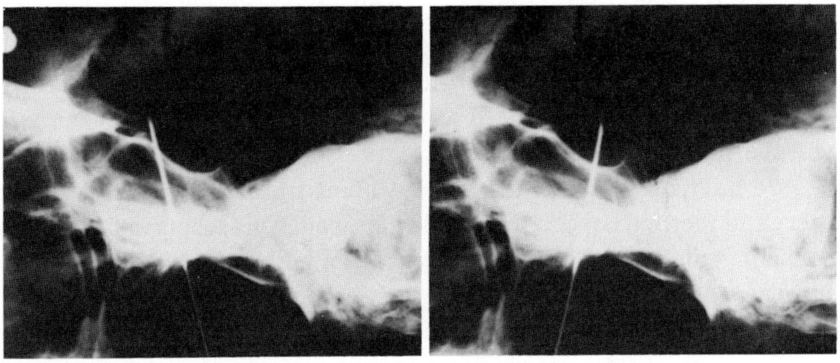

Fig. 1/7. Same skull as figure 1/6. Lateral radiograph with 20-gauge electrode through foramen of Vesalius. On left with maximal forward trajectory and on right with maximal backward trajectory permitted by foramen in this skull.

likely it is to be behind aberrant ganglion cells among the rootlets [Schmidek, 1968; Stibbe, 1939] and the less likely is recurrence from this cause. With so small a 5-mm bare needle it may not always be possible with one trajectory to make an adequate lesion; a second fluoroscopically guided placement may be needed. Possibly the tactic of Brisman [1987a] of combining heat with glycerol may prove helpful in such cases. The earlier view of Sweet that a freehand approach based on external landmarks was safe has required modification.

Use of an Electrode Protruding beyond the Tip of the Sharp Needle

The instrumentation of a small, curved, dull-tipped electrode protruding beyond the end of the entering 18-gauge needle described by Zervas [1965] — early favored by Nugent and Berry [1974] and Rovit [1985] and more recently by Tew [Tobler et al., 1983] — has the advantage of permitting improvement in the electrode position simply by withdrawing only the electrode, rotating it and reprotruding it. Nugent finds that he need give no general anesthesia during the lesion making with this small electrode, a tactic which allows prompt termination of the lesion if first-division analgesia is imminent as is often the case. Numerous observers agree that as one is gradually deepening second-division analgesia a total first-division anesthesia may suddenly appear. The use of this small electrode has enabled Nugent and Rovit to keep corneal anesthesia to the low level of 2 and 4%, respectively, for the better part of their series. Nugent lost the corneal reflex in only one of his last 172 patients. Tobler and Tew have drawn attention to another advantage of this curved protruding electrode, i.e. that whereas they had 5% masticator paralyses in 700 procedures with the straight nonprotruding needle, this figure was reduced to 0.66% or one patient in 150 procedures with the curved electrode.

We have been concerned lest the blunt tip of the electrode indent an artery and thermal coagulation weaken its wall. This seems in fact to be a rare problem. Apfelbaum [1977] has described a patient who drifted into stupor during lesion-making with such an electrode, 5 mm beyond the needle, and became comatose and hemiplegic with a fixed dilated pupil before the neurosurgeon could remove an apparently intratemporal hematoma. The hemiplegia persisted. One of Nugent's patients developed a subarachnoid hemorrhage the day after operation but had fully recovered in a week. Ipsilateral bruits from a carotid-cavernous fistula in 3 patients of Nugent and Rovit were presumably due to indentation of the intracavernous internal carotid; all healed spontaneously. Sekhar et al. [1979] describe 2 such fistulas which did require surgery; one resulted after use of the Nugent type of electrode with an 18-gauge sheath, the other followed a single bupivacaine injection which was preceded by a recognized intracranial venepuncture (probably cavernous sinus) with a 19-gauge needle. Kanpolat et al. [1982], using the same 18-gauge sheath with protruding electrode, have also had, in 294 procedures, one carotid cavernous fistula requiring surgery.

Another potential hemorrhagic hazard is the patient with a symptomatic trigeminal neuralgia due to an arteriovenous malformation. We have had one such patient successfully treated without incident. Especially because of this lesion, or a small tumor or aneurysm, a high-resolution CT scan with contrast might be advisable in the workup.

Trigeminal Motor Weakness or Paralysis

Tew has emphasized the value of minimizing the sequela of masticator weakness and has also found trismus to be more troublesome than weakness. He has succeeded admirably in reducing both to one case in his last 150 by using a protruding type of dull-tipped electrode he developed with the Radionics Instrument Company. Table 1/II shows a marked variation in the incidence of this loss, with the Sweet figures being among the highest. In the comprehensive report of Frank et al. [1985a] from three major independent neurosurgical services there was a masticatory deficit averaging less than 1% with one service describing no such loss in 309 cases. Campos et al. [to be published] noting masticator weakness in 51% of their cases, record a mean time to recovery of 9 months. Perez Calvo et al. [1983] and Sweet find that but few patients have complained of the unilateral temporary loss of this function. Sindou and Keravel [1979] and Sindou et al. [1987] though, report that the paralysis was lasting in 2% of their patients. Pertuiset et al. [1977] had 2 patients with 'chewing troubles' lasting for 6 months and Siegfried [1981] describes masseter weakness at 5–8 years in 1.5% — 2 of 135 patients.

However, in those with a threat or the fact of the disorder becoming bilateral, i.e. especially those under 50 years of age or with multiple sclerosis, one should also concentrate on saving the motor root. If the response to single shocks of a square wave signal is a masticator jerk at a threshold less than thrice the sensory threshold at that site, we recommend shift of the electrode more laterally until this response is eliminated. Thus far, these patients of ours have had no problems related to masticator weakness.

Paralysis of tensor tympani and/or tensor Veli palatini has in the view of several observers given rise to such symptoms as roaring, popping or fullness in the ear [Tobler et al., 1983] or impaired hearing [Menzel et al. 1975; Lahuerta et al., 1985]. Schürmann and Schürmann [1975] suggest that slight hearing disturbances in 9% of their patients may be due to hematomas in the vicinity of the Eustachian tube.

Contralateral Neuralgia Developing in the Postoperative Period

Sindou et al. [1987] describe this curious behavior in 1.6% of their cases without any relation to the primary neuralgia.

Minor Sequelae

Various secretory disturbances have been noted. Menzel et al. [1975] list increased tearing in 17% and too dry an eye in 3%, increased nasal secretion in 23%, increased salivation in 17% and a decrease in 3%. Rifkinson [1987] has a remarkable case of bilateral trigeminal neuralgia whose open rhizotomy with analgesia and anesthesia on the first side was followed by an RF lesion 6 years later on the other side. This produced analgesia without anesthesia in all three divisions. Although the tic pains were gone both eyes began to tear profusely much of the time.

Atypical Trigeminal Neuralgia

A constant or long-lasting background pain on which the provokable paroxysms are superimposed is the commonest reason for classification in this category. This was the case in 185 of our 790 patients, in 86% of whom both the constant pain as well as the paroxysms were completely relieved. In the remaining 26 patients modest constant pain persisted. The feature of a continuing background pain often appeared after paroxysms only had been present for some years, and might occur after a recurrence following an initially successful invasive procedure.

Penzholz's [1986] experience with the constant pains occurring after destructive operations for the typical neuralgias — 'principally electro-coagulation of the old type' — has been much more discouraging. He states that they can 'practically never be eliminated by thermocoagulation'. Menzel's [1986] experience has been similar.

Other atypical features of trigeminal neuralgia included minimal sensory loss, protracted bouts for 30 min to 2 h of intense steady pain, ipsilateral trigger zones outside the trigeminal domain or even on the other side of the face. With the exception of one patient with multiple sclerosis these features did not negate a good result from an RF lesion.

Multiple Sclerosis

The facial pains in this disorder are usually indistinguishable from those of clear-cut tic douloureux but a substantial number fall into the atypical category. Thus, 4 of the 12 such patients described by White and Sweet [1969] had atypical features and in my present series of 44 patients with multiple sclerosis out of 702, 16 or 36% were atypical in one or more respects. In the 31 patients who are remaining unilateral, we have ventured to make denser lesions; recurrences in 2 of them led to operations elsewhere; we are treating the lesser recurrences in a third by low doses of medication. Since most of these with multiple sclerosis are likely to have their other symptoms of this disorder worsened by average doses of the drugs, they may require a denser lesion to completely eliminate the need for such drugs. The 13 bilateral patients of W.H.S. have been handled in a more cautious fashion to avoid both masseter weakness and loss of touch sensation on the oral mucosa. Three or more procedures were needed in 8 of the relieved 12 and 9 of them needed medications at the last follow-up. One of them, after another lesion elsewhere, must eat before a mirror because of intraoral sensory loss.

We have failed to provide adequate relief in only one case who was unusual on three scores. (1) In addition to short electric shocks there were 15-min to 2-hour intervals of steady pain of agonizing intensity in the temple; (2) later in such an attack the steady pain or 'shocks' would appear in the ipsilateral shoulder and skipping the arm appear in the ipsilateral outer forearm; (3) there was not the slightest tendency for a local stimulus to provoke pain anywhere. Toxic doses of tegretol controlled the pain. Nonprovokable pains in the first two divisions appeared after a third-division trigeminal RF lesion was made. Despite a total of three RF lesions in a month producing complete analgesia in all three divisions of skin and mucosa, he still had the episodes of intense pain in the analgesic areas of the face and in the upper limb. The patient's weight of 340-lb, gross rigidity in both legs and pain in the arm have discouraged open operation.

Rovit [1985] has excellent results in 18 patients; he notes that the recurrence rate is higher especially if the first division is affected. Of Broggi et al.'s [1985] 14 cases 3 were bilateral. They did a total of 26 procedures on them including one patient with 3 procedures on each side. Their final result was 100% relief in the whole group with no analgesics required. Brandt and Wittkamp [1983] are especially encouraged by their results in the 11 of 257 patients with multiple sclerosis. Their average of 9 years of freedom from pain was longer than any other group of their patients. Ipsilateral reoperation was needed in 4 of Brisman's [1987a] 16 patients, in 5 of whom the attacks were bilateral; all patients were relieved. Of the 20 cases of Siegfried [1977b] 19 had excellent results, the only failure being in a patient with an inadequate lesion who refused reoperation. His lone bilateral operation was without complications. Similarly, Brett et al. [1982] had 8 happy patients after lesions which produced transient masticator paresis in 2 with only one recurrence after an average follow-up of 26 months.

Bilateral Trigeminal Neuralgia without Multiple Sclerosis

Brisman [1987b] has sought since December 1983 to reduce the intratrigeminal complications of bilateral RF lesions by combining a mild electrical lesion with a small dose of glycerol up to 0.25 ml. This course of action, pursued in 10 of the 37 operations on 32 patients, was carried only to the level of less than 50% hypalgesia in all of them. He made this mild lesion on the second side of those with profound denervation on the first side. W.H.S. thinks he controls the site and degree of sensory loss better with RF heat only.

Conclusion

The numbers of patients being treated by this method indicate that many neurosurgeons find it acceptable as the first invasive procedure to use.

Retrogasserian Injection of Glycerol

Synonym: Percutaneous Retrogasserian Glycerol Rhizotomy

Historical Note

During the development of a stereotactic technique for γ-irradiation of the trigeminal ganglion and root in the treatment of trigeminal neuralgia, glycerol was used as a vehicle to introduce tantalum dust into the trigeminal cistern [Leksell, 1971; Håkanson and Leksell, 1979]. Quite unexpectedly, it was observed that the intracisternal injection of glycerol alone rendered the patient completely free from the paroxysmal pain without producing any significant sensory loss. This fortuitous observation led Håkanson to the development and evaluation of the injection of glycerol in the subarachnoid space behind the trigeminal ganglion in the treatment of tic douloureux [Håkanson 1981, 1982, 1983].

Methods and Results of Håkanson

Methods. The patient is seated in a rotatable chair with radiography available both by fluoroscopy and films. Premedication is with 1 ml oxicon and 1 ml scopolamine plus 5 mg droperidol (Dripdol). Half this dose is used for older or debilitated patients. He gave only local anesthesia to 74 of his first 75 patients. A 22-gauge lumbar puncture needle penetrates the skin well lateral to the labial commissure. CSF must be obtained. If fluoroscopy and films show the needle tip to be approximately in the correct position but no CSF appears, he leaves that needle in position and places another in what he thinks is a more correct spot. Figure 1/8 illustrates a position that is too far lateral for the original needle.

Usually the shaft must go through the medial half of the foramen ovale. This film also illustrates the next step of his procedure, in which he injects less than 1 ml of concentrated metrizamide (300 mg I/ml). Later fluoroscopy shows the contrast medium filling the cistern and running back through the porus trigemini into the cerebellopontine angle. The relationship of the CSF space with the rootlets to the subdural space in the trigeminal cistern and to the subarachnoid space beneath the temporal lobe is demonstrated by Håkanson's diagram in figure 1/9. Films taken after the injection of the metrizamide may demonstrate that the needle is in the subarachnoid space below the temporal lobe or in the subdural space of the cistern. Placement in the subdural space is more evident as the metrizamide passes through the porus trigemini and lines the subarachnoid space behind the clivus (fig. 1/10). He found that previous open trigeminal operations in the middle cranial

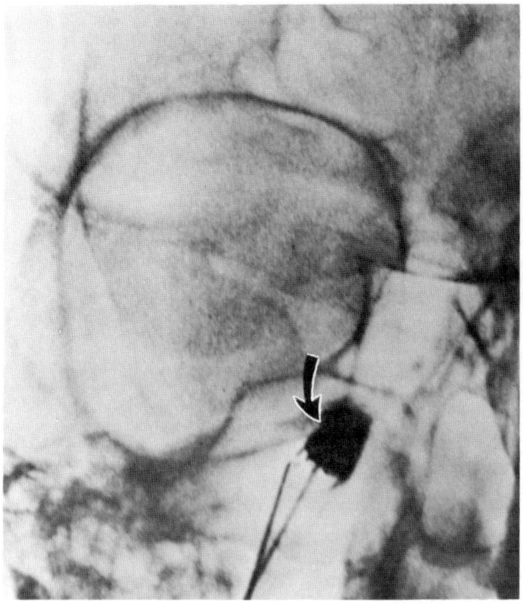

Fig, 1/8. Håkanson technique of needle placement and use of metrizamide. When the first 22-gauge needle was placed too far laterally in Meckel's cave to enter CSF, a more medial placement succeeded and metrizamide (curved arrow) was injected. (Courtesy Håkanson: unpublished).

fossa often damaged the trigeminal cistern so that the metrizamide would leak out of it. When, as rarely occurred, he is unable to secure CSF, he makes a selective thermal lesion. Having verified the proper position of the needle tip, he then empties the metrizamide into the posterior fossa by removing the syringe and extending the patient's head for several minutes. If the patient has no third-division trigger zone, however, he seeks to leave a little of the heavy metrizamide (specific gravity 1.329) which will in turn form a layer below the CSF (specific gravity 1.007). He adjusts the amount of glycerol to the volume of the cistern, estimating from the metrizamide picture that the total amount of glycerol to be injected into the cistern varies from 0.2 to 0.5 ml. (In one of his cases the metrizamide film revealed a small benign tumor here.) In cases with first- or second-division neuralgia he injects up to 0.25 ml. His 22-gauge needle shaft contains about 0.05 ml. He does not examine facial sensibility during or immediately after the procedure. Once an injec-

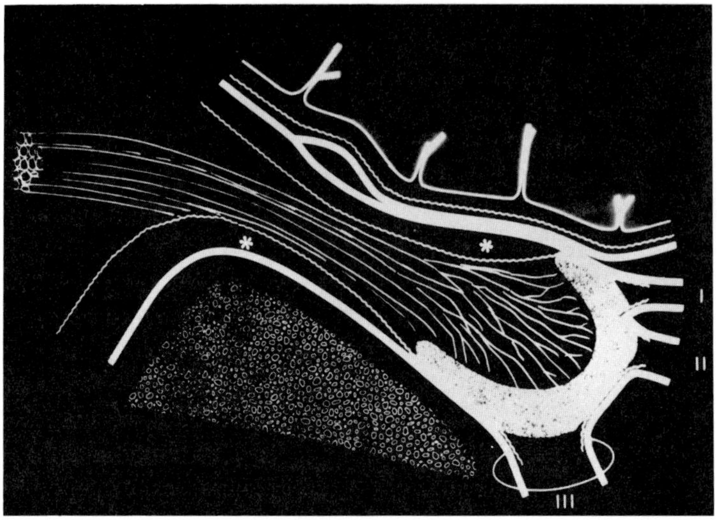

Fig. 1/9. Håkanson's diagram illustrating possibility of injecting into the subdural space. Arachnoid membrane indicated by wavy lines, dura by dense white lines, subdural spaces by asterisks. From Håkanson [1981].

tion is complete the patient is kept sitting in bed with the head flexed for another hour in order to keep the glycerol mainly in the cistern. He has mixed tantalum dust with the glycerol before injection in most cases so that later films show the exact size of the cistern in order to facilitate a future injection therein.

Whisler and Hill [1972] and Apfelbaum [1978] also recommend routine fluoroscopy to which Apfelbaum has added the tactic of speeding up penetration of the foramen ovale by placing a small radiopaque marker 3 cm lateral to the labial commissure at the site of needle penetration of the skin. The marker is projected to overlie the foramen ovale. This facilitates directing the needle straight down toward the foramen aided by intermittent fluoroscopic feedback. We have also found it simpler to use an electrode with a radiolucent hub.

Results

In his first 100 patients Håkanson achieved early complete pain relief in 96. In about half of these pain relief was delayed for 4–6 days, during which paroxysms of pain, occasionally severe, occurred. At 1- to 6-year follow-up

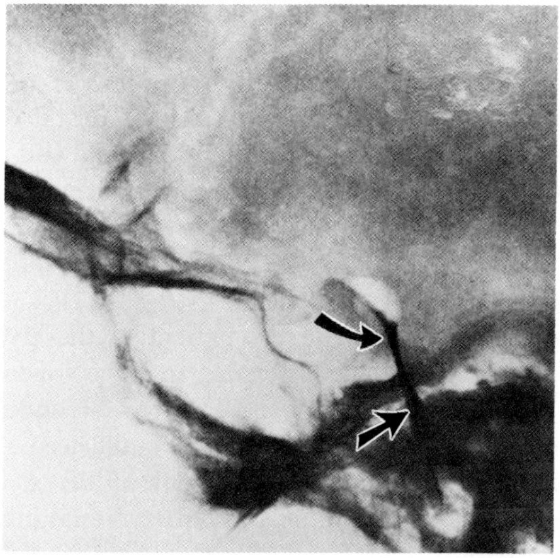

Fig. 1/10. Subdural injection of metrizamide proven by its close apposition to the full length of the clivus following extension of the patient's head. (Courtesy Håkanson: unpublished.)

relief did not persist in 35 but only 16 of the recurrences were severe enough to require reinjection. This rendered 12 of them pain-free — only 4 requiring further surgical therapy. A further dramatic feature was the complete absence of any complication. There was no significant sensory loss, no corneal anesthesia, facial dysesthesia nor involvement of other cranial nerves. No one else has such a perfect record of no complications.

Mechanism of Action of Glycerol

As already discussed under RF lesions evidence is conflicting as to whether or not there is a nonselective or a selective destruction of nerve fibers of various sizes, and if selective which fibers are preferentially destroyed [Håkanson, 1982; Sweet et al., 1981; Rengachary et al., 1983; Lunsford et al., 1985].

Another Technique

In an effort to decrease the numbers of early failures, dysesthesias and corneal anesthesias we have modified the technique in three ways:

(1) With the electrode intracranial we test for physiologic responses to electrical square wave and heat stimulation in order to place the tip to the best advantage just as we do for making an RF lesion. The electrode is adjusted so that the reference of sensation is confined to the lowest division harboring a trigger zone, i.e. the third division if both the second and third divisions contain trigger zones. We try to ensure that the CSF is coming from the trigeminal cistern by adjusting the tip until the threshold for sensory response to pulses of 1 ms at 50 cps is 0.03–0.2 V and that to gentle RF heating it is from 40–48 °C — the lower the better.

(2) We use the physiologic responses of the patient to the glycerol injection as evidence that the agent is actually going into the trigeminal cisternal CSF rather than the cisternal subdural space or the CSF under the temporal lobe. (We inject only if a drop of CSF emerges from the needle with the patient sitting immediately prior to the placement of the glycerol syringe.) The sensory responses are either of nonpainful paresthesias in a few patients or more frequently painful sensations usually evoked by the first intracisternal drops of glycerol. In the sitting position in which the injection is made it is not easy to maintain the needle electrode immobile so that no portion of the bevel lies in the subdural space, precluding a subdural locus of some of the glycerol. In fact, in one of our early patients the flabby facial tissues allowed the needle to slip below the foramen ovale when she sat up with her head flexed. Now the surgeon holds the needle-electrode in its desired position for the several minutes needed to complete the injection.

In our experience the glycerol has penetrated more readily into the first than the third division, consonant with Henderson's [1965] postmortem studies which showed that alcohol had a tendency to skip from the third to the first division, apparently due to a circular venous sinus in Meckel's cave which facilitates this type of spread. Keeping the patient's head fully flexed and leaning markedly toward the side of the lesion has not solved this problem of securing third-division involvement. In the lone patient in whom facial sensations did not occur during injection, the preinjection thresholds upon electrical stimulation were high; there was no immediate sensory loss and no relief of pain. We had almost certainly failed here to inject into the trigeminal cisternal CSF. Varying degrees of early trigeminal sensory loss did occur in the other 11 failures. In the 72% of our 74 cases with early relief it was complete within less than one day and in 24% more it occurred in less than 5 days. Hence we conclude that these were properly placed injections. In 2 patients only was relief deferred until 3 and 6 weeks later. In a few patients severe pain has been provoked during or shortly after the glycerol injection.

We keep the needle of a syringe loaded with brevital lying in the side-arm of the intravenous line, ready for instant use. When we are seeking to avoid first-division loss we use first-division reference of sensation as an indication to withdraw the electrode a bit so that subsequent increments cause sensation only in lower divisions.

(3) The promptness with which some sensory loss usually develops has led us to do a sensory examination to pinprick after each drop of glycerol injected from 0.15 to the maximum 0.4 ml (the 10-cm shaft of a 20-gauge needle holds almost exactly 0.1 ml, and that of a 22-gauge needle about 0.05 ml).

Many of the patients in whom glycerol is left in the cistern for an hour have major fading of their analgesia within the first weeks. The corneal sensation was initially lost to cotton in 13 (14%) of our patients and was graded 1–2/10 in another 7 (9%). By the next day or within a few months 8 of these 17 patients had recovered some corneal sensation. Although 5 others lost some corneal sensation from levels of 5–10/10 early postoperatively, it dropped to zero in only one of these. We hoped that pouring the glycerol out of the trigeminal cistern by placing the patient horizontal within 20 min from the development of first-division analgesia would eliminate this corneal anesthesia. However, of 4 patients with prompt first-division analgesia in whom glycerol was kept in the cistern for only 20 min, there was recovery from the associated corneal anesthesia in only one; all 4 had only 0.2–0.25 ml injected. Of the 24 subsequent procedures at which the glycerol was left in the cistern less than 15 min after the development of analgesia in the trigger areas or in the first division, one had lasting corneal anesthesia after such a 12-min exposure. We are now limiting glycerol exposure after first-division analgesia to 5 min. A decision as to the dose and time of exposure of glycerol is in our view more soundly based on the evolving sensory loss than on an estimate of the size of the trigeminal cistern.

As noted under RF lesions we monitor blood pressure during the procedure, using i.v. sodium nitroprusside to prevent dangerous rises. We agree with Lunsford and Bennett [1984] that preoperative atropine to counteract vasovagal reactions and the anxiolytic and anti-emetic droperidol are advisable.

Various Modifications of Technique

Of those reporting recently only Shetter and Hadley [1986] and Thurel [1987] do not regard it as essential to obtain CSF before injection. The use of metrizamide is giving way to the use of nonionic contrast media such as iopamidol (isovue 300) by those who prefer radiographic demonstration that

Table 1/IV. Trigeminal glycerol rhizotomy — 17 services

Author, year	Number of patients	Initial failure, %	Time to relief	Relief 1st op., %	Relief 2nd op., %	Average follow-up
Håkanson, 1983	100	4	4–6 days in half the patients	96		1–6 years
Dieckmann et al., 1985	51					78% relief at 1 year
Igarashi et al., 1985	27		up to 1 week			
Lunsford, 1985	225					
Lunsford and Apfelbaum, 1985	73	14	av. 5 days up to 21 days	86	90	up to 3 years av. 15 months
Takusagawa et al., 1985	122	10		79		1–3 years
Arias, 1986	100	5	2–4 days in 6%			6–36 months
Beck et al., 1986	58	17		69	72	2–40 months av. 18 months
Shetter and Hadley, 1986	64	14		86		2–45 months av. 18 months
Slettebo et al., 1987	60	10		90		av. 24 months
Burchiel, 1987	48	12				

the needle is in the trigeminal cistern. Aseptic meningeal reactions described by Arias [1986], Beck et al. [1986], Lunsford [1985], Lunsford et al. [1985], Apfelbaum [1977, 1978], Rappaport [1986], and Waltz et al. [1985, 1987] have encouraged this change. Beck, Lunsford and Rappaport continue to use a contrast medium to estimate the volume of the cistern; others only to establish that the tip of the needle is in the cistern. Lunsford and Apfelbaum find the cisternal volumes to be less than 0.35 ml in 90% of the patients with no cistern greater than 0.5 ml. It would seem to us useful to adhere to the original maximum of 0.4 ml recommended by Håkanson. Any amounts less than this which overflow a small cistern will simply be diluted at once in the large posterior fossa pools. Only Beck and Sweet describe securing the

Table 1/IV. (cont.)

Recurrence reop. not needed	Recurrence reop. needed	Corneal anesthesia	Sensory loss
16%	15%	0%	never more than mild
			no dysesthesias
			40% (mild); anesth. dol. 2% (marked)
		decreased with more than 0.4 ml	hypalgesia at 8 weeks in 30% 3 high-grade dysesthesias
65% pain-free at follow-up			
10% of 73 patients; 19% of 62 patients	13% of 73 patients; 15 % of 62 patients		6% dysesthesias (moderate) 0 anesthesia dol.
58% pain-free; 17% improved; 25% in pain			anesth. dol. 2 patients 1.5%; hypesthesia 80%; dysesthesias 35%
		0%	never more than 30% loss in any division
16%	9%	1%	17%–? intraganglion inj. in 1; 1 lasting total analgesia
61% pain-free at av. 18 months		3%	analgesia 1 of 64; dysesthesia bothers about 5%
11%	28%		
	30% at av. 2 years		higher proportion sensory deficits 'than in earlier articles'
mean time to recurrence 5 months in 43% of 46 operations		7%	sensory loss >1 month in 72%

response to electrical stimulation to guide precise placement of the needle tip before injection.

Arias [1986], Igarashi et al. [1985], Shetter et al. [1986], Waltz et al. [1987], Young [1987] and Sweet [1988c] emphasize the importance of securing a sensory response to the glycerol as the most reliable evidence of its presence at the rootlets and of following this with further sensory appraisals as the drop-by-drop injection continues. Arias, in a comparative study of 100 cases, 50 injected by each method, has demonstrated that sensory examination during the procedure is preferable to metrizamide cisternography. His tempo of injection is even slower than ours with a wait of 1–5 min for sensory testing after each 0.05-ml increment of glycerol. He

Table 1/IV. Trigeminal glycerol rhizotomy — 17 services (continuation)

Author, year	Number of patients	Initial failure, %	Time to relief	Relief 1st op., %	Relief 2nd op., %	Average follow-up
Rappaport, 1986	60		relief at once 54%; 46% rel. in av. 3 days – max. 14 days	81	90	
Saini, 1987	552 469 followed			96 after up to 3 injections		1–6 years in 469 patients
Thurel, 1987	50			75		av. 15 months
Waltz et al., 1987	184	18		70	81	1–52 months
Young, 1987	157	6				
Sweet, 1988c	88	18	relief <1 day in 72%; 1 day to 1 week in 24%	82		av. 2.9 years 1–8.5 years

adds the useful feature of testing for correct position of the needle tip by insisting on trigeminal paresthesias or pain after the first 0.05 ml into the cistern, presumably correcting the position until this occurs. He seeks to place the needle tip at the profile of the middle third of the clivus as seen in the lateral radiograph. He finds the preferable position of the head is a 40° flexion for first-division pain, 25° flexion for the second division and almost erect for the third division, the reverse of what seems logical to Håkanson and Sweet. He keeps the patient in the appropriate position usually for an additional hour after the final drop of glycerol, decreasing this, however, if the sensory loss is greater than 30%. There have been only 2 aseptic meningeal reactions in our 93 procedures and none in his 56 without metrizamide cisternography.

Shetter and Waltz have occasionally injected more than 0.4 ml glycerol. We have seen one patient in whom a neurosurgeon had injected 1.5 ml in 0.1-

Table 1/IV. (cont.)

Recurrence reop. not needed	Recurrence reop. needed	Corneal anesthesia	Sensory loss
mean time to recurrence 14 months	recurrence rate 28% at 1–4 years		hypalgesia 38%; of 7 recurrences 6 did not have sensory deficit; 5% dysesthesias after 1st injection; 14% after 2nd injection
recurrences increased annually from 28% at 1 year to 96% by 6 years			dysesthesias 13%; anesthesia dolorosa 5%
	15%	2%	1 anesthesia complete VI, 2 at 5 months but no major dysesthesias
12%	17%		hypesthesia 67%; 'sensory deficit mild with 1 exception'
pain-free 79%		5%	67% significant sensory loss; 0 anesthesia dolorosa; 2% dysesthesias
	22%	14% (7) 50% of 14 V1 trigger zones	27 hyp.; 49 analg.; 4 anesth. (2 anesth. dol.); 1 hyp. dol.; 0 hyp. dol. since 1983; 0 analg. dol. since 1980; 0 anesth. dol. since 1983

ml increments over 10 min, producing minutes later total ipsilateral trigeminal hypalgesia which was followed by severe hypalgesia dolorosa in V2 and analgesia dolorosa in V3 persisting 2 years later.

Results of Proponents

Since Sweet's relatively discouraging appraisal of the literature and experience recorded in 1985 [Sweet and Poletti], nine services have published accounts, on the whole happy as to their results. Special satisfaction is reflected by the accumulation by Waltz et al. [1985, 1987] and by Young [1987] of respectively 184 and 157 cases in a relatively short time. Table 1/IV presents summary data from 17 reports of those continuing to use the procedure to varying extents. Waltz et al. [1987] had the curious experience of about 15 consecutive failures after success in over 100 previous patients. These failures proved to correlate with their pharmacy having changed to a brand of glycerol of different viscosity and osmolarity. Their excellent results resumed upon reversion to the original brand. When the earlier cases of Sweet included so many with more dysesthesias and sensory loss than Håkanson described, our pharmacy tried two other sources without eliminating these problems.

The column 'Time to relief' indicates one of the major problems when the patient comes from a long distance away. He usually prefers not to wait away from home to see if he will fall into the initial failure category of 4–18% or have delayed relief in days to one week. Since the average follow-ups are shorter than in those articles reporting many cases of RF rhizotomy, the data regarding recurrences in the 2 groups are not directly comparable. No one quite confirms the original contention of Håkanson that the sensory loss is never more than mild with no dysesthesia.

Although Rappaport [1986] continues to favor glycerol, he points out disadvantages brought to light in his 14 patients (23%) requiring reinjections for recurrences. Of these 14% developed 'painful' dysesthesias and 43% new sensory deficit as compared with 5 and 14%, respectively, after the initial injections. This was correlated with evidence for arachnoidal adhesions in the cisternal trigeminal rootlets upon comparison of cisternal volumes and appearances on the 2 occasions.

Qualified Endorsements

Saini's [1987] extensive experience of 552 cases with follow-up in 469 of them has yielded 13% with dysesthesias, 8% with anesthesia dolorosa and 5% with keratitis. The recurrence rate was 28% at one year rising annually to 96% after 6 years. The method is of special value in India and other countries where it is much cheaper than tegretol or an RF lesion. (Of interest is the fact that one fourth of these and other Indian series were under 40 years of age.) In Hamada et al.'s [1985] 136 cases there was relief in only 58%.

Reports of Dissatisfaction

At least 9 services have become dissatisfied for some combination of the following reasons:

(1) Too many early failures and later recurrences [Fraioli and Cantore, 1985; Fraioli et al., 1987; Laitinen, 1985; Maxwell, 1985; Price, 1985; Siegfried, 1985; Rhoton, 1985; Takusagawa et al., 1985; Sweet, 1988c]. In the experience of Siegfried and Rhoton the results are so clearly inferior to theirs

with RF lesions that they have not reported them and use no glycerol. Recurrence rates at 3 years were 40% for Fraioli, 57% for Price, and 20% at 1–3 years for Takusagawa. In Sweet's series 17% with initial failures were supplemented by 24% with significant recurrences; 2% required medication and 22% reoperation at from 4 months to 4 years with an average recurrence time of 1.9 years. Burchiel et al.'s [1981] and Burchiel's [1987] recurrence rate was 43% at an average postoperative time of 5 months after operation.

(2) Dysesthesias and major sensory loss. Corneal anesthesia occurred in 7% and dysesthesias in 21% of Price's [1985] cases. Corneal sensation to cotton, initially normal, was reduced as a late finding in 10 (12%) of our patients to a level of 0–2/10. In one patient the sensation dropped from 5/10 early postoperatively down to zero at one month where it remained. One of Fraioli et al.'s [1984] patients also had the delayed development at 3 months of a complete ipsilateral trigeminal anesthesia with keratitis. The worst experience regarding 'painful dysesthesia' was that of Takusagawa et al. [1985] — this occurred in 35% of 136 patients with a successful injection; in 2 it reached the level of anesthesia dolorosa; 3 had neuroparalytic keratitis. Igarashi et al. [1985] injected 0.15–0.6 ml of glycerol in 27 patients producing initial dysesthesias in 81%; these persisted with hypalgesia at 8 weeks in 30%. Of Laitinen's [1985] patients 2 had the bitter experience of hypesthesia and dysesthesia in all three divisions plus no relief of the original pain; one of them had two injections. The horizontal position and intermittent general anesthesia for an RF lesion seemed preferable to the 1-hour head-flexed, sitting position for glycerol in many of the patients of Maxwell [1985] and of Sweet.

Complications

Blood pressure fluctuations during the procedure have included a patient of Fischer [1985] whose level went to 240/100 at once after glycerol was placed in the cistern. Subsidence to a normal level took 20 min. Young [1987] also noted marked blood pressure rises with glycerol; in one of his patients the first drop of glycerol provoked such severe periorbital pain that he discontinued the procedure. Contrariwise, a burst of pain in the sitting position in one of Patrick's [1985] patients led to a marked fall in blood pressure. Bradycardia and hypotension at operation occurred in 15% of the Lunsford-Apfelbaum [1985] series.

Postoperative extratrigeminal morbidity has been minor or controllable. Three services have reported temporary extraocular palsy. Beck et al. [1986] had one facial palsy develop after 3 weeks and Waltz had one severe trigeminal and facial motor deficit which cleared entirely in one week. Bacterial meningitis without permanent sequela has been reported in 3 cases [Waltz et al., 1987; Young, 1987].

Comparison between Radiofrequency Heating and Glycerol

The most cogent comparative data we have are in our 45 patients in whom, after RF heat or glycerol lesions were made at the first session, the other modality was used either for the recurrence or after failure of the first method. Seven patients called the sensations worse after the heating; they were worse after glycerol in 17. No difference was noted by 7. The first glycerol injection failed to give initial relief in 10 of these 45, the heating in 2. Of our 88 patients treated with 93 glycerol sessions initial relief of pain occurred within 2 weeks after 74 procedures, i.e. 12 (13%) were failures.

Table 1/III p. 28 compares the incidence of paresthesias and dysesthesias between the RF and glycerol groups of Sweet. The persistent dysesthesias requiring medication after glycerol have not been eliminated in subsequent cases by using small doses of glycerol for shorter periods. Thus, 4 of the patients in this category were limited, respectively, to 0.15 ml for 6.5 min, 0.2 ml for 23 min and 2 patients each with 0.25 ml for 4 and 5 min. In each instance, exposure to glycerol was stopped after analgesia had been present throughout the skin of the first 2 trigeminal divisions and in 3 of the 4 in the third division as well for the specified number of minutes after the final drop of glycerol. These data point to more difficulty in controlling the dysesthesias than in reducing the incidence of corneal sensory deficit by detailed sensory testing and reduction of the exposure time to glycerol. Although the loss of corneal sensation once produced is not as likely to recover after an RF lesion, the locus and initial extent of sensory loss are more controllable with the RF heating.

Lunsford has suggested that our higher percentage of dysesthesias may be due to our injecting into the ganglion. We regard this as unlikely inasmuch as we have injected with the needle point at or behind the profile of the clivus in 58% of our procedures, and always only after CSF is obtained from the sitting patient's needle immediately before injection. Moreover, there has been minimal resistance to the injection. Fraioli et al. [1987] attribute 4 of their 6 initial failures to achieve relief to an intraganglionic injection.

Multiple Sclerosis

Of Lunsford and Bennett's [1984] 12 patients there was a poor result in only one, whereas 3 of 4 of the multiple sclerotics of Beck et al. [1986] were failures. Sweet had failures in only 3 of 11 patients, with 5 recurrences at 6 months to 2 years (average 1.3 years) and 3 with continuing relief from 3.2 to 6 years. Fraioli et al. [1987] failed to relieve either of 2 patients. Burchiel's [1987] 9 procedures, all successful at first, have been followed by recurrences in 6 at an average of 11 months.

Conclusion

Longer follow-ups may be required before the place of the procedure is established. At present we offer the glycerol option only to those with trigger areas in the first division, bilateral multiple sclerosis, or a desire to repeat glycerol when recurrence develops after an otherwise happy result from the first procedure. However, we take care to point out that even with short periods of glycerol in the cistern some patients may be very annoyed by the new sensations; we leave the glycerol in the trigeminal cistern for no more than 10 min after clear-cut hypalgesia develops.

Percutaneous Compression of Trigeminal Ganglion and Root

Historical Note

Mullan and Lichtor [1983] have converted to a percutaneous procedure the open compression of the trigeminal ganglion and roots in the middle fossa initiated by Shelden et al. [1955] whose method was given an extensive trial by many surgeons. White and Sweet [1969] summarized the reports of relatively few initial failures and recurrence rates varying from 8 to 25%. Mullan's excellent description of the details of his closed method involves inserting a No. 4 Fogarty balloon catheter to the tip of the standard 14-gauge liver-biopsy needle under general anesthesia. Guided by radiography he passes this into but not beyond the foramen ovale. The catheter is then pushed in 1 cm beyond the needle into Meckel's cave. The balloon is inflated with 0.5–1.0 ml of diluted 50% Conray under fluoroscopic control to assure correct position. Inflation is maintained for from 3 to 10 min, the balloon deflated, and the whole assembly withdrawn. This relatively simple gesture gave initial relief in all but one of his first 50 patients. Since the first case in 1978 there have been 6 recurrences in the first 26 cases; a repeat balloon compression relieved 3 of them and one required only a little carbamazepine.

Significant sensory loss 'almost analgesia' occurred in only 4 patients. Persistent 'distressing dysesthesias' occurred in 3 patients, one of whom also had a temporary trochlear palsy. Technical difficulties and how to avoid them were described. He concludes that the lesser inflation will eliminate dysesthesias at the price of more recurrences whereas more inflation will be followed by the converse situation. In Mullan's [1987] recent report no patient to date has had severe dysesthesias.

Bricolo and Dalle Ore [1983] used 0.6 ml in the balloon for 6 min; they had a 100% initial success rate in their 51 patients with no subjective complaint. Only a few had mild to moderate sensory loss. Of the 11 recurrences in the first year 6 required reoperation.

Fraioli et al. [1987] have treated 125 patients by this method, preferring it to RF lesions or glycerol because of the minimal sensory loss in 57%, early pain relief in 90% and recurrences in only 10.6% after an average follow-up of 2.5 years. Fraioli et al. [1984] used the smaller 2 or 3F Fogarty catheter in 6 cases; all were failures.

Lobato et al. [1987] also have a large series of 100 patients. Although they kept the balloon inflated only 50–60 s they have had only 3 recurrences at 7–11 months postoperatively. Patchy areas of sensory deficit persisted for one year after operation in 29%. 'Minimal' dysesthesia in 18% and 'significant' dysesthesia in 3% were noted.

Meglio et al. [1985] compared the results of 25 RF lesions with those of 25 microcompressions. There were 2 with dysesthesias in the RF group; none was seen after the Mullan operation but this was followed by more recurrences.

Recently, Belber and Rak [1987], who leave the balloon inflated close to 10 min, reported complete relief after every one of 33 procedures. There were 8 recurrences all medically managed in a 6-month to 7-year follow-up. There was only one mild dysesthesia. They emphasize the elimination of first-division pain with complete preservation of corneal sensation. Multiple sclerosis, present in 2 patients with bilateral pain, was successfully managed by 8 procedures, 2 on each side in each patient. One bilateral procedure at the same sitting was followed by severe weakness of mastication for 8 days before recovery set in. A 13-gauge needle was used.

Dan [1988] reports an instance of deliberate production of the numbness in the first and second trigeminal divisions thought advisable in a patient with pain after major facial injuries. The balloon compression to achieve this lasted 12 min and was followed 8 h later by complete blindness in the ipsilateral eye which persists with optic atrophy 2 years later. Ophthalmic, angiographic and CT studies have not revealed the cause of this loss.

Some of us are concerned about lasting pain from thrusting a 13- or 14-gauge needle into the mandibular division; this has apparently given rise to no problem, although Mullan suggests methods for controlling supra- as well as infrazygomatic hematomas.

Conclusion

These enthusiastic accounts may initiate much wider use of the method.

Subcutaneous Injection of the Neurotoxin Stilbamidine

A few of the many substances which are transported from nerve terminals via their axons to neuronal cell bodies will kill the cell soma when they reach it. Borges has found the least poisonous of these to the whole animal to be stilbamidine. Moreover, this agent injected intravenously is selectively toxic to trigeminal neurons to whose peripheral terminals it is carried in the plasma and thence by their axons to the neuronal soma. A trial of the agent by systemic administration in trigeminal neuralgia often resulted in control of the pain but at the unacceptable price of diffuse facial dysesthesias [Smith and Miller, 1955; White and Sweet, 1969, pp. 169–171]. Borges et al. [1988] are experimenting with the possibility of confining the toxic effect to the specific fibers involved in the pain by small subcutaneous injections only into the trigger zones. This is the most precise tactic yet evolved which may possibly stop the pain at the price of minimal deficit and risk.

Microvascular Decompression

Historical Note

As early as 1932, Dandy [1932a] wrote that tic douloureux could be due to a lesion that compressed the trigeminal nerve in the posterior fossa. In 66 out of 215 patients, this compression was of a vascular nature, but not much attention was paid to these findings of Dandy, because it was in some cases difficult without microsurgical techniques to explore the anterior part of the cerebellopontine angle and modern photography was needed to document findings. However, Gardner [1962] explored this area in 18 patients with tic douloureux and found that in 6 an arterial loop compressed the nerve; he separated the two structures and interposed a gelatin sponge. Jannetta, while using a binocular dissecting microscope, observed in 5 consecutive patients that the trigeminal nerve was mildly to severely compressed by one or more small tortuous arteries. In one patient with first-division tic and decrease of the corneal reflex, he freed the artery from the nerve at the pons and did a small inferolateral section of only the portio major of the trigeminal root. The patient was pain-free with normal corneal reflex postoperatively, light touch totally intact, and a small area of hypalgesia in the lower face. On the basis of these observations, Jannetta and Rand planned for a future series of patients 'this possibly definitive procedure, namely release of the artery without nerve section' [Jannetta and Rand, 1966; Jannetta, 1967b]. This 'future series' comprised in 1980 [Jannetta, 1980] 411 patients and more than 900 in 1985 [Jannetta, 1985]. Several large series by other authors have been published. The procedure has also given rise to a remarkable controversy, some considering microsurgical decompression as the invasive treatment of choice while others think 'there is no place' for this operation in the treatment of trigeminal neuralgia [Morley, 1985].

Mechanism

Jannetta states that the primary etiology of trigeminal neuralgia is vascular pulsatile compression of the junctional area of the central trigeminal myelin (within oligodendroglia) and peripheral myelin (within Schwann cells), in the cerebellopontine angle adjacent to the brain stem [Jannetta, 1985]. It is therefore important to consider the anatomy of the root entry zone of the trigeminal nerve in the pons and how this zone can be compressed by vascular elements.

The trigeminal nerve at the pons is described as consisting of a cephalic motor root (portio minor) and caudal sensory root (portio major). Dandy further described a number of small 'accessory fibers' lying between the major sensory and motor roots entering the pons, and noted that the 'accessory fibers' might be concerned with the perception of light touch [Dandy, 1929, 1932b].

In anatomical dissections on cadavers using the binocular surgical microscope it was observed that the major sensory root fibers fuse into a soft, rather gelatinous mass about 5 mm in diameter before entering the pons. This mass has a thin, tough outer layer and is described as the 'fibrous cone' region of the portio major. Just distal to the coalescent area, a group of five or more small bundles arise from and leave the portio major. These fibers may lie closely adjacent to the 'fibrous cone' region. They enter the pons in the gap between the other roots and have been termed 'intermediate' fibers [Jannetta and Rand, 1966; Jannetta, 1967a; Rand 1976]. It was postulated that the anatomical position of the fibers of the portio major, minor and intermedius could be correlated with the location of the major sensory, motor and descending spinal nuclei of the trigeminal system within the brain stem and that the preservation of the portio intermedius should preserve light touch when the portio major is cut. From the anatomical evidence, it appears that gross somatotopic representation of the three major peripheral trigeminal divisions is more or less maintained in the portio major, although rotational movement and overlap of one division with respect to the others do occur as fibers progress from the periphery centrally. The varied patterns of sparing of facial sensation seen after partial rhizotomy of the portio major are explicable in terms of the loose somatotopic organization and variable degree of rotation of the sensory root [Gudmundsson et al., 1971] (fig. 1/11). There is also electron microscopic evidence that up to 20% of the fibers in the human portio minor are unmyelinated fibers [Young, 1978b] which are potentially sensory in function and, therefore, cannot be considered exclusively motor in function. There is electrophysiological evidence in monkeys that sensory proprioceptive fibers lie in the portio minor [Pelletier et al., 1974]. Intermediate root fibers are, according to Pelletier et al. [1974], not different from portio minor fibers; their course on macroscopical examination is rather variable [Gudmundsson et al., 1971] and they find no anatomical and physiological evidence to support the suggestion that the afferent fibers in the intermediate (accessory) rootlets subserve a specific sensory modality. Jannetta describes neurovascular compression of the root entry zone in 395 of 411 patients. In 242 the compression was arterial, in 57 venous and in 96 mixed arterial-venous. Most commonly, in lower facial tic douloureux, there was compression by a loop of the superior cerebellar artery on the anterosuperior aspect of the entry zone of the root; in first-division tic douloureux, a vessel was seen to compress the inferolateral side of the trigeminal root entry zone with a normal horizontal loop of the superior cerebellar artery. Note that this is the reverse of the somatotopic disposition described by Gudmundsson. Jannetta [1981a] found the most common cause of isolated V2 neuralgia to be compression of the trigeminal vein along the nerve. Similar findings of vasculo-nervous compression have been confirmed by others although the frequency of the findings varies substantially [van Loveren et al., 1982; Breeze and Ignelzi, 1982; Zorman and Wilson, 1984; Kolluri and Heros, 1984; Sindou et al., 1987].

One of the criticisms of the concept of neurovascular compression as an etiological factor in tic douloureux is that such a compression might be

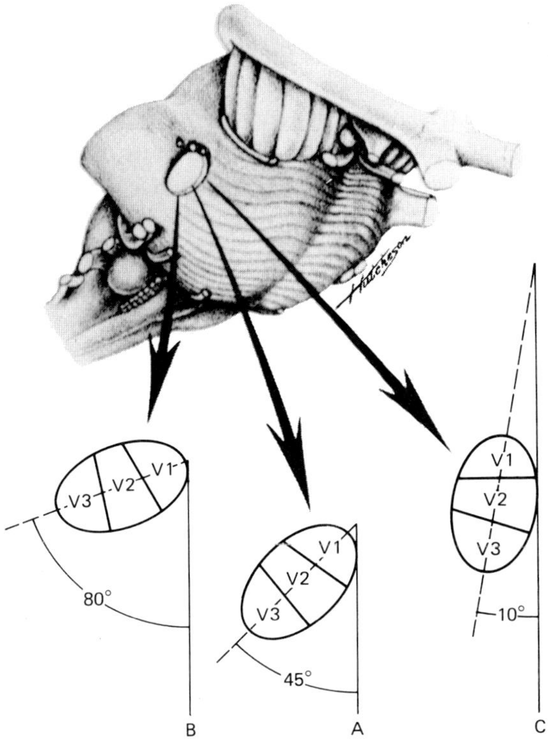

Fig. 1/11. The variability of the longest axis of the elliptical cross-section of the trigeminal nerve at the pons (broken line) to the longitudinal axis of the body (solid line). The long axis of most nerves makes a 40–50° angle with the longitudinal axis of the body (A); however, this can vary from 10° (C) to 80° (B). In B, the third division (V3) is almost directly lateral to the first division (V1), and in C it is almost directly caudal. From Gudmundsson et al. [1971].

coincidental and found in a large proportion of the normal population. The best control data regarding neurovascular relations come from postmortem studies of individuals without facial pain (table 1/V). Comparison of the data from the 4 available articles reveals that Klun and Prestor [1986] studied their cases only after removal of the brain stem and cerebellum as a separate specimen. Hardy and Rhoton [1978], Haines et al. [1980] and Mehta et al. [1981] removed all CNS structures rostral to a midcollicular section studying cerebellopontine angle relationships in situ before fixation. Mehta et al. [1981] found in 30 adult cadavers (60 sides) only 8 arteries in contact with

Table 1/V. Anatomy of the microvascular relations of the trigeminal nerve

Author, year	Nontic cadavers					With tic in vivo				
	N	A. cont., %	V. cont., %	A. comp., %	V. comp., %	N	A. cont., %	V. cont., %	A. comp., %	V. comp., %
Hardy and Rhoton, 1978	50	52		'often'						
Haines et al., 1980	40	25	23	10 SCA: 53.8% AICA: 25.6% pontine branch of basilar A: 20.6%	10	40	5	23	80	
Piatt and Wilkins, 1984						103	31	30	37	5
Tarlov, 1985						64	5	10	72	
Klun and Prestor, 1986	130	23	9	7	1					

N = Trigeminal nerves; A. cont. = arterial contact; V. cont. = venous contact; A. comp. = arterial compression; V. comp. = venous compression; SCA = superior cerebellar artery; AICA = anterior cerebellar artery.

the trigeminal root and no distortion of nerve by artery. Since the number of contacts, arterial or venous, occurred much more often than frank compressions in these pain-free patients described by all 4 groups, the logical study is to determine the outcome regarding pain relief in the various types of neurovascular relationship. The first neurosurgeon to do this, Wilkins [Piatt and Wilkins, 1984], has come up with the fruitful data that when an artery has caused distortion of the root or is wedged between the root and the pons (37 cases) microvascular decompression (MVD) yielded an 'expected cure rate' of 83%; this dropped to 62% of 31 cases when there were only contacts with arteries. In those with only venous contact or distortion or no abnormality (30%), the expected success rate fell to 42%. When 3 of 5 MVD's in patients with gross distortion of the root by a vein were followed by recurrence Wilkins, on these and other patients with no arterial contact, subsequently did a partial sensory rhizotomy. This (in 21 patients) gave the highest percentage of excellent and good results. Zorman and Wilson [1984], on the other hand, saw no difference between outcomes after MVD for venous versus arterial cross-compression or after partial sensory rhizotomy. Adams et al. [1982a] classified only 11% of his 55 patients in this category of vascular distortion of the root. It may be that those with only arterial contact should have posterior root section. This appears to be the view of Tarlov [1985] who did vascular decompression in the 48 of 64 patients in whom he described arterial wedging between root and pons or distortion of root from above or below an artery. Only 8% of these failed to get initial relief. In the remaining 18 patients submitted to posterior root section 6 failed to get relief. We need more data correlating neurovascular relationships with results. The problem regarding significance of what the surgeon sees is intimated by Wilson's (to us dubious) statement: 'Veins and arterial loops not in direct contact with the root were presumed to be causative if they were in close proximity to an anatomically deformed nerve root because retracting the cerebellum could displace the pons and trigeminal root away from an offending artery or vein'. Those relying on partial sensory rhizotomy would do well to bear in mind that Dandy performed subtotal sensory rhizotomy by his approach only rarely in his later years because of the increased recurrence rate [White and Sweet, 1969, p. 202].

The most puzzling set of facts continues to be the similarity of results between minor maneuvers confined to the middle cranial fossa and those confined to the posterior fossa. Table 1/VI illustrates this point. It may be that the least equivocal situation — gross distortion of the nerve by an artery or tumor — will often be demonstrable in the recently available high-quality magnetic resonance imaging (MRI) scans which might come to be of crucial help to us.

Technique

The technique has been described in detail [Jannetta, 1976, 1981a; Apfelbaum, 1982]. The intervention involves a displacement of any arteries and coagulation and division of veins in contact with trigeminal root usually at the entry zone via a retromastoid craniectomy and a superolateral approach, avoiding stretching of the acousticofacial bundle. The compressing artery is transposed to an innocuous position, and usually kept separated from the root by placing a prosthesis (muscle, periosteum, polyvinyl foams,

Table 1/VI. Comparison of some of the large series

Authors, year	Number of patients	Initial failure plus significant recurrence (%)	Mortality (%)	Follow-up
Microvascular decompression in the posterior fossa				
Jannetta, 1980	411	83 (20)	4 (1)	1–10 years
Breeze and Ignelzi, 1982	51	23 (45)	0	1–53 months
Taarnhøj, 1982	86	17 (20)	1	up to 10 years
Apfelbaum, 1983	289	60 (21)	3 (1)	av. 55 months
Barba and Alksne, 1984	37	10 (27)	0	av. 42 months
Kolluri and Heros, 1984	72	16 (22)	0	av. 60 months
Piatt and Wilkins, 1984	81	21 (26)	1 (1)	av. 48 months
Zorman and Wilson, 1984	92	11 (12)	0	av. 26 months
Sindou et al.,1987	113	16 (14)	1	1–6 years
Totals	1,232	278 (22.5)	10 (0.8)	
'Decompression', compression or other minor manipulation in the middle cranial fossa				
Gardner and Miklos, 1959	102	48 (48)	2	3 1/4 to 5 1/2 years
Rowe, 1959	96	14 (15)		
Bohm and Hojeberg, 1960	111	24 (22)	0	2–4 years
Hamby, 1960	88	7 (8)	1	up to 6 years
Graf, 1963	100	26 (26)		up to 8 years
Shelden, 1964	200	50 (25)		up to 10 years
Taarnhøj, 1982	230	93 (40)	3	up to 29 years (av. greater than 12 years)
Totals	927	239 (26)	6 (0.6)	

Teflon fibers, Dacron, radiopaque synthetic sponge, etc. . . .) between them. The procedure requires an experienced microneurosurgeon. If feasible the surgeon may tether the artery to the tentorium by a fascial sling or the adhesive effect attributed to Teflon fibers.

Results

Usually the majority of the patients will be free of tic douloureux after awakening from the intervention but some will continue to have postoperatively attacks of tic douloureux for a few days, which will usually gradually disappear.

In table 1/VI are summarized the results of several of the largest series. As can be seen, the long-term failure rate of posterior fossa MVD at 22.5% is similar to the 26% failure rate of minor manipulations at open operation in the middle fossa. Although the rationale of MVD is to eliminate the cause of the pain rather than to replace it by numbness, the clinical course appears to be about the same when the minor surgical gestures likewise conserving sensation are confined to the middle cranial fossa. We think it most unlikely that these latter manipulations could change neurovascular relations near or at the root entry zone of the pons. These results seem to us to refute the conclusion that neurovascular compression in the posterior fossa is the major cause of trigeminal neuralgia. Both operations offer then the advantage of maintaining normal sensation in the face and therefore avoid the complications of dysesthesias including anesthesia dolorosa and corneal anesthesia. It will be noted that Taarnhøj's [1982] middle fossa series, followed for up to 29 years, have by that time nearly double the failure rate of the shorter follow-ups at either site.

Complications

The reported complication rate is low. However, our Neurosurgical Poll [Sweet and Poletti, 1988] brought to light problems of disturbing frequency and magnitude. We have reports by letter from 55 services in only 9 of which 70 or more MVD operations had been done. No deaths and only moderate lasting sequelae were described by 28 services, but 27 services reported 32 deaths or permanently disabling sequelae. The 5 largest series were of 97–150 cases; the next largest was of circa 70 cases. There were 2 especially tragic series compiled by 3 technically competent distinguished neurosurgeons; 4 of their 60 patients were postoperative deaths, all healthy individuals aged 31–59; all of their operations had been 'smooth and uneventful'. The only clue to avoiding such outcomes we found was that a major infarct in 4 cases was probably due to coagulation of essential veins draining the brain stem. However, the nondisabling complication of ipsilateral deafness has been sharply reduced by acting on the warnings obtained by monitoring auditory evoked potentials. We think the few major complications and deaths from percutaneous operations can be almost eliminated in all age groups by the precautions described earlier. We can justify no such optimistic conclusion anent MVD, and regard the risks as a major drawback in the treatment of so nonlethal a disorder as trigeminal neuralgia. We also think the decision to take such risks with the likelihood of relief accompanied by minimal if any dysesthesias is the prerogative of the patient. The less experienced neurosurgeon would do well to describe greater risks than have been seen in the best series. Usually transient 4th, 6th, 7th and 8th nerve palsies, facial numbness, intracranial hematomas and ataxias have been seen in the large series. Many minor complications such as CSF leak and aseptic or bacterial meningitis may occur [Jannetta, 1981a; Swanson and Farhat, 1982; van Loveren et al., 1982; Breeze and Ignelzi, 1982; Zorman and Wilson, 1984; Kolluri and Heros, 1984]. Apfelbaum [1983] described 88 transient complications in 13 different categories in his 289 patients — many more of course than occur with the percutaneous procedures.

Since MVD is a major operation with possibly severe complications, since alternative treatments do exist, and since the recurrence and failure rate total about 20%, it is important to recognize prognostic factors in MVD. In a thoughtful study in which 20 factors were analyzed, the presence or absence of a constant background pain proved to be the only factor significantly related to prognosis. In patients with paroxysmal pain only, a cure was obtained in 95% (44 patients) whereas in those with paroxysmal plus constant pain only 58% (24 patients) were fully relieved [Sindou et al., 1987]. This contrasts with the figures for percutaneous lesions, i.e. relief in 99% of 605 patients with only paroxysmal pains versus a drop to only 86% in the 185 with constant pain as well (p. 42).

Other Intervention for Tic douloureux

Posterior Fossa Rhizotomy

Partial trigeminal root section through a posterior fossa approach is now usually performed during MVD when no vascular pathology is found or the vessel cannot be safely moved [Jannetta, 1976]. Where and how much to cut when a partial trigeminal sensory section is performed is not wholly clear, and depends of course on the locus of the trigger zones. Variations in the orientation of the V rootlets to the pons are well illustrated by Gudmundsson and give perhaps the best available guidance to the surgeons. The greater the number of rootlets cut the more likely are major dysesthesias. Swanson and Farhat [1982] have combined this procedure with MVD in all of their 14 patients.

The recurrence rate of tic douloureux was higher in patients who had a partial trigeminal rhizotomy than in those who had an MVD [Tarlov, 1985;

Burchiel et al., 1981]; it was the same in the experience of Zorman and Wilson [1984] and lower in the series of Piatt and Wilkins [1984].

Other Indications for Trigeminal Rhizotomy than Tic douloureux

Percutaneous trigeminal rhizotomy is now the main operation we use initially for pain due to cephalofacial neoplasm. The extensive open rhizotomies of cranial and cervical roots are now rarely done for such pains. Other types of facial pain at times successfully treated with RF lesions include other trigeminal neuropathies than multiple sclerosis, such as post-herpetic neuralgia, very atypical questionable trigeminal neuralgia in which the constant pain is worse than the paroxysms, and constant post-traumatic pains. We deal with these complex problems in a later publication. Patients with constant nonprovokable pains unrelated to any demonstrable focal cause, i.e. atypical facial pain, are not fruitfully treated by any invasive trigeminal procedure.

Conclusions

The intensive review undertaken for this monograph confirms numerous lines of evidence that the mechanism responsible for essential trigeminal neuralgia is often mysteriously labile. The peculiar propensity for the pain in this nonlethal disorder to stop on minimal and even presumably unrelated maneuvers demands an unusually conservative surgical approach in the first instance because of the amazing likelihood of its success. It is crucial to recognize that the debate as to the cause or causes of the disorder need not be resolved in order logically to lead to this decision. It is immaterial whether the cause is abnormal myelination of sensory trigeminal fibers or extensive pressure against them, or both or neither. We conclude from an analysis of the available results that performance of a conservative percutaneous lesion represents the best tactic as the first invasive procedure. Specifically, we mean RF lesion carried only to hypalgesia, glycerol in small amounts for brief intervals once sensory loss occurs, or balloon inflation in Meckel's cave for less than a minute. These procedures are likely to be virtually free of dysesthesias or corneal anesthesia as well as the many minor and major complications which may follow open operation in the posterior fossa. We usually prefer RF heating to the other two methods since the site of the minor lesion is under better control. These highly conservative approaches involve a change in thinking of Sweet, but have been the policy of Gybels for over 10 years. Incidentally, the low morbidity of these tactics should lead to earlier referrals by physicians for such procedures. When such initial efforts fail there are reasonable, more aggressive tactics to pursue.

Chapter 1.B. Periodic or Chronic Migrainous Neuralgia — Cluster Headache

An early dramatic description, Opperman's [1747] doctoral thesis, is of a 35-year-old woman suffering from 15-min. attacks of hemicrania of agonizing intensity recurring every hour day and night for 5 years. At the onset there had been 2 periods of 4 weeks of such attacks with a 6-month remission between them. The remissions and the intensity and duration of the attacks, but not their location, were typical of this syndrome. A general physician, Muller [1813], first described the full-blown picture with typical frightful episodes in himself continuing for 34 years with onset at age 20. The spontaneous attacks lasting a few to 30 min began in the eyebrow and included photophobia, 'inflaming' of the conjunctiva and tearing, and a pounding temporal pulse [Isler, 1987].

Harris [1926] gave an excellent comprehensive description of this disorder under the rubrics of migrainous neuralgia, periodic migrainous neuralgia and ciliary neuralgia. He emphasized the differential features between this and essential trigeminal neuralgia. His last publication on the subject [Harris, 1940] describes briefly complete relief after 19 of 29 alcohol injections of the Gasserian ganglion with 5 other patients much improved and 'less violent recurrences' in the remaining 5. 'Cluster headache', the term introduced by Kunkle et al. [1952], has become the more popular designation for the disorder.

Clinical Features

These include as differing from trigeminal neuralgia: (1) spontaneous onset of the pains rather than provocation by local stimuli to specific facial areas; (2) a constant rather than paroxysmal character; (3) a duration of minutes to many hours; (4) a tendency to occur at a specific time of the day or night for a period with spontaneous changes in this schedule; (5) a greater tendency to waken the patient from sound sleep; (6) usually origin around orbit, forehead or temple, but often with radiation not only elsewhere on the face but also to ear, back of head, side or back of neck and shoulder; (7) tendency to remain unilateral in any one attack, but more frequent involvement of the second side in other attacks; (8) ipsilateral autonomic features are much commoner, mainly of parasympathetic hyperactivity appearing as ipsilateral redness of eyeball or cheek; dilation, pounding and tenderness of the superficial temporal artery, ipsilateral profuse tearing; watery rhinorrhea or nasal congestion and mucus; less often swelling of eyelids, cheek or nasal mucosa and rarely excessive salivation.

Sympathetic paresis is common in the form of miosis and ptosis. These signs may occur associated, oddly enough, with hyperhidrosis of the ipsilateral forehead when the pain is referred mainly to cheek and jaw, 'the lower syndrome' of Ekbom [1970].

Of 416 cases reported in 10 publications the pain spread to the other side during an attack in only 7, and three quarters of the patients were males. Roughly half of them [White and Sweet, 1969, pp. 348–354] provoke their attacks by drinking an alcoholic beverage. A small amount may suffice to do so promptly. The clinical features may change to those of classical migraine and vice versa.

Although these attacks tend to occur in 'clusters' for weeks or months and then stop for a time, the onset in a few patients is primarily chronic without remissions from the beginning. A larger group of patients stop having remissions, becoming secondarily chronic as the disease continues. On the basis of at least two attacks per week for a year Ekbom and Olivarius [1971] placed 10% of their 167 patients in this chronic category. It is mainly from this group that the surgical candidates are drawn, although in some patients each attack is so devastating that they are unwilling to await a remission and seek surgery.

The panoply of drugs now available for this disorder results in medical control in the great majority, e.g. Graham has needed to refer for surgery only 4% of his circa 550 patients. Having worked with him for the last 20 years, W.H.S. has a surgical series confined to the medical truly intractable cases. Indomethacin, which so promptly controls the variant described by Sjaastad and Dale [1976] as chronic paroxysmal hemicrania, should not be forgotten. However, as we shall be commenting frequently in this book, medical management is all too often being carried to undesirable lengths and the opportunity lost to return the patient to productivity by timely surgery. Thus, one of our patients persisted in taking the lone agent which relieved him, cafergot, until the coronary arterial disease it provoked required 2 open heart operations. He is now a cardiac invalid despite neurosurgical complete control of his pain.

The distinguished neurologist Sir Charles Symonds [1956] has stated that in these patients there is 'no evidence . . . that psychological factors were operative'. Although this may well be true of the dramatic attacks themselves there are patients whose personality traits and social situations make the chance of surgical success too small to justify it. One of us cites details of 4 such examples in a forthcoming publication [Sweet et al., 1989].

Neural Pathways Activated during These Pains

Present data point to at least two afferent pathways in the cranial roots which may be taken by the impulses related to this pain: (1) trigeminal, and (2) nervus intermedius and conceivably glossopharyngeal and upper vagal. No one has as yet proposed any clinical feature which characterizes one route more than the other. Mayberg et al. [1984] have depicted afferent fibers from dural and cerebral arteries and venous sinuses in the cat which traverse the trigeminal first division; these could account for vascular pains related to intracranial vessels being referred to this area of the face as so commonly occurs in this disorder.

Temporary Trigeminal Denervation

Retrogasserian Lidocaine Block

The trigeminal pathway seems to be involved oftener than the intermedius-greater superficial petrosal alternative; hence we begin by trying to determine if the former is implicated by a selective block of the pain fibers in the trigeminal rootlets. The severity and relatively short duration of many attacks usually preclude placement of the needle to try to abort the attack once the pain has started. However, we think that the state of partial sensory loss of analgesia without anesthesia is not as well tolerated by patients with cluster headache as by those with trigeminal neuralgia. Moreover, first-division analgesia is more likely to lead to major dysesthesias in both groups of patients than is second- and third-division loss. Hence we think it advisable to let the patient sample the sensations both of analgesia only and as well that combined with loss of appreciation of touch. We seek also to provoke an attack once the needle is placed and then try with lidocaine to stop it, the crucial test of the value of differential or total rhizotomy. We have done such blocks on 36 patients, twice in 4 of them with a less equivocal result the second time in 2 of the 4. In 4 others, whose attacks were readily provoked by drinking alcoholic beverages, we have given oral whiskey or i.v. alcohol without ever initiating an attack. Ekbom's 1968 suggestion of using sublingual nitroglycerin has worked better, with 2 of 8 patients developing typical clinical attacks. Recently the second of two doses of i.v. naloxone totaling 0.11 mg in one and a combination of increasing doses to a total of 0.33 mg i.v. naloxone and 1.7 mg nitroglycerin sublingually in another patient provoked an attack. In 16 other patients a major attack began during the needle placement or during electrical stimulation to correct the placement. If feasible, the whole procedure should be timed just to precede an expected attack. In the 19 who developed an attack it was clearly arrested in 13 of them by the lidocaine-produced analgesia. Only 24 of the 36 patients found the new sensation of analgesia acceptable. The remaining 12 were not submitted to any form of trigeminal rhizotomy.

We think this diagnostic procedure helps select the type of surgery; in those who have found the sensation of analgesia acceptable no patient has developed major facial dysesthesias after a subsequent trigeminal rhizotomy.

A longer temporary trigeminal denervation advocated by Harris [1940] consisted of peripheral injections of alcohol into supra- or infraorbital or temporal areas. Neurectomy of the appropriate peripheral branches may be tried when an attack cannot be provoked at the lidocaine block.

Radiofrequency Rhizotomy

As we have already commented these patients have a greater tendency to develop anesthesia or analgesia dolorosa after trigeminal lesions than those with trigeminal neuralgia. Hence these patients especially benefit from the fact that the control of the locus and degree of sensory loss is better with percutaneous RF heating than with open operations in the middle or posterior fossa. Usually the reference of pain is to the first two divisions to which consequently we confine lesions, extending them to the third division of course for pain in this zone. Because of so many recurrences when only hypalgesia was present we have been more aggressive about producing full analgesia in the areas of pain than we have in trigeminal neuralgia, using a 5-mm bare 20-gauge electrode heated to 100 °C for 4 min if needed. Much lower temperatures have usually sufficed, and we start about 5 °C above the threshold temperature for pain. In one patient in whom at 46 °C there was a 'burning' in the eye, the first lesion at 50 °C for 1 min with a 5-mm bare electrode yielded the desired analgesia of the first and upper half of the second division.

We have now carried out 28 RF procedures on 20 patients. Watson et al. [1983] with the next largest series have done 27 RF procedures on 13 patients. Both groups have had the disappointing result of inadequate or no relief from a presumably appropriate trigeminal sensory loss. Of our 6 such patients 2 had analgesia throughout all three trigeminal divisions and 4 had analgesia in much or all of the first two divisions in the zone of the worst pains; yet they had pain referred to these areas. Only one of these had had an attack aborted by a lidocaine block. Another, after an open rhizotomy elsewhere, had had 4 years of relief until recovery of pinprick sensation. We have found it advisable to secure analgesia throughout all areas of pain before classifying the result as a failure. Thus, in one patient it took us three procedures before we achieved sustained useful relief by rendering analgesic and anesthetic all of the second division's painful oral mucosa. Another patient's pain predominantly in cheek and temple was stopped by a V2, V3 lesion. Attacks then gradually built up over 18 months in the typical orbital area and were eliminated by a V1,2 lesion. In 3 other of our patients two or three lesions were required to deal with initial failures to secure adequate analgesia or later recovery of algesia. Relief continues in 11 of our 20 patients followed from 10 months to 20 years for an average of 5.3 years; 4 of these require supplemental medication. Two others were relieved for 3 and 10 years before recurrence and one other with early relief was lost to follow-up. Of these 14 patients with complete V1 analgesia some decreased corneal sensation to touch was retained in 5, another advantage of RF lesion over open rhizotomy.

The experience with RF lesions of Watson et al. [1983] can be summarized as follows: 14 without complete analgesia in V1,2 were unrelieved; 3 with such 'inadequate' sensory loss were relieved. However, one with full analgesia of V1,2 and another with analgesia in V1 continued with pain in the analgesic zone. Of 8 with analgesia throughout V1,2, relief continued in 4 and was maintained until recovery of sensation in the other 4. Relief continues in 7 from 10 to 36 months with an average of 24 months. Anesthesia dolorosa developed in one patient who was nevertheless glad he had the operation.

The series of Onofrio and Campbell [1986] includes 24 RF procedures on 22 patients. The analgesia they produced was incomplete in 12 procedures with 11 early failures and a recurrence at 6 months in the 12th. In 6 of these patients they proceeded directly to open rhizotomy in the posterior fossa. Of the 12 RF procedures followed by good to excellent relief 11 had complete V1,2 analgesia and the 12th severe hypalgesia in V1 with analgesia in V2 confirming the thought that full analgesia in the painful zone is usually necessary. Follow-up ranged from 12 to 32 months with an average of 21 months. Some corneal sensation to touch was retained in 3 of the 12 patients with relief. These authors also describe a successful outcome in one patient following bilateral RF lesions for attacks on both sides. Tew et al. [1982] comment briefly that their V1,2 lesions gave 'satisfactory relief' to 6 of 8 cluster headache patients.

Maxwell [1982], with the preliminary criterion of stopping an attack by retrogasserian lidocaine, has compiled the perfect record of 8 initial successes after RF lesions. His objective of producing only hypalgesia is, judging from the results of the three groups just described, likely to be followed by more severe late recurrences than the 3 mild ones he has described.

Glycerol Rhizotomy

The results of 13 injections of an average of 0.4 ml of glycerol in 6 severely afflicted patients followed 5–47 months (mean 16 months) were described by Ekbom et al. [1984]. In 3 patients a total of 7 injections yielded slight V1 sensory loss and poor relief. In 3 others immediate complete relief was followed after 2, 6, and 11 months, respectively, by recurrence and a repeat injection. Complete relief was again achieved in 2 followed for 9 and 18 months and 90% relief in the third was maintained at 4 years. In these 3, analgesia around the eye and loss of corneal reflex also ensued. Waltz et al. [1985] treated 5 patients by glycerol injection with no benefit in one and with enough improvement in the other 4 to render them 'more easily managed medically'. The attacks were not stopped in any of them. We think the lidocaine-RF lesion sequence is more logical and effective.

Open Trigeminal Rhizotomy

Dott [1951] and White and Sweet [1969] have described relief following this operation. In the 2 cases of the latter authors this result persisted at 4 and 15 years. Mazars and collaborators [1976] in an extensive experience from

1948 to 1975 sought to limit their rhizotomy to first-division rootlets. They used electrical stimulation at operation to identify 'those rootlets responsible for meningeal sensation' and cut only this 'meningeal contingent' in 11 of their 31 patients. They describe only 3 failures — one apparently after relief for one year.

The Toronto group [Watson et al., 1983] did 8 open rhizotomies on 8 patients with initial cessation of the pain attacks in 5. There was a recurrence at 30, 36, and 44 months in 3. Relief continued at 48 months and 8 years in the other 2. They achieved anesthesia at the site of the main pain in these 5 — only one of whom had the result marred by anesthesia dolorosa. Noteworthy are 3 failures despite adequate sensory loss. One of them with pain only in the upper gum was not relieved by complete V2,3 anesthesia. These emphasize again the importance of a temporary procedure to assess the value of trigeminal analgesia during an attack. The brief accounts of O'Brien and MacCabe [1984] and of Campbell [1984] tell us of 6 more encouraging results; there is no indication that either group preceded the rhizotomy by a temporary block.

Onofrio and Campbell's [1986] 11 posterior fossa rhizotomies included 6 carried out only after prior failures of an RF lesion, 4 more as the primary procedure and the 11th operation when the first open operation produced only minor sensory loss. There were 5 excellent results and 2 failures to control the pain correlated in one with incomplete V1,2 analgesia and in a second despite complete anesthesia including the cornea. There were 2 other results classified as poor even though relief of pain was achieved associated with complete anesthesia. One patient went into a severe depression and deserted his family; the other with anesthesia dolorosa became totally disabled and vindictive.

Of Hitchcock's [Wake and Hitchcock, 1987] 4 patients treated by open rhizotomy with extensive anesthesia, 3 have maintained complete or good relief at 12, 15 and 25 years. One of the 3 was not relieved by a prior lesion producing only complete hypalgesia. The 4th patient was unrelieved despite production of complete trigeminal anesthesia, again pointing to the utility of temporary trigeminal loss as a preliminary procedure.

We conclude that production of any necessary analgesia without anesthesia in order to decrease the incidence of major dysesthesia is an objective best achieved by differential thermal rhizotomy or by bulbar tractotomy of the descending cephalic pain pathway. Our first patient with this disorder treated by a dense extensive RF lesion found the areas of anesthesia dolorosa far worse than her neuralgic pains (which never recurred). When sensory recovery set in she was grateful only to the physician whose medication made her hypalgesia dolorosa more tolerable. The course in 3 of our patients treated by other neurosurgeons by open rhizotomy reemphasizes its disadvantages. One, although free of his attacks of migrainous neuralgia for 29 months, is infuriated and states he is totally disabled by anesthesia dolorosa associated with the total anesthesia; he is suing and threatening to murder the neurosurgeon. (These patients seem prone to more violent responses to an adverse result than those with trigeminal neuralgia.) The other 2 patients' operations were followed by recovery of sensation and recurrence.

Superficial Petrosal Neurectomy

Chorobski and Penfield [1932] found in the monkey efferent vasodilator fibers to the arteries of the supratentorial pia mater only in the greater superficial petrosal nerve. This nerve also carried secretory and vasodilator fibers to the mucosa of nose, mouth and upper pharynx, as well as secretory fibers to the lacrimal gland. They also identified a distinct bundle of small myelinated and unmyelinated fibers in the nervus intermedius just proximal to the geniculate ganglion passing directly into the greater superficial petrosal nerve without interruption in the ganglion (fig. 1/12). Further on, a distinct bundle of nerve fibers emerged from the greater superficial petrosal nerve passing to the nerve plexus on the internal carotid. These appear to be efferent pathways. Coupling these observations to the evidence that vasodilation causes this type of headache, Gardner et al. [1947] proposed that superficial petrosal neurectomy might be effective treatment, suggesting the term petrosal neuralgia for the disorder. Although at first encouraged by his results Gardner [1951] later lost his enthusiasm for the procedure. Table 1/VII summarizes the results in 13 communications reporting on this operation. It is noteworthy that Gardner's successors at the Cleveland Clinic, Kunkel and Dohn [1974], have persisted with the operation in carefully selected patients, adding 'neurolysis' of the trigeminal sensory root to the petrosal neurectomy. By neurolysis Gardner [1962] meant: 'freeing the sensory rootlets from their dural sleeve, gently brushing them with a cotton pledget and spraying them forcefully with a Ringer's solution using a 21-gauge needle.'

Since section of the greater superficial petrosal nerve is distal to the geniculate ganglion from which its afferent fibers arise, one would expect regeneration with a recurrence of the pain in most of the cases if these

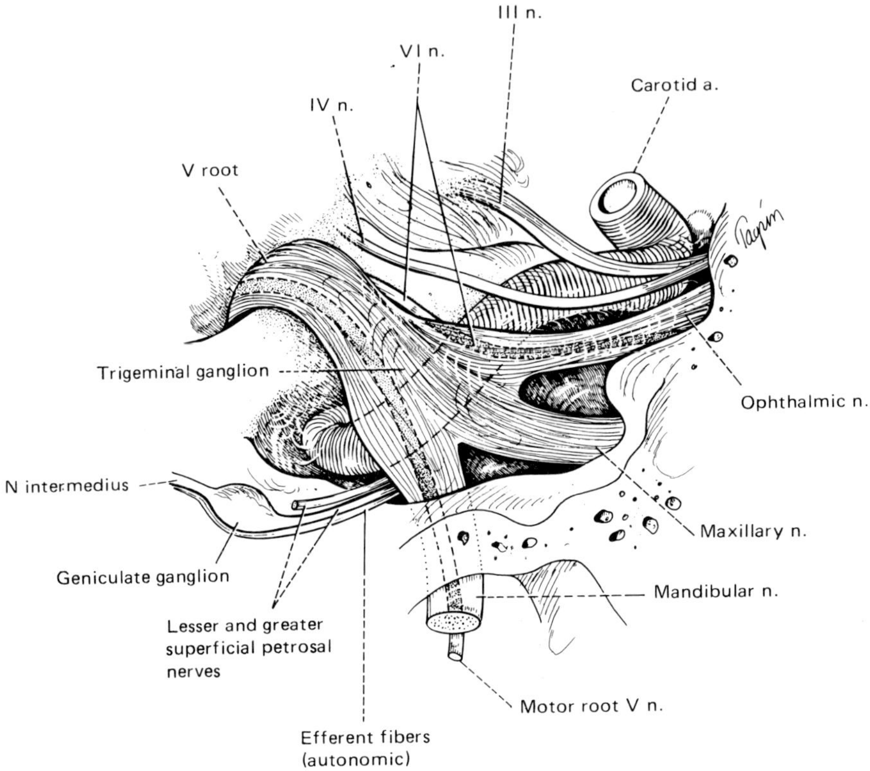

Fig. 1/12. Neuroanatomy medial portion right middle cranial fossa. For clarity the sizes of all nerves but the trigeminal are exaggerated. The geniculate ganglion and neural structures in its immediate vicinity lying within the petrous base are shown as though fully exposed by removal of their bony roof. The only unusual anatomical description is of the autonomic efferent fiber traveling adjoining the nervus intermedius and geniculate ganglion to course antero-medially with the greater superficial petrosal nerve until parting from it to continue on the internal carotid artery.

afferents are responsible for it, just as we see after peripheral trigeminal neural avulsions in trigeminal neuralgia. Hence we now consider this operation to be stage 1 in assessing the likelihood that the more permanent rhizotomy of nervus intermedius, IX and possibly the upper fibers of X or a high bulbar tractotomy may be in order.

In 1955 and 1969, White and Sweet reported on the results of nearly always dividing both the greater and lesser superficial petrosal nerve, and rarely the usually unidentified external superficial petrosal nerve as well, plus the middle meningeal artery in 10 patients. In 3 patients there was no relief;

Table 1/VII. Chronic migrainous neuralgia

Authors, year	Number of patients	Petrosal neurectomy	
		good initial results	longer term results
Gardner et al., 1947	13 (16 sides)	12 (of 16)	follow-up 4–48 months — av. 16 months; recurrence in 5 of the 12 at av. 25 months
Gardner, 1951	'Only half the patients get enough relief to justify operation'		
Trowbridge et al., 1953	4	3	follow-ups only at 5, 6, 8 months
Ponti and Valerio, 1960	6	6	1 mild recurrence at 4 months 5 no recurrences at follow-ups 2–5 years in 4
Durán-Obiols, 1961	6	6	recurrence at 6 months and 2 years in 2 patients; duration follow-up not stated.
Stowell, 1963	21	18	duration follow-up not stated.
White and Sweet, 1969	9	7	recurrence in 4 after gratifying relief 1.5–3.5 years; good long-term results at 10.5–14 years in 3
Kunkel and Dohn, 1974	12 (13 sides) combined with neurolysis trigeminal sensory root	9	recurrence in 3 patients; no recurrence in 6 followed up to 4 years
Alvarez-Garijo et al., 1975	9	9	recurrence at 2 months and 2 years in 5 patients; relief at 2–12 months in 4
Denecke, 1977	3	3	no recurrence but no follow-up more than 1 year
Watson et al., 1983	4	3	2 recurrences at 12 months and 4 years; 1 no recurrence at 5 years
Wake and Hitchcock, 1987	6	4	3 complete relief with no recurrence at 1, 1, and 20 years; 1 petrosal neurectomy + V rhizotomy — control with medication 15 years
Sweet et al., 1989	13	5	no relief 7; 50% relief 1; relief then recurrence at 6–27 months (av. 18 months) 5

Table 1/VIII. Petrosal neurectomy

Correlation between pain relief and responses to stimulation greater and lesser superficial petrosal nerves

Stimulation with tiny concentric bipolar electrode

Patient certain clinical pain reproduced by stimulation

6 patients — 4 relieved, 2 unrelieved by petrosal neurectomy

Patient certain of either no pain or no reproduction of clinical type of pain

5 patients — 4 no relief, 1 relief

Patient uncertain if clinical pain reproduced

2 patients —both no relief

Conclude: Fair correlation between response to stimulation and likelihood of relief by neurectomy

Bony roof carotid canal deficient in 2 patients permitting stimulus to int. carotid artery

1 patient — no pain at 7V to superficial petrosal nerve but at 2V to int. carotid pain at sites of and like clinical pain but 'sharper' (no neurectomy this patient but useful relief persisted 3 years)

1 patient — 2V to int. carotid — pain only V3 not like clinical pain

in them stimulation of neither superficial petrosal nerve at operation reproduced the patient's pain. In the remainder the results were gratifying as described in table 1/VII. The subsequent experience of W.H.S. in 13 patients has been much less favorable with no relief in 7 patients, temporary '50% relief' in one, and full or good relief varying from 6 to 27 months with an average of 18 months in the remaining 5. Complete recurrence has taken place in all 5. Hitchcock [Wake and Hitchcock, 1987] also cuts both lesser and greater petrosal nerves. Other authors describe cutting only of the greater superficial petrosal nerve.

W.H.S. has always awakened the patient after the nerves were exposed and stimulated them electrically. In the cases since 1968, the use of a tiny concentric needle electrode has permitted greater precision than with earlier larger electrodes. Both the two intact nerves and then their central and peripheral cut ends were stimulated. At times gentle suction to the nerve or cutting it gave a more decisive reproduction of the patient's pain than the electrical stimulus. Table 1/VIII summarizes the results, including those in 2 patients whose absence of a bony roof over the carotid permitted stimulation of the neural plexus on the intrapetrous internal carotid artery as well. Hitchcock also stimulated the exposed petrosal nerves in the awakened patient. In one patient he cut the trigeminal root when petrosal nerve stimulation failed to reproduce the pain — securing relief supplemented by medication for 15 years. The possibility that the mechanism of evoking the pain induced an autonomic effect or an effect in the periphery which then excited nociceptive afferents was assessed by stimulation of the cut medial (peripheral) end of the nerves before they passed beneath the Gasserian ganglion. In only 2 patients and only in the greater superficial nerves did low voltage elicit pain like the clinical pain. In one of them stimulation of the lateral cut end of both nerves also provoked the same response. All the rest, upon stimulus to the medial cut end of the nerves, experienced no facial contraction and either no pain or pain referred to the medial part of the third trigeminal division's zone, hence clearly related to spread to these nearby trigeminal nerve fibers.

We conclude, as did White and Sweet [1969, p. 363] from earlier studies on other patients, that these two nerves contain pain fibers and that when their section relieves pain this is a consequence of cutting an afferent nociceptive pathway.

Division of the Nervus intermedius

In their first monograph on pain, White and Sweet [1955, p. 501] proposed that patients deriving clear-cut relief from petrosal neurectomy should, upon recurrence of severe chronic pain, have division of the n. intermedius (the sensory rootlets of the geniculate ganglion). Dr. E. Sachs, Jr., is the pioneer who first actually carried out this operation in patients with chronic cluster headache, doing his first operation in 1952 and reporting his first 4 patients in 1968 (fig. 1/12). In his first case stimulation of the n. intermedius with a forceps reproduced the patient's clinical pain. However, when this nerve was cut similar stimulation of the VIIIth cranial nerve also reproduced her pain, so with her assent this nerve was also cut. The second patient also had a complete hearing loss on the side of the cut n. intermedius after operation. Two previous operations for section of the greater superficial petrosal nerve had relieved him for 3 and 2 years, respectively. Both patients, after complete lesions of n. intermedius and VIII, had remained pain-free at the last follow-ups 16 and 11 years later [Sachs, 1969]. By 1971 [Sachs, 1976], he had done rhizotomy of n. intermedius in 8 patients with this disorder with excellent very long-term results in 4. One recurred promptly on the 3rd postoperative day; in another relief persisted on the operated side but the pain recurred on the opposite side a year later. In 2 the pain spread during the attacks out of the usual fronto-facio-aural area to the back of the head and side of the neck. In these 2 'who also had unstable personalities' and 'were poor candidates for the operation', it failed. Sachs [1976] also reports a patient of C. Drake in whom initial good result was followed by recurrence.

W.H.S. has cut the n. intermedius in 3 patients (2 women and one man); in all 3 we first did greater and lesser superficial petrosal neurectomy, at which operation, in all 3, stimulation of the intact petrosal nerves and of their cut central ends reproduced the clinical pain. This report was especially striking in the man in whom cutting the greater nerve provoked a grade 3/4 attack of his clinical pain. The petrosal neurectomy gave only 50% relief to Janice D., but had yielded complete relief for 19 and 17 months, respectively, to the other 2. In Janice D. n. intermedius section bilaterally at a 4-month interval between the two sides was soon followed by a major recurrence equally severe on the two sides with up to 12 attacks per day by the following year. A lidocaine block with V1,2 analgesia had also failed to stop her pain. In the man it was especially disconcerting at the posterior fossa operation to have him report that stimulation of n. intermedius caused only aural pain, not at all like his clinical pain. His n. intermedius consisted of three unusually large fibers, but cutting them gave him no relief despite the good result for 19 months after petrosal neurectomy. In Maureen L. we cut the glossopharyngeal as well as the two well-developed rootlets of n. intermedius. Pain in her ear had been particularly prominent. She was completely relieved of the original attacks for over 4 years until December 1980. Since then infrequent less severe groups of attacks have been well controlled by nontoxic doses of medication. In another of our female patients with poor relief from retrogasserian lidocaine block we concluded that her personality and environment made her a poor candidate for surgery. Subsequently she had three sections of n. intermedius elsewhere, first on the left side, then on the right and finally on the left again with only a few months of benefit following each.

A problem with the anatomy of the n. intermedius is its propensity to have some of its fibers incorporated into either the VIIth or VIIIth cranial nerves as beautifully depicted in Bischoff's [1865] dissections and republished in small part by White and Sweet [1969, p. 626]. The clinical importance of such disposition was clearly demonstrated in Sachs' first 2 patients in whom the VIIIth nerve function was sacrificed but with excellent sustained relief. Although cranial n. IX and the upper fibers of X also supply

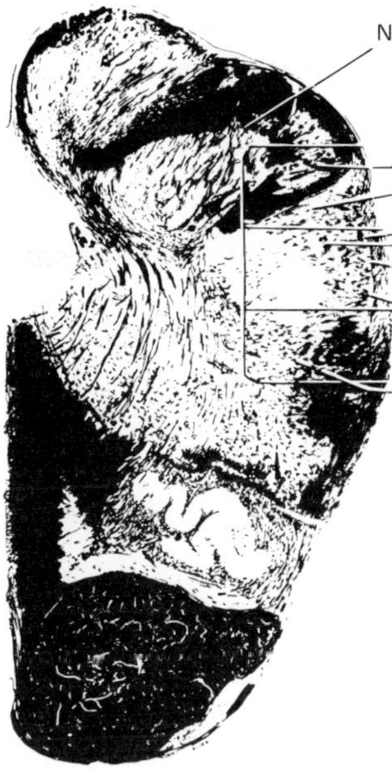

Fig. 1/13. Cross-section of the bulb just below the obex. Site of incision which surrounds descending trigeminal tract indicated by faint continuous lines. From Krieg [1942].

the ear and pharynx we are not certain that dividing those at the time of an operation on n. intermedius would help in this disorder, having divided IX in only one of our 3 patients. However, our failure in Janice D. suggests that the operation about to be described would have been preferable.

Tractotomy of Bulbar Descending Cephalic Pain Tract

The initial observations of one of us (W.H.S.) in 1942 and 1943 [White and Sweet, 1955, pp. 463–466] revealed that all cephalic pain fibers from V, VII, n. intermedius, VIII, IX and X travel in what was originally denoted the spinal or descending trigeminal tract. Extensive incisions into this tract in the medulla oblongata at about the obex were likely to give the full analgesia of inner head and face indicated above. Our first operation which deliberately achieved such analgesia was carried out on June 8, 1945 [White and Sweet, 1955, pp. 476–478]. However, analgesia of the first 2 trigeminal divisions requires a less extensive incision placed more caudally. Figure 1/13 shows that if one deliberately divides a dorsal bit of the spinothalamic fibers ventral to the descending tract and produces some V3 as well as V1,2 analgesia at operation, one can be reasonably certain of having divided all of the upper two thirds of the trigeminal fibers, which are the most important for the management of chronic migrainous neuralgia in the usual picture. We have done the more rostral operation with an incision extending dorsally into the fasciculus cuneatus in 2 patients with migrainous neuralgia, both of whom had extensive reference of their pain, and in whom we wished to divide as much as feasible of the descending cephalic pain pathway.

Patient Eric M. Born 8/57, had his first attack at age 12. The pain involved left periorbital area, temple, ear and the whole lateral and posterior neck. He had had only 7 attacks of right-sided pain. He was totally disabled from work or social activities by the severity of his pains uncontrolled after 4 years of a thorough trial of medications by a cluster headache specialist (J. Graham). A lidocaine block 10/16/80 yielded V1,2 analgesia and stopped an attack; this hypersensitive man thought the numbness was probably acceptable. On 10/17/80 an RF lesion produced an initially excellent analgesia which soon faded to hypalgesia with recurrence of attacks. On 11/26/80 a bulbar descending cephalic pain tractotomy was carried out to a depth 3 mm in the transverse plane 1 mm caudal to the obex. Extensive intraoperative testing revealed and postoperative testing confirmed in more detail analgesia of the opposite distal lower limb from mid calf on down as well as throughout trigeminal skin and mucosa, both walls of the external auditory canal, tympanic membrane and tonsillar fossa but not oral pharynx. Temporary ipsilateral lateropulsion confirmed an adequate dorsal extent of the incision.

In the 86-month period since operation he has had many mild attacks controlled by modest doses of medication, but he works full time having only an occasional bout of pain and has contracted a successful marriage, in contrast to preoperative total disability.

Patient John B. Born 6/43. Pain attacks in left temple radiating to left jaws and lateral neck since 1970. Cafergot, the only useful drug, controlled the attacks but led to 3 episodes of congestive heart failure and in 1977 an aortic and mitral valve replacement. On 3/2/82 left greater and lesser superficial petrosal neurectomy was done with no relief. On 5/7/82 a bulbar lesion in the plane 2 mm rostral to the obex was made deeper than in the previous patient, in the hope of destroying ascending fibers within the nucleus of the descending cephalic pain pathway. Analgesia of the ipsilateral trigeminal zone and opposite limbs and torso has controlled the facio-cephalic reference in the attacks of pain, but they resumed within 3 months in a zone about 36 cm^2 in an area in the left side of the neck with the same time course and disabling intensity as the original attacks. They remained under control only with massive doses of cafergot, which he refused to give up despite its leading to another open heart operation in November 1983. On 7/11/84 right C2–3 posterior rhizotomy was done (C. Poletti) yielding anesthesia of posterior scalp and upper two thirds of neck. Complete relief of pain persists at 3.5 years follow-up.

Patient Eric M.'s original extensive cervical reference of pain has not required rhizotomy of this region.

Patient Stephen H. Born 2/51. First attack left cluster headache 7/83 superimposed on bilateral migraine attacks since age 8 years. Pain in left posterior scalp as well as face. Two retrogasserian glycerol injections, the 1st with V1,2 numbness and inadequate relief; the 2nd with V2,3 denser numbness and relief 6 months — the numbness 'extremely unpleasant' — same for 1 h numbness after a lidocaine block 5/86. At Massachusetts General Hospital 6/11/86 analgesic, then anesthetic lidocaine block during attack of pain — no benefit. 6/24/86 — bulbar descending cephalic pain tractotomy and C1,2,3 posterior rhizotomy (Poletti) producing analgesia all V, VII, IX , X zones but no cervical analgesia; tested 6th postoperative day. Although the cluster attacks have been greatly relieved, the patient is disabled by analgesia dolorosa — a constant severe burning throughout left V2,3 and behind eye. Not realized was the hope that the more complete preservation of touch associated with bulbar tractotomy than with RF rhizotomy would avert dysesthesias. These have been helped only temporarily by Dr. R. Tasker's implantation of a stimulating electrode in the area of the trigeminal ganglion and root. In retrospect since the glycerol injections had also provoked dysesthesias we should have cut VII, IX and upper X posterior roots.

Autonomic Activity vis-à-vis Attacks of Pain

Although the frequent linkage between the manifestations of autonomic activity and the episodes of pain led to Gardner's performance of petrosal neurectomy, numerous observers have noted that after surgical treatment, episodes of pain may be stopped while the autonomic signs continue and vice versa. Thus, Dott [1951] states: 'After trigeminal rhizotomy in some cases periodic watering and suffusion of the eye and throbbing in the temple (continue) with no pain or even discomfort.' Mazars [1976] noted after his rhizotomy confined to the trigeminal first division that although the attacks of pain disappeared, 'vasomotor and secretory episodes may persist — decreasing over several months.' One of Maxwell's [1982] thermally rhizotomized patients, though relieved of pain continued with attacks of mild tearing, hemicranial flush, and nasal fullness. Campbell [1984] too had a pain-free patient in whose first year after open trigeminal rhizotomy there was a painless episode of unilateral tearing and ptosis. We have had 2 patients with persistent pain relief but dramatic attacks of autonomic manifestations. In one patient trigeminal V1,2,3 analgesia and V1 nearly complete anesthesia with elimination of all symptoms was followed 32 months later by the sudden recurrence with clock-like regularity of these features of the original attacks; right-sided profuse tearing, watery rhinorrhea, flaming red face and eyeball, miosis, and ptosis with nausea, generalized weakness and sweating on both sides of the face and all limbs. These attacks occurred at 3–4 p.m. or awakened him at 3–4 a.m. — all now 'with absolutely no pain whatsoever'. The second patient's total trigeminal anesthesia and complete cessation of all symptoms was followed 5 years later by episodes beginning with drooping of the right corner of the mouth, then miosis, ptosis and profuse ipsilateral watery rhinorrhea without tearing, but generalized weakness so striking that he must lie down for the 25- to 35-min duration of the episodes. These, persisting for 8 years, include only minor initial stabs of pain ipsilaterally behind the right eyeball and in the right ear canal.

Conversely, Kunkel and Dohn [1974] describe 3 patients whose pain recurred after greater superficial petrosal neurectomy and trigeminal sensory 'rhizolysis' but without lacrimation, conjunctival injection or other such symptoms. In 3 more of their similarly treated patients the attacks of parasympathetic discharge were stopped but the pain persisted without a period of relief. Wake and Hitchcock's [1987] case 8 showed the same behavior. We have a patient whose tearing and rhinorrhea stopped but the pains continued despite excellent V1,2 analgesia.

These observations all make it clear that the impulses regarding the pain may travel by grossly disparate routes from those for the autonomic discharge which probably travel via the fiber bundle described by Chorobski and Penfield as bypassing the geniculate ganglion.

Summary

Pain in this disorder may be transmitted over trigeminal, n. intermedius, glossopharyngeal and possibly upper vagal afferent paths. We recommend as initial evaluation for possible invasive therapy a retrogasserian needle placement followed by a sustained effort to provoke an attack and to ascertain if analgesic block of rootlets will stop the attack at the price of an acceptable denervation sensation. The great majority of the successful surgical cases have had appropriately sited trigeminal analgesia. If the attack is not stopped or the numbness is not tolerated, petrosal stimulation and neurectomy is the next step. Should this peripheral neurectomy yield relief but be followed by recurrence, section of the roots of nervus intermedius, IX and perhaps upper X may yield longer relief. Section of the bulbar descending cephalic pain pathway may be advisable in severe cases with widespread neural involvement or poor tolerance of sensory deprivation. The rare case may require supplemental cervical posterior rhizotomy.

Conclusions

Although far fewer patients with this disorder require surgery than do those with trigeminal neuralgia and the management is more complex, the desperate medically intractable patients who are benefited are truly grateful even for a degree of relief which requires medical supplementation. Since we have not been able to identify features indicative of the specific neural pathways involved we favor the sequence of diagnostic and therapeutic procedures we have described.

Chapter 2. Cranial Nerves VII, IX, X, XI

Historical Note

We owe to Ramsey Hunt's [1915] series of studies, mainly on the location of the eruptions of herpes zoster, a determination of the cutaneous and mucosal areas supplied by the geniculate ganglion of the nervus intermedius, and the two pairs of ganglia related to the glossopharyngeal and vagus nerves. However, as Hunt points out, mild inflammatory reactions in adjacent ganglia could blur the validity of some of his conclusions. Our most useful data as to which of these nerves may play a role in various loci and types of faciocephalic pain come from neurosurgical clinical reports which have been but little amplified from those in chapter VII of White and Sweet [1969].

Anatomy

The n. intermedius of Wrisberg is the sensory root of the facial nerve (fig. 2/1). It consists of the proximal afferents of the unipolar cells of the geniculate ganglion which leave the trunk of the facial nerve in the internal acoustic meatus and pass centrally as one or more slender bundles between the motor root and the vestibulo-cochlear nerve or joining the latter entering the brain stem at the lower border of the pons. The distal afferents from the ganglion cells are the taste fibers which course in the chorda tympani and the greater superficial petrosal nerve, and also a few somatic afferents from the concha and medial surface of the auricle. The details of this cutaneous innervation by the facial nerve, and whether facial fibers reach also the external acoustic meatus and tympanic membrane and anterior two thirds of the tongue remain undetermined [Saunders and Weider, 1985]. The sensory

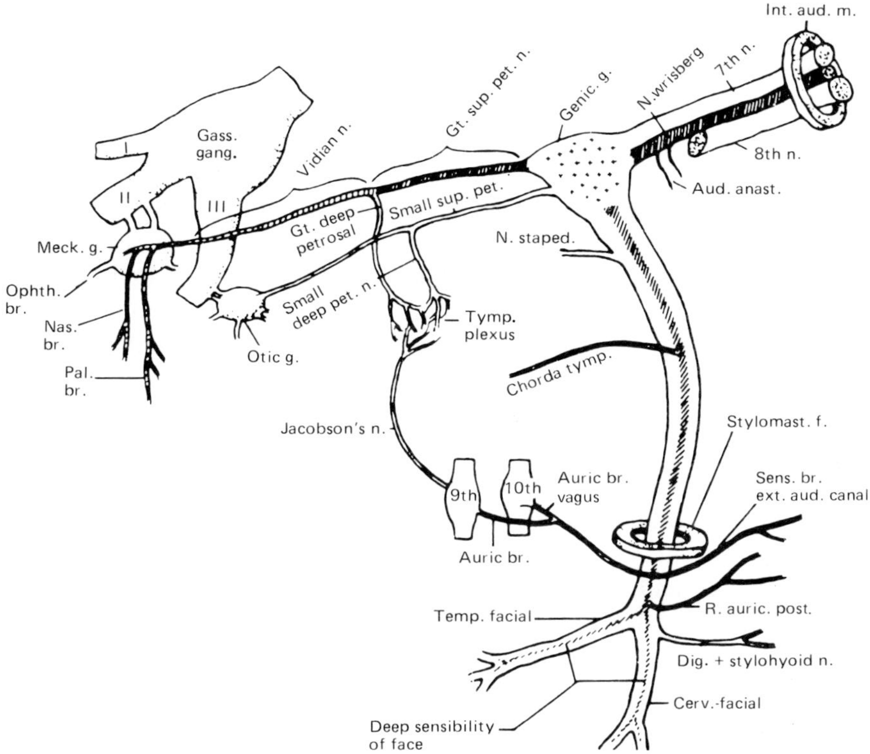

Fig. 2/1. Diagrammatic representation of the facial nerve, illustrating the distribution of the sensory components (shaded portions). Note branches associated with deep sensibility of the face. From Hunt [1937].

root of the facial nerve also contains the efferent preganglionic autonomic fibers for the salivary glands. Because of the variable dispositions of the pain fibers as a single or several independent filaments (nervus intermedius) or as travellers with vestibular or auditory components of VIII, White and Sweet [1969, pp. 288, 368] recommend awakening the patient in order to identify by electrical stimulation the rootlets which are causing pain. Those coursing with the vestibular component can be cut without permanent adverse sequela. If the pain fibers are interspersed with auditory fibers it may be well to secure the patient's verbal approval of unilateral deafness in the hope of relief of pain, before cutting them.

The glossopharyngeal nerve supplies motor fibers to the m. stylopharyngeus, secretomotor fibers to the parotid gland and sensory fibers to the pharynx, the tonsil and the posterior part of the tongue and the tympanic cavity; it also contains taste afferents from this part of the tongue. It emerges as three or four rootlets from the cranial part of the medulla and is separated in the jugular foramen from the tenth by a dural septum. The spinal accessory cranial nerve is usually regarded as a purely efferent nerve, supplying the sternocleidomastoideus and trapezius muscles. We have, however, found that an occasional tiny rootlet on stimulation in the awakened patient gives rise to pain in the zone of the patient's clinical complaint and have cut such rootlets with impunity.

A study of the connections between dorsal root C1, C2 and the spinal accessory nerve showed that the posterior root of the first cervical nerve is inconstant and that its anatomy presents four types of variation. Depending on the type of variation, often the only pathway for the sensory fibers of C1 to reach the spinal cord is through the rootlets of the eleventh cranial nerve [Ouaknine and Nathan, 1973]. Usually it is assumed that the posterior root fibers of C1 participate in the innervation of the meninges, the atlanto-occipital joints, and the area of the occipital foramen. Knowledge of the variation of the rootlets of C1 and its possible anastomosis with the eleventh nerve is important for adequate denervation of these same head regions especially when they are involved in a cancerous process.

N. intermedius (Geniculate) Neuralgia

There are relatively few clinically proven patients in this category if one excludes those with chronic or periodic migrainous neuralgia. They have all had pain mainly in the ear canal, some with pain in the pinna as well and some with radiation beyond these sites. They rarely have brief provokable paroxysms with trigger zones. Commonly constant pains occur lasting for hours and changing in site and type as the disorder continues. Cutting of the chorda tympani has relieved 2 patients; in 2, cutting of n. intermedius only and in 4 cutting of this nerve along with some of VII, VIII or IX gave relief. In one patient cutting n. intermedius failed, but bulbar tractotomy at the level of the obex stopped the attacks [see White and Sweet, 1969, pp. 257–265, for details]. Pulec [1976] has by far the largest series (15 cases) all relieved he says by excision of the geniculate ganglion and adjoining n. intermedius plus at times a small part of VII (without producing facial weakness). Bruyn [1984] in a comprehensive review article challenges the whole concept of a geniculate neuralgia on the basis of an untenably restricted definition of a neuralgia. A recent decisive postmortem study of Ouaknine et al. [1979] described a patient who had had tinnitus and episodes of stabbing pains without trigger zones in one ear plus intermittent dizziness, ipsilateral hypoacusis and trigeminal hypalgesia and hypesthesia for 6 years. These then subsided but were correlated at autopsy (cause of death unrelated) with striking cross-compression of VII and VIII by a redundant loop of the posterior inferior cerebellar artery.

Conclusion

'Essential neuralgias' in which the pain is confined to the ear canal are rare but should not be forgotten when such a problem presents. The intricacies of the relevant anatomy should be carefully studied before surgery is undertaken thereon.

Vagoglossopharyngeal Neuralgia

Synonym: Glossopharyngeal Neuralgia

The sensory fibers of cranial nerves IX and the upper third or more of the fibers of X transmit the impulses causing bursts of pain in the throat including the back of the lower jaw and tongue, the area of the auditory canal or a combination of these zones. This involvement of both nerves has led White and Sweet to adopt the term vagoglossopharyngeal neuralgia. In the first successfully treated cases Sicard and Robineau [1920] cut extracranially in 3 cases not only IX and the pharyngeal branch of X but also the cervical sympathetic trunk. In the following year Harris [1921b] and Siebert [1921] independently described some cases and gave the disorder the incomplete name glossopharyngeal neuralgia. This has gained general acceptance because: (1) open rhizotomy of this nerve only despite incomplete denervation of the area has often sufficed to relieve the pain, and (2) Dandy [1927] published a detailed picture depicting a most unusual extensive anesthesia from the roof of the nasopharynx to the bottom of the oral pharynx and pyriform recess after his rhizotomy of IX which stopped the pain in both reported cases.

Clinical Features

We summarize here the longer more fully documented account of White and Sweet [1969]. This disorder's manifold features display a much richer range of symptoms than does trigeminal neuralgia. It occurs about equally in both sexes, with a left more than right preponderance of 3:2, contrasting with trigeminal neuralgia in which females and the right side are in the majority. Bilateral occurrence was recorded in only 1.4% of the 175 cases tabulated by White and Sweet. The clinics these days treating many patients with trigeminal neuralgia are seeing less than 1% of that number with vagoglossopharyngeal neuralgia. Because of the greater difficulty in making the latter diagnosis, and the sustained success of current medical treatment the incidence may actually be greater.

Site of Pain

This may be referred to any of the domains described under anatomy. The throat is affected more often than the ear, but radiation from one of these areas to the other is common, and unlike trigeminal neuralgia, the pain may radiate well beyond both the cutaneous and deeper zones of IX and X.

Modes of Provocation

Swallowing is the commonest provoker of attacks but any movement of head or face may suffice. Chewing, eating, talking, laughing, yawning, coughing, sneezing, straining, blowing the nose or head turning have all been described. Infrequently some movement may be helpful, e.g. Kunc's [1960] case 6 dared swallow only when his head was bent forward, and Bohm and Strang [1962] had 2 patients with left-sided pain alleviated by head turning, in one to the right and in the other to the left. Some cutaneous trigger areas in the neck may overlie hyoid bone and laryngeal areas supplied by the superior laryngeal branch of the vagus. Characteristics of food or fluid such as temperature outside a tepid range or specific tastes such as spicy, salty, bitter or acid may set off an attack. Spontaneous attacks with no identifiable stimulus are also common.

Onset, Type and Duration of Attacks

Mild dysesthesias or unusual sensations may be forerunners of sharp stabs of pain which in others mark the onset of the disorder. Thus, one of our patients described vague persisting discomfort below the angle of the jaw 'like a gland beginning to swell' for 2 months before her typical stabs came on. Sometimes the premonitory sensations come in bursts of such feelings as a 'clicking', a 'bang' or a little noise 'in the ear', 'something sticking in the throat', 'nonpainful electrical tremors'. Later when the paroxysms begin they may be immediately preceded by a burst of the old sensations. Bohm and

Strang had 2 patients with initially puzzling onsets — one with dysphagia for a year and another with nearly constant mastoid pain and ipsilateral complete facial paralysis, before more characteristic pains appeared. The intensity, duration and frequency of the attacks may be so low that the patient does not bother to consult a physician. Some patients may be awakened by attacks many times a night and Bohm and Strang had 2 patients whose attacks were almost always at night, when they were also at their worst. A refractory priod after an attack during which another cannot be provoked is usually brief. However, one of our intensively studied patients soon became refractory to all provocation except hyperventilation with his mouth open. As in trigeminal neuralgia spontaneous remissions of greatly variable duration occur in most patients especially during the earlier years of the disease.

Special Variability in Clinical Manifestations

Unusual features far exceed the number seen in trigeminal neuralgia. These are almost the rule rather than the exception. We describe them under nine headings:

(1) Constancy of an aching, pressing or burning pain lasting an hour to days or weeks occurs in up to 25% of the patients in various reports.

(2) Trigger zones or onset of pain outside the pharyngeal and aural zones. Small trigger areas activated by light touch may be more obvious outside the IX, X domain such as periphery of pinna, the neck near the jaw or shaving areas of the face. The pain itself may start in the 'anterior two thirds of the tongue', 'the gum of the lower jaw', 'the entire half of the face', 'throughout the side of the face and neck', 'in front of the ear, cheek and jaw to the chin', '2 lower back teeth, side of jaw and a little on upper lip and eyelid' and 'both sticking pain and itching in the neck radiating to the ear'. In 5 of these cases the pain was relieved by cutting the rootlets of IX and/or the upper rootlets of X so the diagnosis of coincidental trigeminal or other neuralgia may be invoked in none of them. The right diagnosis in all of these was achieved only after a critical history and examination. For example, an ultra-sensitive trigger spot between the back of the tongue and the tonsil was the clue to the correct diagnosis in one. Radiation into the auropharyngeal zone was helpful in others. In another 2 of these cases the correct diagnosis was made only after the failure of trigeminal rhizotomy; in the later history of onset of all attacks with a stabbing pain deep in the ipsilateral ear led to the correct operation. Perhaps those who have failed to relieve paroxysmal facial pains after trigeminal rhizotomy would do well to restudy their cases regarding the diagnosis of IX, X neuralgia.

(3) Pain starting within but radiating outside the anterior cervical and auropharyngeal zone has occurred 'into the ipsilateral 4th and 5th fingers', 'the ipsilateral shoulder', 'the eye', 'much of the ipsilateral trigeminal field', 'down the neck, the front of the nose and rarely to the opposite ear'. In the larygneal forms the radiation may be up to gums or zygoma or down to shoulder or upper thorax. These unusual references of sensation should not lead to the diagnosis of hysteria.

(4) Elicitation on palpation of localized soreness only rather than a frank paroxysm has been reported in at least 10 cases including ours with tenderness over masseter, cheek and lower jaw.

(5) Sensations other than pain during the attacks, especially when these were severe, have included illusion of swelling in the soft palate, dizziness and vertigo, or this plus unsteadiness, unilateral or even bilateral tinnitus.

(6) Preoperative sensory loss somewhere in the IX, X zones has been described in at least 5 patients whose later course makcs thc diagnosis of tumor unlikely. Bues [1963] reported 2 of these cases with small hypalgesic, hypesthetic areas in front of and/or behind the pinna. The necessary sensory study of these areas is not carried out by most of us.

(7) Involuntary motor accompaniments of attacks include coughing and/or vomiting. These may be especially distressing when they exacerbate the pain, cannot be inhibited, and are associated with a sense of choking or suffocation. Another patient would cry out with his attacks of pain despite maximal self-control and had the impression his vocal mechanisms automatically went into action. The reverse effect on the vocal cords of a brief hoarseness after an attack has also been described. This paralysis has also been much more protracted in a patient of ours. Others have had a brief run of hiccups after the pain began. The dramatic onset in one patient was of mysterious attacks for 5 months of a severe cramp in the throat and a sensation as though food were passing into the larynx with impending death from suffocation. There was a 7-month remission whereupon attacks of burning pain in the tonsil radiating to the ear led to the successful rhizotomy. This is perhaps the most remarkable example of a general feature of this disorder, namely a frequent major variability in the manifestation in the same individual.

(8) Autonomic phenomena. Excessive salivation both between and during attacks has been observed and in several instances has been measured from each parotid gland with a photoelectric sialometer. Mucoid content, specific gravity and concentration as well as total volume were elevated from

the ipsilateral parotid during an attack in one patient, whereas between attacks the parotid on the normal side secreted 3–5 times as much as that on the side of the pain. The reverse state of marked dryness in the mouth has been reported by at least three others. Various combinations of lacrimation, sweating, mydriasis and a hot, flushed face and neck, usually but not always only ipsilateral to the pain, have occurred in a few cases, and could lead to confusion with chronic migrainous neuralgia.

(9) Cardiovascular and/or cerebral reflex responses mediated by the carotid sinus nerve of Hering. These are the most spectacular symptoms associated with this disorder and can have a fatal outcome. The sinus nerve of Hering issues from the carotid sinus containing specialized receptors for cardiovascular regulation at the base of the bifurcation of the common carotid artery. Higher in the neck this nerve joins the glossopharyngeal nerve which communicates there with the vagus. Hypersensitivity at the sinus causes a syndrome of bradycardia, hypotension and syncope which may lead to convulsions — or convulsions may occur as a direct cerebral effect without disturbance of the general circulation. Exactly the same symptoms can occur in especially severe attacks of vagoglossoparyngeal neuralgia without hypersensitivity of the sinus proper. The mechanism may be an ephaptic transmission of the intense action potential burst to the sinus nerve fibers provoking bradycardia and hypotension. This may progress to cardiac arrest, syncope and convulsions. If only severe bradycardia, e.g. 5–10 cps, comes on during the attack of pain when the patient is lying down, the decreased cerebral blood flow may not even cause clouding of consciousness or subjective dizziness. The longer the asystole especially in the standing patient the more likely it is that syncope and convulsions will be added to a faintness, mental confusion and blurring of vision. Since Riley et al. [1942] first described this syndrome many cases have been reported. The patients usually have lesser attacks of pain for months or years before their intensity and frequency lead to this additional syndrome. It is rare in these patients for the region of the carotid sinus itself to be hypersensitive to digital pressure or head turning; only if there is intense pain do the cardiovascular symptoms appear. We have found only one case of the cerebral seizure form without bradycardia or hypotension. However, the abrupt loss of consciousness and/or convulsions are so dramatic that their provocation by the pain may not be obvious and a number of patients have been treated for epilepsy before the diagnosis was made. This is especially understandable if the seizure has focal characteristics. We have not seen a report of an abnormal resting EEG in this disorder. We have had one patient with a malignant tumor and radiation

sclerosis in the throat in whom dangerous bursts of extreme hypotension without major bradycardia were provoked by bursts of pain.

Differential Diagnosis

A focal lesion in the infracranial auropharyngeal area may give rise to paroxysmal pains; the more dominant any steady component the more likely is a clear-cut focal lesion. The commonest are tumors, often malignant, but some advancing so slowly that months of agonizing pain all too often precede the diagnosis.

If careful appraisal by an ENT specialist and neurological examination disclose no abnormality, it is well to study the neck, base of skull and intracranial cavity by both MRI and high resolution CT scan with contrast enhancement. Since tiny lesions can be causative the slices should be of minimal thickness and of appropriately varied projections and special parameters.

Medical Treatment

The cardinal therapeutic drugs used for trigeminal neuralgia, carbamazepine, phenytoin and baclofen have similar efficacy in this disorder and their thorough trial will usually precede any invasive procedure.

Surgical Treatment

Open Rhizotomy. Section of the IXth and upper rootlets of the Xth nerves is required, performed through a unilateral suboccipital craniectomy. Failing to cut vagal rootlets will often lead to inadequate relief. As formulated by White and Sweet [1969) the fundamental question is not whether vagal rootlets should be sectioned but how many may be cut before provoking undesirable sequelae. To decide this, one lets the patient wake up, stimulates the rootlets to determine where pain is felt, and cuts these rootlets until the patient becomes somewhat hoarse. To date the paretic vocal cord has always recovered.

During operative manipulation of the IXth and Xth rootlets, one may note a decrease in blood pressure or a sudden tachycardia [Nagashima et al., 1976; Rushton et al., 1981]. The reverse may occur on cutting the glossopharyngeal nerve, i.e. a temporary sharp or gradual rise of the blood pressure because of the interruption of afferent vasodepressor impulses originating from the carotid sinus [White and Sweet, 1969]. This rise may persist for hours so that the surgeon's hemostasis must be meticulous to avoid postoperative bleeding.

This neuralgia responds well to root section. In a study of 217 such cases seen between 1922 and 1977, 129 patients were operated; mortality in the immediate postoperative period was 5.4%. In the first 15 years rhizotomy was confined to the IXth nerve; some failures to achieve relief led to many operations in which upper vagal rootlets were cut as well. However, even rhizotomy of IX and the 3 upper vagal rootlets rarely produces complete analgesia in the oral pharynx, much less in the tympanic membrane and posterior wall of the ear canal [White and Sweet, 1969, pp. 290–291]. In one patient with cancer individual stimulation of each of the 8 isolated rootlets of the vagus nerve gave rise to pain in the throat and tongue [White and Sweet, 1969, p. 900]. Despite what might be inadequate denervation for trigeminal neuralgia these patients nearly all remain pain-free. About 20% of Rushton's patients had difficulty with swallowing and many complained of having a foreign body or a tickling sensation in the throat [Rushton et al., 1981].

Although Rushton et al. [1981] describe relief by rhizotomy in 110 of 123 patients they do not indicate how many if any vagal fibers were cut in the failures.

In the rare patients in whom the pain is referred low in the throat superior laryngeal neurectomy is likely to be successful.

A review of several important series, compiled in 1976, and comprising 254 cases of deep and/or extensive cervical cancers and cervicofacial cancers treated by different combinations of cranial nerve sections, combined most often with high cervical rhizotomies showed 53% good results, with generally short survival and 18% mortality [Sindou et al., 1976], in part due to the precarious state of the patients operated upon. Since alternative treatments have become available, these operations are now rarely performed.

Percutaneous Rhizotomy. The relative ease of carrying out a percutaneous (RF) rhizotomy at the pars nervosa of the jugular foramen makes this the invasive procedure of first choice for all of the variants of vagoglossopharyngeal neuralgia. Tew [1977] and Lazorthes and Verdie [1977] were independently the first to make successful RF lesions here. The external landmarks we use after penetration of the skin 5–10 mm lateral to the labial commissure are, as seen from laterally the upper border of the tragus, and from sagittally 9–10 mm lateral to the medial border of the lacrimal caruncle. However, we rely heavily on films and fluoroscopy with superior equipment providing a standing image and a small focal spot of circa 0.6 mm. Sweet has

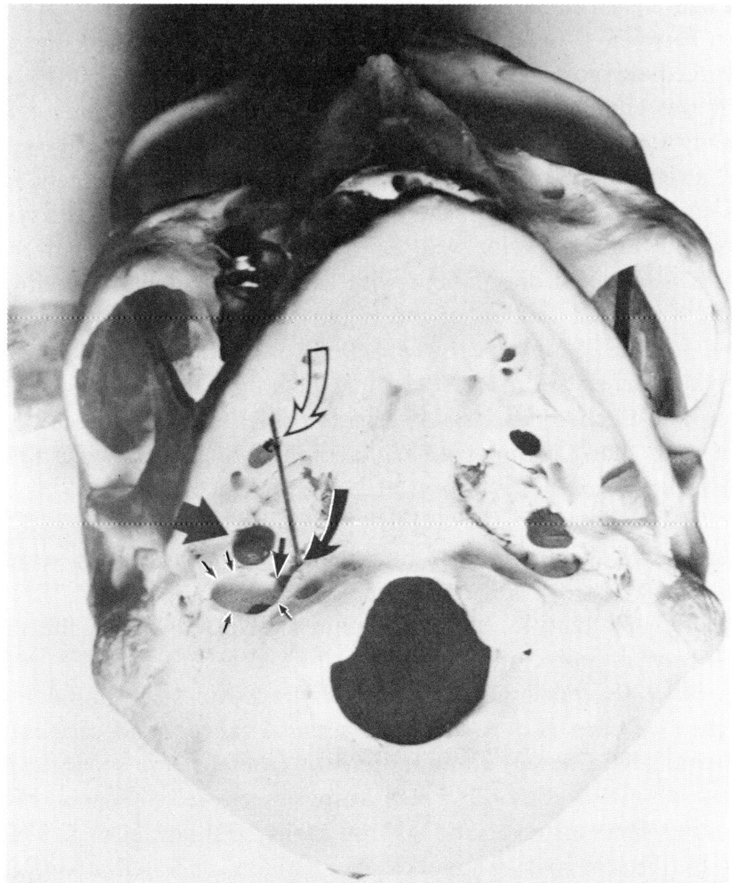

Fig. 2/2. Basal view of the skull with an electrode tip in the pars nervosa of the jugular foramen. Slight rotation of the skull away from the side of the electrode in the head-extended position. Open curved arrow = electrode shaft overlying the medial corner of the foramen ovale; closed curved arrow = electrode tip in medial corner of the pars nervosa; large black arrowhead = internal carotid artery; small black arrowhead = bony spur separating the pars venosa for the jugular venous bulb from the smaller pars nervosa for the ninth, tenth, and eleventh nerves and associated ganglia. From Sweet [1982b].

needed the constant collaboration of an experienced neuroradiologist to identify the pars nervosa which is usually not seen with the clarity shown in figure 2/3a, b. Figure 2/2 illustrates that one can pass medial to the foramen ovale, although when the electrode's trajectory transects the shadow of this foramen (passing below it), this has caused no problems (fig. 2/3a). It may be necessary to use this more lateral path to pass by the lateral pterygoid plate. One does well though to be medial to the internal carotid artery as it passes upward to enter the petrous bone. The broad undersurface of the body of the sphenoid bone medial to the jugular foramen can be struck harmlessly; hence we begin with a more medial placement and correct under radiologic control to enter pars nervosa. The bony spur projecting from anteriorly into the jugular foramen indicates the dividing line between the larger lateral opening for the jugular bulb and the smaller medial opening for the IXth, Xth and XIth nerves. The bony spur may be more evident if the skull is rotated a little to the opposite side. Once the jugular foramen is identified a variety of projections will show it, as portrayed in the third edition of 'Operative Neurosurgical Techniques' [Sweet, 1988c]. That dural sleeve may enclose the rootlet bundles down into the pars nervosa has been revealed by the securing of CSF at this site in 3 patients. It is impossible from the anterior approach to enter the intracranial cavity via the jugular foramen. Consequently, no intracranial hemorrhages from needle puncture can occur. The lower or petrous ganglion of IX and the lower or nodose ganglion of X lie below the jugular foramen. Hence one's lesion is central to the cells of origin of nearly all of the primary afferent fibers in both nerves. This may explain the low recurrence rate in the idiopathic group. A further attractive feature in contrast to trigeminal rhizotomy is that denervation dysesthesias probably do not occur.

One aids final placement of the electrode by electrical stimulation both with a square wave signal, and with gentle RF heatings. Readjustment of position continues until the threshold is preferably 0.2 V or less of a square wave or less than 48 °C of heat. One seeks to secure reference of sensation to ipsilateral throat, ear canal or central pinna. Typically the glossopharyngeal fibers lie anterior and lateral to the upper vagal fibers so that replacement of the electrode closer to the jugular venous bulb may be necessary if vagal or spinal accessory motor responses occur.

As with trigeminal rhizotomy by RF heating or glycerol, continuous electrocardiography and intraarterial monitoring of blood pressure are advisable. Dangerous hypertension is much less likely than bradycardia and hypotension because of stimulation of the carotid sinus nerve of Hering or motor vagus. Decrease of blood pressure or heart rate to less than half the preoperative level occurred during 6 of the 11 procedures described by Ori et al. [1985]. Syncope occurred in 2 of them, one of whom had a convulsive seizure and required cardiac massage because of asystole. There were no lasting sequelae. These surgeons used only fentanyl and no i.v. anesthetic

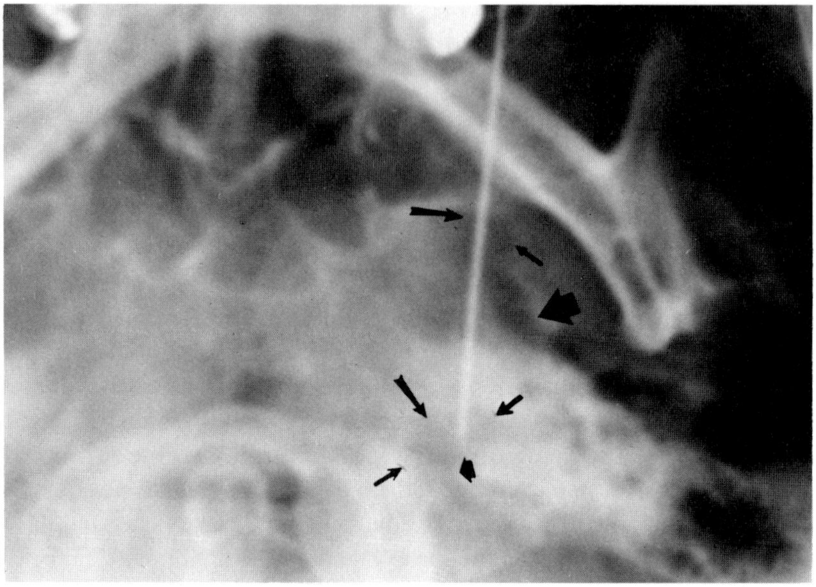

a

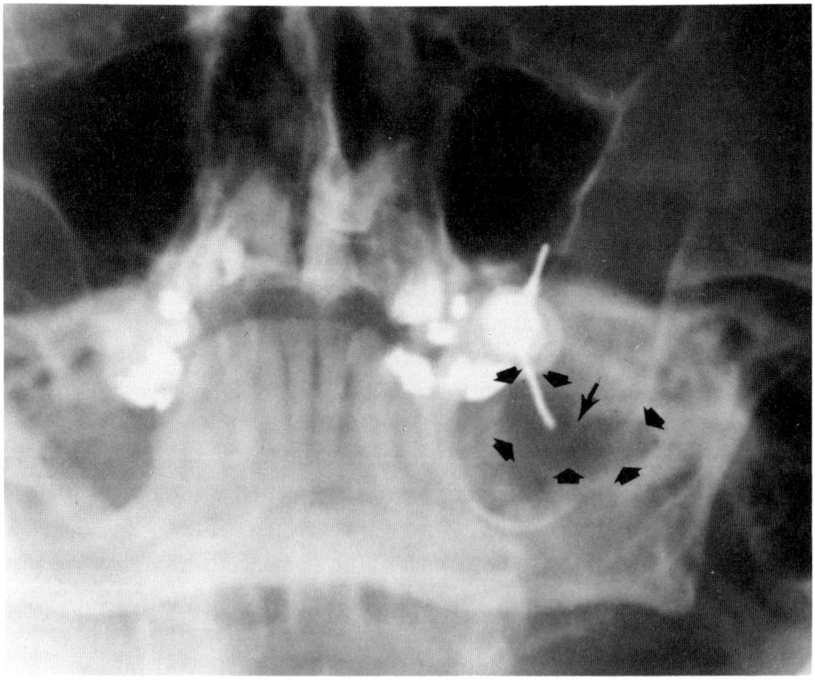

b

agent. We have avoided these more dramatic responses by using brevital i.v., heating in small increments, stopping this before asystole and severe hypotension and using i.v. atropine as needed.

Ori et al. [1985] prefer the lateral approach from below the external auditory meatus and in front of the mastoid process. If tumor lies in front of the jugular foramen this may be the best route available.

Tew et al. [1982] had 2 cases of vocal cord paralysis in the idiopathic disorder and prefer open rhizotomy for these patients. Lazorthes and Verdie [1977] also have an early report of 3 cases of temporary vocal cord paralysis and dysphagia. These results have led many of us to make these lesions in smaller increments under lesser anesthesia. This permits one to check for hoarseness and dysphagia during as well as after lesion-making. Following this tactic we have in one patient finally raised the temperature of a 20-gauge electrode with 5 mm bare to 105 °C for 3 min. Earlier lesions had produced enough sensory loss so that no brevital was required for the last lesion. Even so only hypalgesia of soft palate and posterior wall of oral pharynx developed — not of the tonsillar fossa. Slight hoarseness and dysphagia did not appear until the next day, were never severe but did not disappear completely until 6 months. She remains completely relieved at 105 months, despite recovery to normalgesia upon pinprick. Other surgeons usually settle for lower temperatures.

Table 2/I describes encouraging results from 8 services in vagoglossopharyngeal neuralgia with no patient needing to advert to open rhizotomy although several recurrences were again successfully treated by the same method. There have also been many good results in the tumor group.

Open Exploration; MVD or IX–X Rhizotomy. Jannetta [1981b] has reported finding an 'offending vessel' at the IX, X rootlets in 15 of 17 cases of 'glossopharyngeal' neuralgia. He describes seven different vascular types of

---

Fig. 2/3. Electrode position for RF lesion IX–X rootlets at jugular foramen. The electrode tip unchanged in position and correctly placed for a lesion in the lateral part of pars nervosa, shown in two different projections. *a* With marked extension of head shows shaft underlying the foramen ovale (with no third-division trigeminal irritation). Anterior arrows indicate medial and lateral margins of foramen ovale; large arrowhead opening for internal carotid artery; posterior arrows outline boundaries of pars nervosa. *b* With head not extended shows more clearly boundaries of entire jugular foramen (large arrowheads), and small arrow points to bony spur, indicating boundary between the neural portion and vascular portion of the jugular foramen. From Sweet [1982b].

Table 2/I. Vagoglossopharyngeal pain: percutaneous RF rhizotomy

Author, year	Ear-throat-tumor pain		Neuralgia	
	number of cases	useful relief	number of cases	useful relief
Lazorthes and Verdie, 1977	11	good to excellent, 6; fair, 3; 0, 2	1	pain-free 28 months
Broggi and Siegfried, 1979	2	1 required 2nd RF lesion; both pain-free at follow-up at 1 year; 1 patient dysphagic 3 weeks but lasting XII deficit		
Isamat et al., 1981			3	pain-free at 5–32 months
Giorgi and Broggi, 1984	5	Until death or last seen 3; improved 2	6	3 pain free at 3, 4, 5 years; 1 much better 3 years; 1 recurrence V pain 2 years
Arias, 1986			2	pain-free at 1–2 years
Salar et al., 1986	5	slight pain; no narcotics	3	good
Sweet, 1988d	2	poor	4	pain-free at 1, 3 and 8 years; medication controlled other at 28 months
Tew and van Loveren, 1988	9	5 pain-free until death 4–18 months later	2	pain-free but vocal cord paralysis in both

compromise of the rootlets. Nerve section was carried out originally in 2 patients and in 2 others after no relief or a recurrence following MVD; 2 died postoperatively. Because major mobilization of an artery is usually not feasible in the tight spaces between artery and rootlets he has more recently used shredded teflon to separate them. Panagopoulos et al. [1987] relieved by

MVD all 4 patients in whom they describe vascular compression — in one case by a vein. There are at least 4 other single case reports in which elimination of compression of the IX, X complex was described with relief of pain at follow-ups from 9 to 15 months [Morales et al., 1977; Haines, 1986; Tsuboi et al., 1985; Yoshioka et al., 1985]. However, since rhizotomy of these nerves carries less risk of recurrence than microvascular decompression and minimal if any risk of denervation dysesthesias, we agree with Onofrio [1975] that rhizotomy is the procedure of choice if open operation is done. As during percutaneous RF lesions one must be alert to a variety of cardiovascular vicissitudes especially while manipulating the nerve roots, stopping dissection or retraction and using appropriate pharmacologic prophylaxis. The evidence for cutting upper vagal as well as glossopharyngeal rootlets, as well as the technique for this rarely used procedure, have not changed since the description by White and Sweet [1969], although the operating microscope has added to its precision.

Conclusions

Percutaneous RF rhizotomy at the jugular foramen both for pain related to tumor and essential vagoglossopharyngeal neuralgia probably can be performed with avoidance of dysphagia and hoarseness by the use of small increments of heating and appropriate testing of the patient during and between lesions. In the patients in whom this fails, open posterior fossa operations should lead to IX, and partial X rhizotomies regardless of neurovascular relationships because of the absence of dysesthesias after rhizotomy of these roots and the greater likelihood of recurrence of pain after MVD.

Section II. Neurotomies

Neurotomy had been used earlier in a number of conditions such as painful neuroma, amputation pains, thoracotomy pains, etc. Owing to poor results, it has been almost entirely abandoned, except in a few conditions, such as occipital neuralgia [Blume, 1976] and particularly pseudoradicular pain, originating from the facet joints.

Chapter 3. Percutaneous Medial Branch Neurotomy

Synonyms: Percutaneous rhizolysis, facet rhizotomy, percutaneous neurectomy, percutaneous facet denervation

Back and leg pain related to a facet syndrome was first mentioned by Goldthwait in 1911 and accurately described by Putti in 1927. Progressively, this mechanism of pain of spinal origin was extended from the lumbar to the cervical spine [Sluijter and Mehta, 1981].

We shall take as an example the descriptions of the surgical treatment of the facet syndrome in the lumbar spine but extensive information on the surgical treatment of this syndrome in the cervical spine can be found in Sluijter and Mehta [1981]. The anatomy of the innervation of the spinal facets has been described in detail [Pedersen et al., 1956; Lazorthes and Gaubert, 1956; Fox and Rizzoli, 1973; Bogduk and Long, 1979]. The posterior primary ramus is related to structures in the posterior compartment of the back which are concerned with the stability of the vertebral column. This branch of the spinal nerve arises just lateral to the intervertebral foramen (fig. 3/1a) and divides almost immediately into medial and lateral branches. From the Ll through L4 levels the medial branch turns dorsally and lies in a groove on the transverse process, at the junction of this structure with the superior articular process and is bridged by the medial edge of the intertransverse ligament. It gives off a small branch to the inferior aspect of the capsule of the facet joint and then continues caudally supplying the superior aspect of the joint below and finally ramifies in the dorsal muscles.

The L5 dorsal ramus is much longer than the dorsal ramus at higher levels and runs along a groove between the ala of the sacrum and its superior articular process. Its medial branch passes the caudal edge of the articular process and supplies the L5–S1 articulation. The lateral branches pass obliquely over the transverse processes and, from the upper three lumbar levels, supply a broad cutaneous band immediately lateral to the facet joints.

a 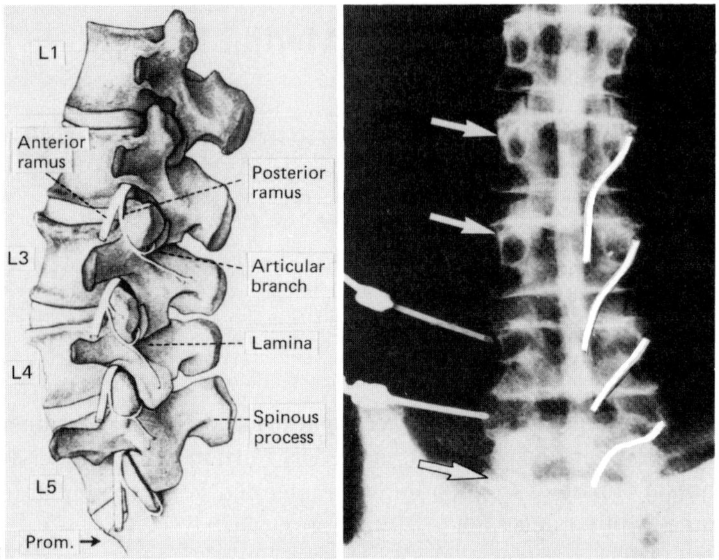 b

Fig. 3/1. a Anatomy of lumbosacral posterior rami [from Pedersen et al., 1956]. *b* Anteroposterior radiograph of lumbar spine illustrating target points for medial branch neurotomy. The target points lie exactly at the tip of either the arrows at L1, L2, and L5, or the guide needles at L3 and L4. Note, at the L3 and L4 levels, how the silhouette of the superior articular process overlaps the target point, demonstrating why electrodes should be introduced obliquely. The overhanging superior articular process covers the target point in a dorsoventral approach. On the right side of the figure the courses of the medial branches of the dorsal rami have been superimposed. From Bogduk and Long [1980].

In 1960, Rees performed the first denervation with a knife, percutaneously introduced; this operation is referred to as multiple bilateral percutaneous rhizolysis, and in 1975 Rees stated that he had performed this 'simple and safe operation more than 6,000 times in all five continents, without major complication and without mortality, on occasion operating on 42 patients in one operating list of 12 hours'. There is still some doubt whether this percutaneous scalpel technique actually cuts the sensory nerves or only performs a myofasciotomy [King, 1976]. Shealy suggested the use of a percutaneous RF thermocoagulation approach, for which he coined the term 'percutaneous spinal facet rhizotomy' [Shealy, 1975] and since that time several modifications of the procedure have been proposed known as 'percutaneous neurectomy' [Fox and Rizzoli, 1973], 'percutaneous lumbar medial

Table 3/I. Sensory responses to stimulation around lumbo-sacral facets [after Lora and Long, 1976]. Stimulation parameters: 0–4 V, 60–100 cs, 1 ms

Facet	Reference of sensation
L5–S1	coccyx, ipsilaterally hip joint, groin, posterior thigh
L4–L5	posterior hip and thigh, less often coccyx
L3–L4	upwards in thoracic area, anterior thigh, flank, groin, coccyx
T12–L1–L2–L3	upper back, thoracic and cervical regions, anterior abdominal wall

branch neurotomy' [Bogduk and Long, 1979] and 'percutaneous facet denervation' [Mehta and Sluijter, 1979].

Several authors have described in detail the technique of percutaneous medial branch neurotomy [Shealy, 1975; Bogduk and Long, 1979; Sluijter and Mehta, 1981]. According to the anatomical studies cited above the target point for medial branch neurotomy at the level L1–L4 is the dorsal surface of the transverse process just caudal to the most medial end of the superior edge of the transverse process. At the L5 level, the appropriate target is the dorsal ramus proper, situated in the groove between the ala of the sacrum and the superior articular process. These targets are identified on antero-posterior radiographs with the patient in ventral decubitus [Bogduk and Long, 1980] (fig. 3/1b)

The target is chosen in accordance with several criteria among which the clinical results of temporary anesthesia are particularly important. The target is approached with an electrode under local anesthesia using radiographic guidance. Electrical stimulation near the medial branch will often reproduce the pseudo-radicular pain distribution. Table 3/I describes the patterns of reference of sensation according to different levels.

The most favorable situation is realized when the stimulus reproduces the pain of which the patient complains. The nerve is then destroyed by raising the temperature of the tip of the elecrode to 80 °C for 90 s. Usually at each level a series of three lesions, two of which are directed, respectively, rostrally and caudally to the target lesion, are performed [Shealy, 1975]. Lesions may be produced in one session at different levels according to the clinical findings. It has been suggested that the electrode should lie parallel to the nerve, which means a posteroinferior approach to the target, since the RF heat lesion forms radially around the electrode and does not extend distal to its tip [Bogduk et al., 1987].

Results of so-called facet denervation in the treatment of chronic low back pain have been severely criticized and much has been written about the placebo effect of these procedures. Not many data are available. However, in a carefully designed study, comprising 149 patients with a follow-up time between 6 and 30 months, 40% of patients achieved satisfactory relief from the procedure. This percentage fell to 26% in those who had had prior surgery and rose to 61% in those with no prior spinal surgery. No patient with arachnoiditis and no patient with a compression fracture due to cancer benefited [Lora and Long, 1976]. Electromyographic control showing denervation of the m. multifidus indicates adequate destruction of the medial branch and correlates positively with satisfactory outcome [Oudenhoven, 1977]. Comparative analysis of radiographs illustrating the target reached by various techniques showed that in some of these techniques the medial branch could not have been reached. This may explain some of the variability of the reported results [Bogduk and Long, 1980]. Complications are minimal [Shealy, 1975; Lazorthes et al., 1976; Lora and Long, 1976; McCulloch, 1976/77; Burton, 1976/77] and include superficial burns and acute radiculitis.

Conclusions

The paucity of publications on the subject in this decade led to an inquiry to Long. He has no follow-up assessment of the patients thus treated at Hopkins since 1980 and consequently is not prepared to make a statement on the indications for or results of the operation. Neither are we.

Section III. Spinal Rhizotomies and Ganglionectomies

Historical Note

Abbe performed the first spinal posterior root section in 1889 in the USA and in the same year Bennett [cited by Abbe, 1889] performed the same procedure in Great Britain. Abbe, in two separate operations on the same patient, cut 'the sixth cervical nerve, both roots (dorsal and ventral) outside, the seventh, both roots outside, and also the posterior root inside, the eighth 'posterior roots only inside the dura'. This then was the first intraspinal procedure developed for the treatment of intractable pain. Abbe, in this same paper, commented: 'In considering the lessons drawn from these cases it is to be remembered that in any path of study knowledge never comes entire at once, but piecemeal. Truth presents herself in fragmentary form, and we put the pieces together; so that, while I do not present the case of cervical operation as a brilliant result as yet, so far as completely relieving the pain goes, I offer it as a unique case making a quick recovery from an operation, as conceived by Dr. Dana, at once simple and scientific.'

Several variations of spinal root surgery have been developed over the years (table 3/II) but on the whole, after a period of rapid expansion, the method has gone through a long decline, initiated by spinothalamic cordotomy.

Anatomy of Spinal Roots and Nerves

The anatomy of the spinal roots and their accompanying arteries is represented in figure 3/2. Anterior roots are formed by three to five rootlets, emerging from the anterolateral sulcus, posterior roots by three to ten

Table 3/II. Landmarks in the evolution of spinal rhizotomy

1	Intradural root section	Abbe, [1889] Bennett, [1889]
2	Extradural spinal root section	Scoville, [1966]
3	Excision of dorsal root ganglion	Smith, [1970]
4	Selective posterior rhizotomy	Sindou, [1972]
5	Percutaneous RF rhizotomy	Uematsu et al., [1974b]

rootlets, which penetrate into the posterolateral sulcus. They are separated by the dentate ligament, and group together before leaving the dural sac. Within the outer arachnoid layer containing CSF, intradurally placed tiny anastomotic branches pass from one rootlet to another; they are readily overlooked by the neurosurgeon. They increase the extent of innervation of the root from which they arise, and failure to cut them may be responsible for some of the postoperative disappointments. Their disposition varies at different metameric levels, and has been described in detail [Hovelacque, 1927; Sindou, 1972].

In the spinal canal, as the roots approach the intervertebral foramen, both anterior and posterior roots are situated in the same common dural sleeve, but remain separated by a fibrous septum. In the intervertebral foramen, the posterior root enlarges to form the spinal ganglion which lies dorsal to the anterior root, but is separated from it by the continuation of the fibrous septum within the same dural sleeve. Here the subarachnoidal space is sealed off by arachnoid trabeculae and usually does not contain CSF [McCabe and Low, 1969]. Just distal to the spinal ganglion outside the foramen the anterior and posterior structures join to form the spinal nerve. The extraspinal nerve is surrounded by epineurium which replaces the dural sheath and quickly divides into several branches. The white ramus communicans which contains preganglionic sympathetic fibers from the anterior root joins the corresponding sympathetic ganglion, and postganglionic sympathetic fibers coming from the sympathetic ganglion join, through the gray ramus communicans, the adjacent spinal nerve. Travelling with each ramus communicans, both gray and white, are afferent fibers including some for pain. White and Sweet [1969] noted repeatedly that stimulation of the central end of each cut ramus elicited pain, whereas from the peripheral cut

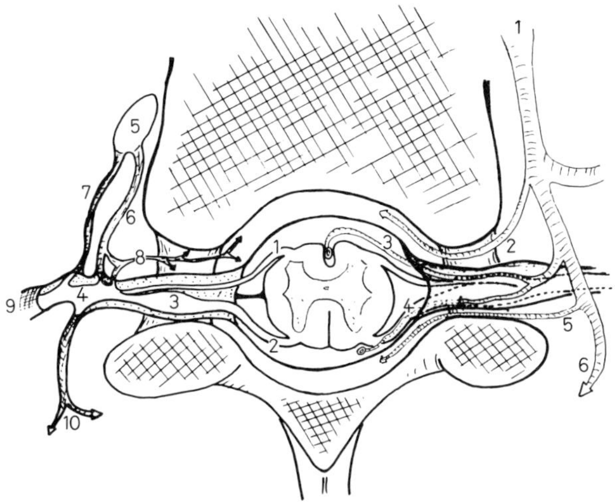

Fig. 3/2. a Segmental organization and vascularization of posterior roots. Left: 1, anterior root; 2, posterior root; 3, spinal ganglion in its opened dural sleeve; 4, spinal nerve; 5, sympathetic ganglion; 6, white ramus communicans; 7, gray ramus communicans; 8, sinuvertebral nerve; 9, spinal nerve in its perineurial sheath; 10, posterior ramus of the spinal nerve. Right: 1, segmental artery (for instance intercostal A); 2, anterior spinal canal A; 3, anterior radicular A; 4, posterior radicular A; 5, posterior spinal A; 6 dorsospinal A. From Sindou and Goutelle [1983].

end no such sensation was evoked. Just after leaving the intervertebral foramen, each spinal nerve gives off a branch which, after anastomosing with another branch coming from the adjacent white ramus communicans, forms the sinuvertebral nerve or ramus meningeus of Luschka. It returns through the intervertebral foramen, lies anterior to the spinal nerve and terminates in the spinal canal, innervating spinal meninges, blood vessels, intervertebral ligaments and vertebral joint surfaces. It probably also contains nociceptive fibers [Mokhtar et al, 1981]. Outside the intervertebral foramen the spinal nerve then bifurcates into a ventral and a dorsal branch.

Each spinal root is accompanied by an anterior and posterior radicular artery, of which only six to eight arteries supplying the anterior spinal arterial trunk and 10–23 arteries supplying the posterolateral spinal arterial trunk are of functional significance in the adult [Lazorthes et al., 1971; Crock and Yoshizawa, 1977].

Chapter 4. Open Spinal Rhizotomies

Intradural Rhizotomies

Rhizotomy has theoretically a great potential for relieving pain in a restricted part of the body since the long held principle of separation of function of the spinal roots implies that sensory information reaches the spinal cord only via the dorsal roots [Bell, 1811; Magendie, 1822]. Posterior rhizotomy spares motor fibers and will therefore avoid paralysis, but complete transection of all sensory roots serving an extremity will lead to a functional paralysis because of the absence of sensory input. There is a dramatic incapacity of an upper limb to make any useful movement whatsoever when all its posterior roots are cut. Section of sacral posterior roots may interfere with sphincter and sexual function. Extensive section of the dorsal roots innervating the upper cervical, thoracic and upper lumbar regions will result in little functional deficit, partly because there is extensive sensory overlap from adjacent dorsal roots. Underlying muscle, bone and joint afferents may also have quite different myotomes and sclerotomes respectively [Foerster, 1933; Dykes and Terzis, 1981] and there is a not negligible interindividual variability. Visceral afferents also enter the posterior roots, but the sensory radicular innervation of the viscera is complex [White et al., 1962; White and Sweet, 1969]. Other theoretical advantages of rhizotomy are that a circumscribed region of the body can be rendered anesthetic, and that the area of sensory loss can be ascertained preoperatively by nerve blocks at the intervertebral foramen.

The technique of intradural posterior rhizotomy is well known [White and Sweet, 1969; White and Kjellberg, 1973; Sindou et al., 1976; Loeser, 1982; Sindou and Goutelle, 1983]. Important aspects from a purely technical point of view include verification of the level of the laminectomy, root identification by anatomical, radiological and physiological means, selection of roots

Table 4/1. Results of relief at least 3 months after posterior intradural rhizotomy.

Author, year	Malignant disease		Nonmalignant disease	
	cases	relief, %	cases	relief, %
Echols, 1969			62	60
White and Sweet, 1969	33	58	19	63
Echols, 1970			9	100
Loeser,1972	7	43	29	25
Onofrio and Campa, 1972	18	28	211	37
Paillas and Pellet, 1972	6	0	42	76
White and Kjellberg, 1973			62	65
Barrash and Leavens, 1973	71	70		
Sindou et al., 1976 (several series cited)	585	47		

by stimulation during a wake-up anesthesia, recognition of anastomoses between roots and sparing of radicular arteries.

As can be seen from the data of a few series (table 4/I), the effectiveness of rhizotomy varies considerably according to different authors. This can be best illustrated by a few statements: 'It is concluded that thoracic rhizotomy for chronic pain, suggestive of nerve root compression, is a highly successful procedure in selected patients [Echols, 1970]. Contrariwise: 'It is our impression that rhizotomy to relieve painful states other than those involving the fifth and ninth cranial nerves has only a poor-to-fair chance of succeeding' [Onofrio and Çampa, 1972]. An intermediate position: 'Our overall rate of permanent success has been 64.5% . . . the initial extent of sensory loss does not tend to contract or fade [White and Kjellberg, 1973].

The reason for these divergent opinions is not clear [Onofrio, 1974], but it is frequently stated that allowance should be made for overlapping of dermatomes, and hence some authors advise cutting two roots above and two roots below the extreme extent of the radicular pain [White and Sweet, 1969; White and Kjellberg, 1973]. This can be achieved in the truncal area but is not feasible in the extremities, for fear of severe motor disability, and in the sacral area for fear of sphincter and sexual dysfunction. Even diagnostic nerve blocks and peroperative verification by electrostimulation of the sensory distribution may not avoid a sharp drop in success rate during follow-up [Loeser, 1972]. Hence the question arises whether there is a new pain-producing mechanism that gradually or after a latent period becomes

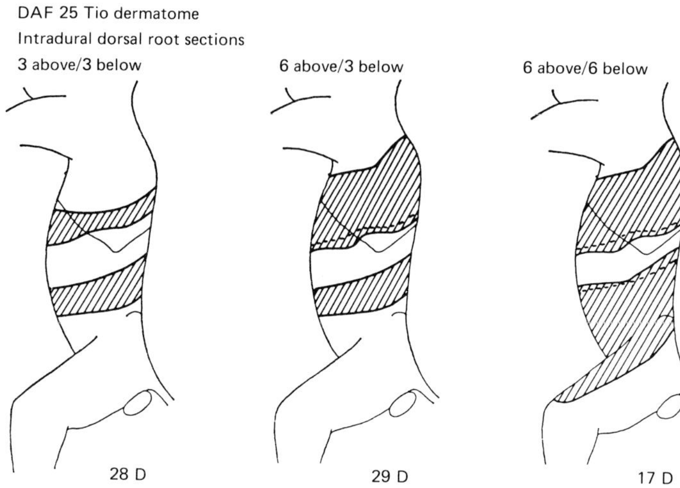

Fig. 4/1. Reduction in dermatome size following scction of additional dorsal roots. The diagram on the left shows the extent of the tenth thoracic dermatome 28 days after unilateral intradural section of three neighboring dorsal roots above and below. The insensitive areas are shaded. The center diagram shows the contraction of the upper border still present 29 days after section of three additional roots above: the dotted line represents the original level of the dermatome boundary. The diagram on the right shows a similar contraction of the caudal border of the dermatome, as seen 17 days after subsequent section of the next three roots below. From Kirk and Denny-Brown [1970].

active after the operation. There is much evidence that dynamic changes do occur after rhizotomy The size of a dermatome of a monkey isolated by intradural section of three dorsal roots above and three below is reduced by subsequent section of three additional roots above and below [Kirk and Denny-Brown, 1970] (fig. 4/1).

After rhizotomy in man areas of relative and absolute sensory loss will decrease upon the administration of *L*-dopa and increase upon the administration of methyldopa [Hodge and King, 1976] (fig. 4/2).

After denervation, abnormal spiking may appear in dorsal horn cells and it is hypothesized that the appearance of these quasi-epileptic foci may be responsible for some forms of post-rhizotomy pain. As early as 1968, high-frequency paroxysmal discharges were recorded in chronically denervated cells in the conus medullaris of a paraplegic patient [Loeser et al., 1968]. How soon and how consistently in man after rhizotomy quasi-epileptic activity develops is not clear.

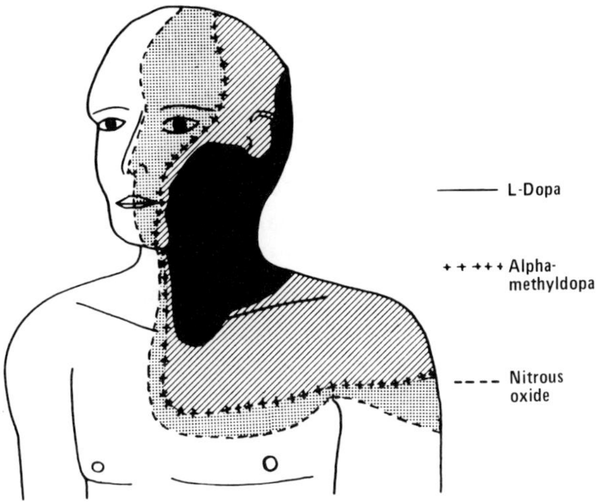

Fig. 4/2. Patient with carcinoma of left middle ear with metastases to left neck who underwent trigeminal tractotomy 5 mm below the obex, section of intermedius, glossopharyngeal nerve, upper rootlets of vagus and C1–C4 dorsal roots. Drawing illustrating the borders of anesthesia while the patient was taking *L*-dopa (solid black), methyldopa (parallel lines), and nitrous oxide (dots). When the anesthetic area was constricted (*L*-dopa) she reported increasingly severe pain in the ear, neck, and head but was quite comfortable while taking methyldopa and during 20% N_2O inhalation. From Hodge and King [1976].

After rhizotomy in rats abnormal spiking appears at the level of a group of cells in the dorsal horn which in normal animals receive convergent tactile and nociceptive inputs. This spiking activity appeared within the first months following the rhizotomy, during which time the animal develops an abnormal behavior, consisting of self-mutilation by eating the distal part of the anesthetic limb ('autotomy') and often destructive scratching of the boundary zone between anesthetic and normesthetic skin [Lombard and Larabi, 1983]. It has seemed reasonable to propose that these abnormal behaviors are due to disagreeable sensations felt in totally and partially deafferented areas and therefore this behavior has been proposed by a number of authors as a model of chronic 'neurogenic' pain in man [Wall et al., 1979; Wiesenfeld and Lindblom, 1980; Lombard and Larabi, 1983]. The most convincing evidence for this is that after traumatic avulsion of the brachial plexus in man, pain in the anesthetic limb usually occurs. Sweet

[1981], however, concluded that from the available data in man surgical posterior rhizotomy rarely, almost never, caused new pain in the anesthetic zone. Hence whether autotomy after posterior rhizotomy in an animal occurs because of pain in the animal is not directly relevant to any form of pain in man for the unassailable reason that the same procedure in man does not cause pain in the anesthetic zone. However, some patients after multiple posterior rhizotomies do complain of severe pain at the transitional zone adjoining the anesthetic skin. Consequently we think it is reasonable to use intense scratching by an animal at this region as a valid model of chronic pain in man. By this we mean that safe measures which stop the scratching in animals might reasonably be tried cautiously in man.

From the anatomical point of view, histological changes are described after rhizotomy similar to those seen in epileptic foci, such as gliosis in the dorsal horn [Kerr, 1983]. The correlation between gliosis and abnormal firing appears to be a close one [Prince, 1978]. New ways of destroying nervous elements without inducing gliosis may therefore be of interest. These include percutaneous iontophoretic application of microtubule inhibitors which induce transganglionic degenerative atrophy of primary central nociceptive terminals [Knyihar-Csillik et al., 1982] or sensory ganglionectomy by way of suicidal axoplasmic transport [Yamamoto et al., 1984].

From the biochemical point of view, supersensitivity is thought to be an important mechanism in the genesis of epileptic foci. Following rhizotomy, supersensitivity to substance P has been demonstrated [Nakata et al., 1979]. Substance P is postulated on the basis of numerous observations to be an excitatory neurotransmitter in primary nociceptive afferent neurons and, therefore, one can hypothesize that perhaps local administration in the subarachnoidal space of substance P antagonists might be useful in certain chronic pain syndromes. Unfortunately, the search for antagonists of substance P has thus far been fruitless.

Disinhibition is another mechanism which is proposed to explain pain after denervation and some neurophysiological evidence of disinhibition and its possible mechanism after nerve section is available [Basbaum and Wall, 1976]. After peripheral neurotomy there is a marked expansion of the receptive fields of the previously studied neurons [Devor and Wall, 1981; Ovelmen-Levitt et al., 1984]. There is some evidence that this disinhibition is due to a loss of presynaptic inhibition, in which the C fiber afferents play a special role [Fitzgerald, 1982]. Together with these neurophysiological changes there are profound biochemical changes in dorsal horn cells, e.g. there is a loss of opiate receptors [LaMotte et al., 1976], substance P and cholecystokinin (CCK), but not of neurotensin [Barbut et al., 1981]. It could be that this reduction of afferent-mediated inhibition following peripheral nerve section contributes to the generation of chronic pain by increasing the excitability of dorsal horn neurons. It is tempting to hypothesize that the abnormal neuronal behavior observed in the above-mentioned experiments and pain states, defined as 'neurogenic pain', is due to such phenomena as denervation supersensitivity, sprouting of aberrant nerve connections, and unmasking of ineffective synapses.

Conclusion

The variability in the clinical results of posterior rhizotomy and the functional changes in neuronal network which follow rhizotomy are obviously a warning for the cautious surgeon not to embark lightly on these denervation interventions and only after having tried alternative reversible procedures, such as neurostimulation and the application of drugs epidurally or subarachnoidally.

Extradural Spinal Root Section

This is a technical variant of root section surgery. It was described in 1966 by Scoville. It can easily be performed under local anesthesia, permitting one to test the source of pain by stimulation. The spinal root ganglion is exposed 'by one bite' with a punch rongeur in the outer edge of the lamina just caudal to the transverse process. The sensory root is identified in its own dural sleeve and the root cut just proximal to the ganglion. This approach avoids opening the dura. Occasionally some drops of spinal fluid appear at the proximal end but this can easily be sealed off by electrocoagulation. The major advantages of the approach are ease of stimulation, avoidance of arachnoiditis and comfort to the patient, who can quickly resume ambulation. In patients with failure of disc surgery, the intraspinal extradural approach through a partial hemilaminectomy allows for direct visualization and permits access as well to those structures known to be causes of the problem such as recurrent discs and cicatricial tissue [Strait and Hunter, 1981].

For pain due to advanced cancer in the pelvis, some authors recommend a simplified method of sacral extradural rhizotomies, in which the S1 spinous process, the overhanging tip of L5 spine and the upper edge of the sacrum are rongeured away. Then two heavy silk ligatures are passed extradurally; one cranially below the axilla of the S1 root and the second as far as possible caudally and both tied tightly. The dural sac with all of its content is then divided between the ties. Use of this technique is of course precluded in patients who still have any useful degree of control of bladder and bowel [Crue and Todd, 1964].

Excision of Dorsal Root Ganglion

Synonym: Trans-Spinal Ganglionectomy

In 1970, Smith proposed for the relief of 'intercostal neuralgia' an intervention which he termed 'trans-spinal ganglionectomy'. This consisted of a lateral laminectomy with rhizotomy through the dural cuff proximal to the ganglion, unroofing of the intervertebral foramen, and division of the rami communicantes at the pleural margin of the pulmonary cavity, followed by section of the intercostal nerve distal to its bifurcation into dorsal and ventral branches. This procedure isolates the proximal intercostal nerve and spinal ganglion from the sympathetic chain and spinal cord (fig. 4/3).

The rationale behind this intervention was that the failures of simple dorsal rhizotomy might be due to afferents conveying impulses for pain from the spinal ganglion to the sympathetic chain and then to enter the spinal cord at higher or lower levels. These assumptions had been made much earlier by Foerster et al. [1929] and Leriche [1939]. Smith's 9 patients could all stop their narcotics after this procedure. Post-thoracotomy pain was the original problem in 7 of them and the other 2 had a thoracic post-herpetic neuralgia. He has not supplemented this brief report.

A ganglionectomy interrupts not only input to dorsal roots but that to ventral roots as well. Long ago Foerster [cited in Sweet et al., 1950] was convinced on clinical grounds that stimuli which give rise to pain are conducted over the anterior roots. In a later study of 9 patients Sweet et al. [1950] showed that in 4 of them stimulation of the anterior roots did not give rise to pain even with signals as high as 100 V; in 5 others it did. However, in 4 of these patients, after cutting the ventral roots and stimulating the central ends, no pain could be provoked. In the 5th patient though in whom the eight anterior roots from T11 through S1 were cut, stimulation of the central cut end of T12, L1, 2 and 5 did evoke pain referred to the appropriate segment.

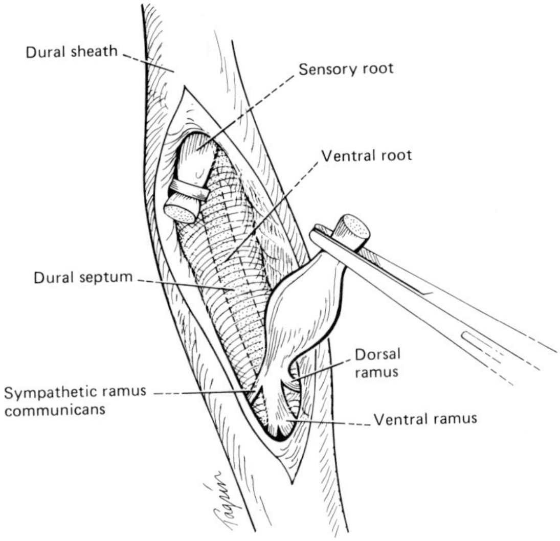

Fig. 4/3. Exposure for thoracic spinal ganglionectomy. Note that the sympathetic rami communicantes can be divided at the same operation and that all connections between ganglion and ventral root are eliminated.

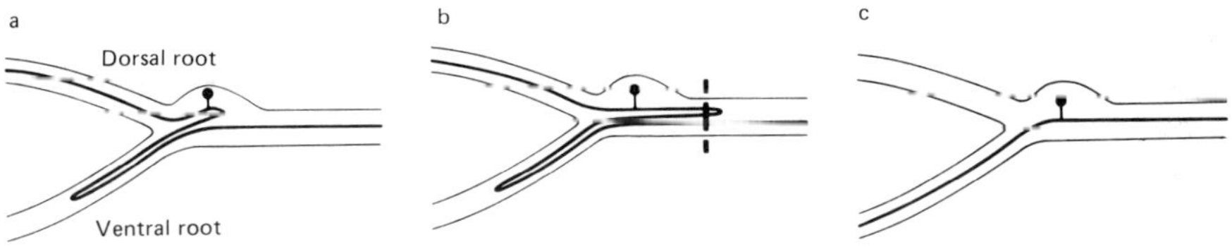

Fig. 4/4. a Dorsal root afferent axon with a recurrent course in the ventral root. *b* Possible course of a recurrent axon within the proximal part of the spinal nerve. *c* Afferent axon entering the spinal cord through the ventral root. From Azerad et al. [1986].

Stimulation of the other 4 roots failed to do so. In recent years, the presence of unmyelinated ventral root fibers has been amply documented [Willis, 1985]. Many of them arise from dorsal root ganglion cells [Coggeshall et al., 1974] and may take several trajectories in the ventral root as schematically shown in figure 4/4.

Electrophysiological evidence also indicates that many of these unmyelinated fibers are sensory [Clifton et al., 1976; Coggeshall and Ito, 1977; Azerad et al., 1986] and that the majority are nociceptors. Moreover, spontaneous activity has been recorded from ventral root axons following peripheral nerve injury [Burchiel and Russell, 1985]. Those fibers that enter the spinal cord directly (fig. 4/4c) through the ventral root could be an explanation for the failure of dorsal rhizotomy to relieve pain completely while those ventral root afferent fibers that enter the ventral root and then curve back to the dorsal root (fig. 4/4a) could be the anatomical substrate for recurrent sensation of pain [Coggeshall, 1985].

These careful studies showing that afferent fibers exist in the ventral root gave a tremendous impetus to the concept that spinal ganglionectomy might improve the results of posterior rhizotomy. However, until 1980 there was still no report in man of any change in the response to objective sensory tests after anterior rhizotomy, as well as no published report of relief by this procedure of pain unassociated with muscle spasm. Finally the crucial datum of relief after anterior rhizotomy of pain persisting after posterior rhizotomy was lacking. Hosobuchi reported the first clear-cut evidence that the human ventral roots may contain unmyelinated afferent axons related to pain [Hosobuchi, 1980b] (fig. 4/5). He removed thoracic dorsal root ganglia in 3 patients after posterior rhizotomy at the same levels had either failed to relieve the original pain or had given rise to hyper- or dysesthesias which were disabling. These 3 patients all had had post-thoracotomy or post-traumatic pain in the chest. After Hosobuchi's last operation (ganglionectomy) the first and the third patient continued relieved for over 5 years. The possibility that uncut posterior root fibers were the critical structures removed at the ganglionectomies remains.

Osgood et al. [1976] reported on 18 patients with a 2- to 20-month follow-up after their effort, the first systematic one, to add ganglionectomy to posterior rhizotomy in man. We were chagrined to learn from Osgood in 1982 that enough of his patients had had recurrence of pain so that he finds pain relief to be about the same as after a posterior rhizotomy without ganglionectomy. However, Hosobuchi [1982b] has gone on to do thoracic spinal ganglionectomies on 17 patients. Only 5 of these have failed to give relief.

The experience of one of us (W.H.S.) has been limited to 5 cases because 4 of them failed to obtain more than transitory relief. Repeated nerve blocks at relevant levels in all 4 had given temporary relief before operation — another illustration of the erratic value of such blocks in predicting the likely

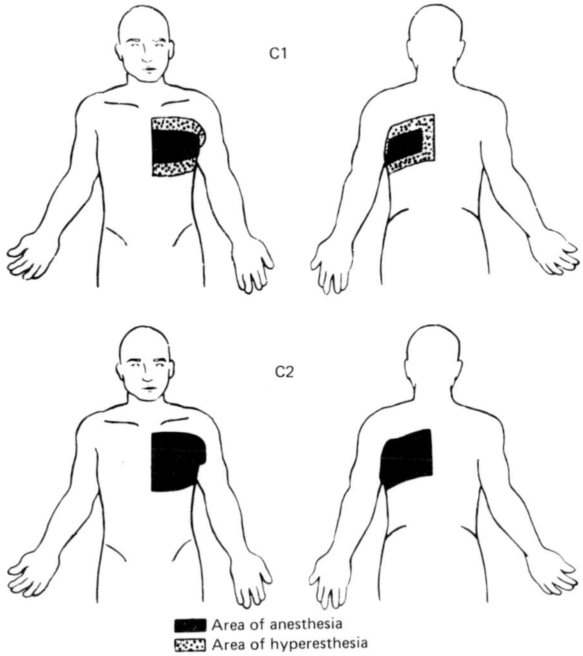

Fig. 4/5. Sensory findings in patient. C1, pre-ganglionectomy (after intercostal neurectomy T2–T5 and dorsal rhizotomy T2–T6); C2, post-ganglionectomy. From Hosobuchi [1980b].

outcome of a more permanent destructive procedure. In the lone patient of these 5 to retain continuing relief for 5 years of his pain, only the C5 ganglion had been removed. At the single level above and below this an intradural posterior rhizotomy was done because even under the microscope the plane of cleavage between ventral root and posterior root ganglion could not be identified. This patient's original pain had been disabling dysesthesias in the first 3.5 fingers. In the other 4 cases the posterior root ganglion was readily separated from the ventral roots T2–T5, T11–T12, L1–L3 and S1 levels, respectively. These were the levels at which the ganglionectomy was done in the 4 failures. The patients were awakened on the operating table after dorsal and ventral roots had been separated from each other extradurally, but the ventral root was left attached to the ventral surface of the ganglion. This would then permit the afferent fibers from the ganglion to continue to enter the ventral root. The patients were all awakened on the operating table and pain in the distribution of the root was elicited by electrical stimulation in three of six extradurally exposed ventral roots. This response required about twice the voltage of the threshold level for pain at the corresponding posterior root. Our first patient was operated on in 1973 when after the nerve was blocked before operation leg movements which had consistently evoked pain were no longer likely to do so. Indeed, following another local block into the S1 ganglion at operation such movements no longer caused pain. However this recurred a few weeks after operation. The fourth patient had RF lesions at the first three left lumbar spinal ganglia which produced crural analgesia without anesthesia of all but the posterior thigh. These lesions however did not relieve the left lateral deep crural pain. Nor did ganglionectomy at these levels which added anesthesia to the analgesia. Scratching this patient's periosteum over the lower third of the anterior femur was still painful, as was squeezing of the left quadriceps. Clearly, even the ganglionectomy had not rendered the deep structures analgesic.

The work of Pawl [1982] and of Taub [1982b] presents a more encouraging picture. The former in 1982 reported on lower lumbar or S1 ganglionectomies at one or more levels in 30 patients who had both a unilateral sciatica and an associated arachnoiditis. They were selected critically from a large number of patients studied at a comprehensive pain treatment center. Final selection of the patients for surgery as well as of the levels for the ganglionectomy was based on responses to stimulation via an electrode inserted into the intervertebral foramina. Of these 30 patients with 'failure of lumbar disc surgery', 63% were able to return to their premorbid activities; all had been followed for more than one year. As in Taub's series to be described next the patients who had only a single root ganglion implicated had the best results.

The largest series has been reported by Taub [1985, 1986]; this is a relatively homogeneous group unusually well studied originally, critically evaluated and carefully followed. Taub selected 55 patients (two thirds of whom were on Workmen's compensation) from about 1,500 patients whose persistent back and sciatic pain was related to disc disease and who had an average of three previous operations. Elimination of any directly treatable residual herniation of disc as well as stenosis or infection and adequate outcomes of psychological assessment were included among the clinical criteria for selection. In every case a totally pain-free state in the painful limb was required upon inducing local analgesia of a single spinal root. In some cases electrically induced paresthesias were also used to spot the appropriate spinal root. The expected neural deficits corresponding to a successful block needed to be confirmed, and absence of significant relief of pain with verified analgesia of the roots above and below was also required. In 53 of the 55 patients the ganglia were at L5 and/or S1; two ganglia were resected in 14 of the patients — usually at two separate procedures.

Marked reduction or elimination of the sciatica occurred in 56% of the whole group; however, it was thought likely before operation that only 34 of them would be able to return to their previous activity should the pain be relieved. Happily, 21 or 68% of the surgially successful group did go back to work; this represented 38% of the total number. Age, persistent back pain and/or other unrelated illness disabled the remainder. If the sciatica were relieved this occurred nearly always on the first postoperative day and was lasting if present. In 48 of the 55 patients follow-up was for an average of 4.8 years.

Post-ganglionectomy dysesthesia: A spontaneous as well as evoked dysesthesia confined to the dermatome of the resected ganglion was the principal postoperative complication. Taub's is the first critical analysis of this phenomenon. It appeared in the domains of 51% of the resected ganglia, usually not coming until 10–14 days after operation. It often began as pain in the calf and hence was confused with thrombophlebitis; but it then spread both distally and proximally. By 7–10 days the pain had gradually risen to a peak. It was graded as 1 to 2+ on a scale of 0 to 4 in 68% of the cases affected and lasted usually 2–3 weeks. In 27% it was graded 3 lasting 3–6 weeks. A rare chronic form has persisted months or years with occasional brief, distal dysesthetic spontaneous bursts and tactile-evoked dysesthesia which is often nocturnal. In 1986, Taub reported that the 5 patients with this dysesthesia in whom he injected subcutaneously 13 ml of 2% lidocaine (150 mg) were relieved totally for 3.3–6 h. Four of these patients then went on a self-injection regime of 150 mg at roughly 4-hour intervals. They experienced no decrease in the relief and no side effects for, respectively, one week, one and 3 months and in a lone patient continuing at 18 months. Incidently, Osgood et al. [1976] mention in their table lasting dysesthesia in 4 of their 18 cases. Three of the 4 had had 2 and one had had three ganglia removed ipsilaterally. In these the dysesthesias were increased upon urination in 2 and during a bowel movement in one. In 2 patients they were mild; in the other 2 they were persisting at 8 and 14 months.

These 2 series contrast with that of Strait and Hunter [1981]. Of their 47 similar patients submitted to spinal extradural rhizotomy of one or two roots sparing the ganglia, only 30% had improvement in activity. The degree of improvement was not specified.

Conclusions Regarding Ganglionectomy

In the rigorously selected cases of Taub and Pawl useful results have clearly been obtained by such critical study of the enormous pool of individuals whose surgery on the low back has failed. We need more data before firm statements can be made.

Chapter 5. Selective Posterior Rhizotomy

Synonym: Selective posterior rhizidiotomy

Selective posterior rhizotomy was introduced in 1972 by Sindou. The aim of this intervention was to interrupt selectively small-diameter nociceptive fibers at their radicular entrance into the spinal cord. Sindou reasoned that such an intervention would suppress nociceptive pathways and at the same time favor the pain inhibitory mechanism as proposed in the Gate Control Theory of Melzack and Wall [1965]. From animal work it is known that the large and small axons in a dorsal root are randomly dispersed but that in some species such as the cat [Ranson and Billingsley, 1916] and monkey [Kerr, 1975a; Snyder, 1977] there is a segregation of fine afferents in the lateral parts of dorsal rootlets. Wall [1962] states that this does not occur in the cat.

In man, each root is formed from a peripheral and a central segment whose supportive tissue is, respectively, Schwannian at the peripheral nerve, and oligodendrocytic at the spinal cord. The junction of the two portions, called Tarlov's pial ring, is, on average, 1 mm from the penetration of the rootlet into the posterolateral sulcus of the cord [Sindou et al., 1974c]. In the peripheral segment, the fibers have no particular localization according to size. On the contrary, at the spinal cord-rootlet junction, large and small fibers are anatomically dissociated. About 1 mm distal to the pial ring, the small fibers migrate to the surface of the rootlet, principally in the lateral area, and then cross the pial ring. The large fibers tend to congregate at the center of the ring. In the central segment, the small fibers are found under the surface of the rootlet, grouped in two small bundles situated on either side of the large fibers, the lateral one being larger then the medial one. On entering the spinal cord, most of the small fibers regroup at the ventrolateral part of the junction, before penetrating into the tract of Lissauer. The large fibers run dorsomedially between the dorsal column and the posterior horn (fig. 5/1).

Sindou has described his technique of selective posterior rhizotomy in several publications [Sindou et al., 1974a, b, 1976; Sindou and Goutelle, 1983] (fig. 5/2). An incision at the ventrolateral region of the rootlets at the medullary junction, 1–2 mm in depth at an angle of 45° to the surface of the columns of Goll and Burdach, cuts preferentially the small diameter fibers. At that level, the large fibers will be relatively spared; the myotatic fibers are situated centrally and the lemniscal fibers dorsomedially. This selectivity of the fibers destroyed by the cut is further aided by the vascularization of the posterior roots and the posterior region of the spinal cord. The vessels which penetrate the dorsomedial region irrigate essentially the external part of the dorsal column and the lemniscal fiber pathway, while those from the ventrolateral region irrigate the tract of Lissauer and part of the head of the dorsal horn.

If the root can be sufficiently mobilized, a continuous incision (sulcotomy) is made in the posterolateral sulcus. If not, a partial ventrolateral cut is made successively at each individual rootlet of the whole root. The results of selective posterior rhizotomy are shown in table 5/I.

The major advantage of selective posterior rhizotomy is that by preservation of the lemniscal fibers, more extensive rhizotomies can be performed with significantly less impairment of the functional capacity of the limbs than is the case with total posterior rhizotomies. Sparing of the lemniscal fibers may also avoid the secondary appearance of pain at the cutaneous boundary zone of sensory loss and leaves intact the substrate for subsequent electrostimulation procedure [Sindou and Keravel, 1980].

Fig. 5/1. Upper diagram: organization of fibers at the posterior spinal cord-rootlet junction in man. Lower diagram: longitudinal axial and cross-section of the rootlet entering the cord. Below this: histologic sections of the spinal cord. Each rootlet is formed from a peripheral Schwannian segment (A) and a central glial segment (C). The junction of the two constitutes the pial ring (B). Peripherally, the fibers are without organization, as the cross-section of the rootlet shows (1). In the region of the pial ring, the fibers of small diameter are arranged under the rootlet surface, predominating at the ventrolateral level (2). They then regroup (3) at the tract of Lissauer (TL) to make their way to the posterior horn. The large diameter fibers are situated in the center of the rootlet, but predominate at the dorso-median level (2); then (3) they move towards the funiculus of Goll and Burdach (GB), after giving off collaterals which run along the internal edge of the posterior horn, ending up in the gray matter of the spinal cord. The selective posterior rootlet incision is represented by the dense black arrow. Lower diagram: Lower left: longitudinal axial section of an inferior cervical rootlet (C5). The small-caliber fibers are found grouped almost exclusively at the ventrolateral level of the spinal cord-rootlet junction (arrow) to penetrate into the tract of Lissauer (TL). Large-caliber fibers pass between the dorsal column (GB) and the posterior horn (PH). From Sindou et al. [1974c]. Lower right: the posterior rootlet entity. Transverse hemisection of the inferior cervical spinal cord, stained with luxol-fuschine, which darkens the myelin, showing 1. The myelinated rootlet

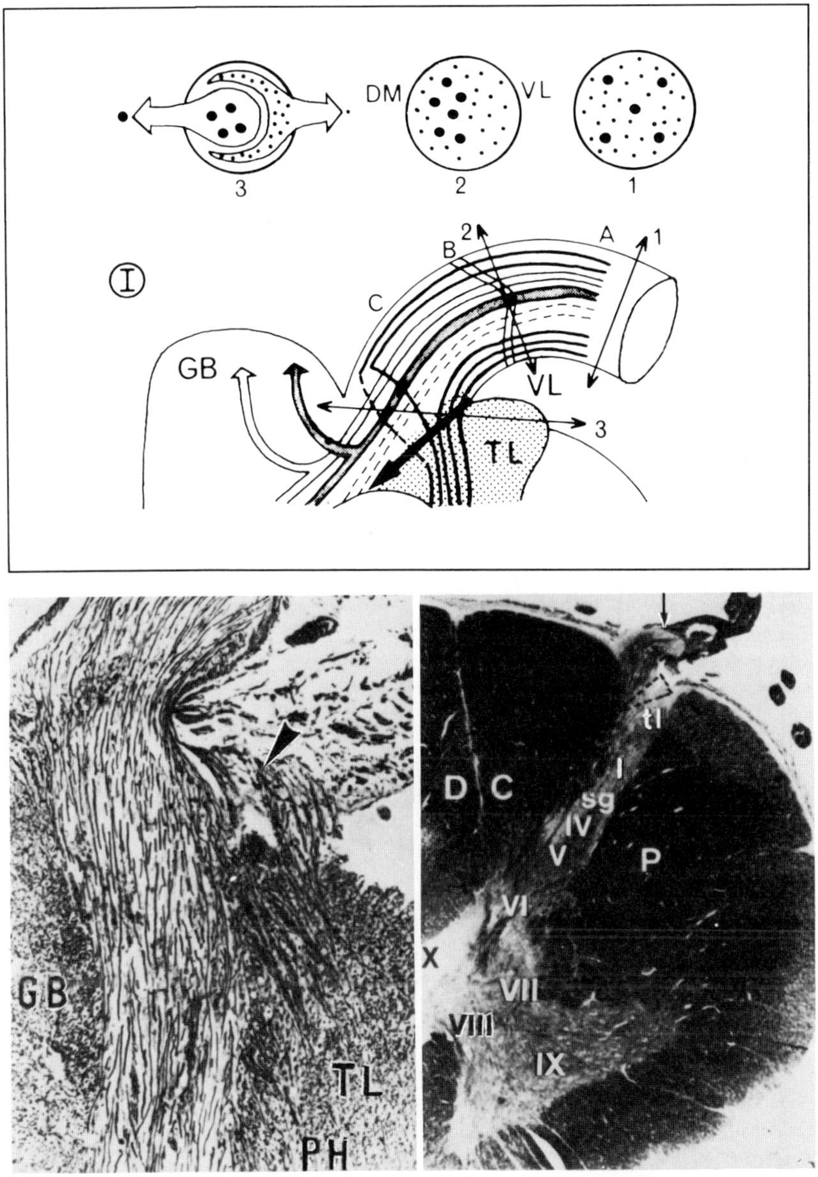

afferents reaching the dorsal column (DC), 2. The Rexed's lamination of the posterior horn. P = Pyramidal tract. The tiny arrow designates the pial ring of the posterior rootlet (diameter: 1 mm). The dotted triangle shows the incision of selective posterior rhizotomy, which makes a 45° angle and extends for 1 mm into the rootlet-spinal cord junction. From Sindou and Goutelle [1983].

Table 5/I. Results of selective posterior rhizotomy in pain and spastic painful syndromes

Authors	Year	Cancer			Spastic painful syndromes				
		n	success	follow-up	n	success for pain	follow-up	success for spasticity	follow-up
Sindou et al.	1974a	20	16	18 1–4 months 1 2 years 1 +	5	5	6–16 months	5	6–16 months
Sindou et al.	1974b				5	5	6–16 months	5	6–16 months
Vlahovitch and Fuentes	1975	5	4	short-term	3			3	short-term
Sindou and Lapras	1982	13	Pancoast 10	3–10 months 1 +					
Esposito et al.	1985	7	Pancoast	6 months					
Sindou et al.	1986				16	total 9/12 partial 3/12	1–12 years	abolished 5 markedly reduced 9	1–12 years
Sindou and Daher	1988*				57	54**	6 months–14 years		
		Neurogenic							
Sindou and Daher	1988*	42	25**	6 months–14 years					

\+ Deceased.
* To be published in Advances in Pain Research and Therapy.
** >50% spontaneous pain relief.

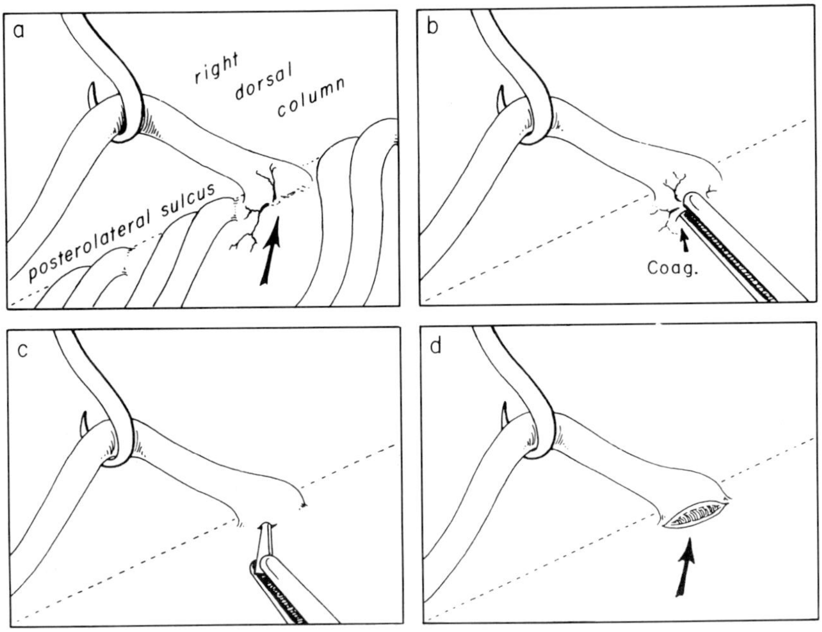

Fig. 5/2. Technique of selective posterior rhizotomy (rhizidiotomy). *a* Right lumbo-sacral-type rootlet, retracted medially by a hook to make the ventrolateral region of the spinal cord-rootlet junction accessible (arrow). *b* This ventrolateral region is the site of a densification of the vascular pial plexus, the small vessels of which are coagulated by means of bipolar forceps. *c* Selective section by ventrolateral incision using a small piece of a razor blade. This incision is 1–2 mm deep and makes a 45° angle with the posterior plane of Goll and Burdach's dorsal column. *d* Postoperative appearance of the incision (arrow). From Sindou et al. [1976].

Clearly the lesion is confined to the lateral part of the dorsal root entry zone (DREZ) and one might describe it as a lateral DREZ. It is obviously much more limited to the entry zone of this root than is the much deeper and broader so-called DREZ lesion introduced by Nashold.

Conclusions

For the reasons we have cited, we think the operation deserves wider use than has thus far been reported.

Chapter 6. Percutaneous Spinal Root Lesion

Synonym: Percutaneous radiofrequency rhizotomy

As an alternative to open rhizotomy, Uematsu et al. [1974b], inspired by the experience obtained with the thermocoagulation of the retrogasserian root, have proposed a technique aimed at destroying the spinal nerve trunk, and the posterior root ganglion or rootlets by a percutaneous method. As in the trigeminal procedure the technique combines the use of a thermistor-monitored electrode, a fluoroscopic image intensifier, a nerve stimulator and an RF lesion generator. The radiological landmarks to introduce the probe into the intervertebral foramen to perform cervical, thoracic, lumbar and sacral rhizotomies, as well as all technical details of the percutaneous RF method, have been well described [Uematsu et al., 1974b; Sluijter and Mehta, 1981; Uematsu, 1982]. Much emphasis is placed on prognostic blocking before performing the procedure, and physiological confirmation by electrostimulation of the proper site of the electrode. As already discussed in the chapter on trigeminal thermocoagulation, the preferential destruction of small-diameter fibers can be achieved by using graded increments of heating. Uematsu et al. [1974b] recommend that these be between 50 and 70 °C for a period of 120 s. For a cervical rhizotomy, the needle should be placed in the posterior part of the intervertebral foramen in order to avoid damage to the vertebral artery. Before heating a thoracic electrode one should verify that the needle is not situated in lung parenchyma.

The published results are summarized in table 6/I. Follow-up has usually been short. Lumping together good and fair results makes a clear-cut appraisal impossible.

Severe complications, such as paraplegia and one transitory paralysis of an arm, have been reported [Verdie and Lazorthes, 1982]. Destruction of essential nutrient arteries to the cord must be a problem.

Table 6/I. Results of percutaneous RF rhizotomy

Authors, year	Nonmalignant				Malignant		
	n	results		follow-up	n	results	follow-up
Uematsu et al. 1974b	17	excellent + good 9	fair + nul 8	1–12 months			
Lazorthes et al. 1976	14	good + fair 13	nul 1	2–23 months	6	good + fair 6	2–23 months
Sluijter and Mehta 1981	45	pain in lumbar region good + fair 30	part.+ nul 15	3–12 months			
	36	pain in cervical region good + fair 28	part. + nul 8	3–18 months			
		Miscellaneous in many categories					
Verdie and Lazorthes 1982	80	good + fair 52	nul 29	up to 6 years			

Conclusions

Although the method is relatively simple for the surgeon and comfortable for the patient, the meager volume of published reports indicates that it has not gained general acceptance. This is probably related to the facts that: (1) trigeminal rhizotomy often need not denervate as completely as spinal posterior rhizotomy; (2) the trigeminal root is more consistently placed vis-à-vis bony landmarks than the various spinal roots, and (3) the trigeminal motor root is less important functionally than many of the spinal motor roots.

Section IV. Lesions in the Spinal Cord

Chapter 7. Lesions, Accidental and Surgical, of Dorsal Root Entry Zone

Anatomical, Physiological and Physiopathological Data Concerning the Dorsal Horn

The anatomy and physiology of dorsal horn neurons is exceedingly complex. The data are still incomplete, difficult to follow and there is a lack of a common nomenclature. The following summary of current knowledge is largely based on a review of Willis [1985], which is chiefly concerned with the neural basis of nociceptive transmission in the mammalian nervous system.

Using cytoarchitectural criteria, Rexed divided the spinal cord gray matter of the cat into 10 cell layers or laminae which extend throughout the length of the cord. Confirmation of this laminar pattern in human material has been provided by Schoenen [1980] (fig. 7/1).

The uppermost is lamina I, also called lamina marginalis or the layer of Waldeyer. Lamina II is synonymous with the substantia gelatinosa. An outer or dorsal and an inner or ventral zone are recognized. The nucleus proprius consists of laminae III, IV and V. At the base of the dorsal horn is lamina VI. Primary afferents enter the substantia gelatinosa from its dorsal aspect. These include fine afferent fibers that originate from nociceptors as well as those from thermoreceptors and certain mechanoreceptors. Other larger primary afferent fibers pass around the substantia gelatinosa to enter its ventral aspect and include hair follicle afferents. As far as nociceptive input is concerned, the C polymodal axons bifurcate T-wise and send rostral and caudal branches for only one or two segments within Lissauer's tract; their collaterals terminate mostly in lamina I and the outer part of lamina II. The myelinated nociceptors bifurcate in the same way and send rostral and caudal branches for one to five segments in Lissauer's tract and have

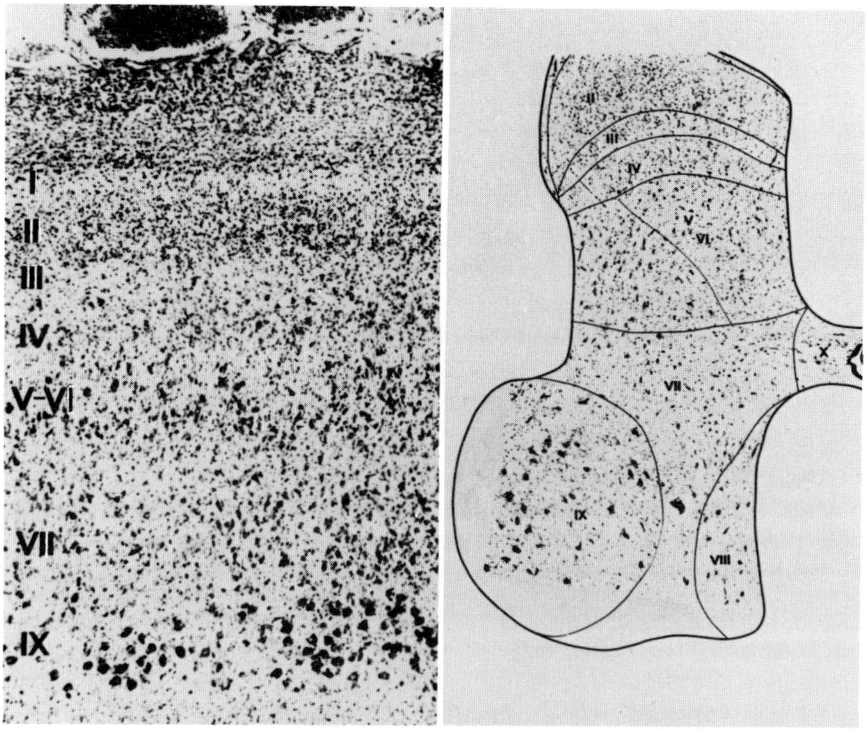

a

Fig. 7/1. Spinal cytoarchitectonic development in human. *a* Lumbar spinal cord section of a fetus 26 weeks old. Nissl. × 48. The lamination proposed by Rexed is clearly visible. *b* Five months old. Cresylviolet. × 20. The laminar organization can still be observed but the limits between the different layers become less distinct. From Schoenen [1980].

collaterals which likewise terminate mostly in lamina I and the outer part of lamina II. However, these afferents also send a branch to terminate in laminae V and X [Light, 1988] (fig. 7/2). Many or perhaps all of the neurons in the marginal layer are projection neurons. Some contribute to long ascending tracts, whereas others are propriospinal neurons. Many neurons in the marginal layer respond specifically to noxious stimuli whereas others are activated by thermal stimuli and both innocuous and noxious stimuli. The latter class of neurons are called 'wide dynamic range cells' or 'multireceptive' cells. The axons of some neurons in the substantia gelatinosa project to other regions of the nervous system, so that this area should not be regarded as a closed system. Many of the neurons in laminae III and IV respond

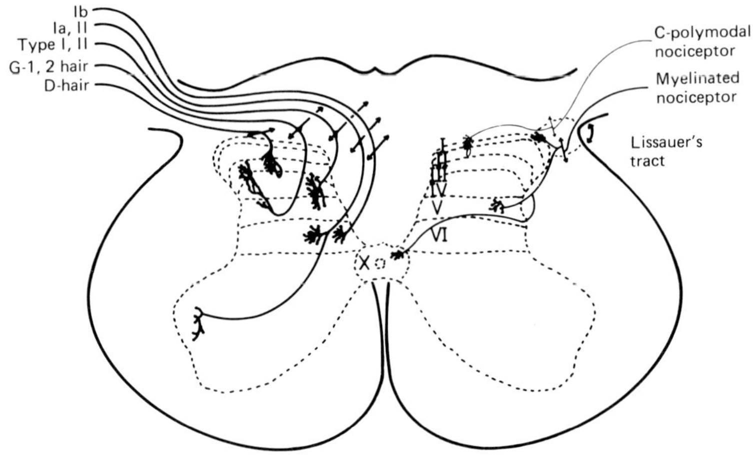

Fig. 7/2. Schematic diagram indicating the spinal termination regions of various primary afferent axons. Left side shows terminations of nonnociceptive afferents. Ib and Ia and II indicate Golgi tendon organ afferents, Ia spindle afferents and II spindle afferents. Type I and II indicate cutaneous type I and II afferent receptors. Laminae are indicated on the right half of the cord. Nociceptor terminations are indicated on the right half of the cord. From Light [1988].

specifically to innocuous stimuli, although some respond additionally to noxious input. Neurons in lamina V are often classified as 'wide dynamic range' neurons. However, there are both tactile and nociceptive specific cells in this lamina as well. Neurons in lamina VI often respond best to proprioceptive stimuli, but here too there are nociceptive specific and wide dynamic range neurons. Nociceptive cells can also be found in the intermediate region and ventral horn, but their role in nociception is as yet unclear. There is also probably a relation of cells in lamina X to nociception. The response of dorsal horn neurons to input from nociceptors in muscle, joints and viscera is so far incompletely characterized. Only rarely have neurons been found that have a visceral but not a cutaneous input, and this common occurrence of convergent inputs may be important in the mechanisms of referred pain.

Finally, a number of pharmacological agents have excitatory or inhibitory actions on nociceptive dorsal horn cells. Excitatory actions have been observed for glutamate, substance P, CCK and neurotensin; inhibitory actions for glycine, gammaaminobutyric acid (GABA), serotonin, norepinephrine, dopamine, enkephalin, substance P, somatostatin and CCK.

The cells of origin of the spinothalamic tract in monkey and rat are located in the marginal zone, deeper layers of the dorsal horn, intermediate region and ventral horn. Spinothalamic tract cells to the VPL (n. Ventralis Posterior Lateralis) thalamic nucleus are concentrated in laminae I and V, while cells projecting to the thalamic central lateral nucleus are more heavily concentrated in the ventral horn. Most spinothalamic tract cells are contralateral to the thalamic target, but concentrations of ipsilaterally projecting spinothalamic cells are found in upper cervical segments and in the sacral cord. Spinothalamic cells can be activated by volleys in A-delta and C fibers including high threshold muscle and visceral afferents. The responses of spinothalamic tract cells to graded intensities of stimuli to the skin allow a classification into low threshold, wide dynamic range and nociceptive-specific cells. Spinothalamic cells activated best or exclusively by receptors located in deep tissue, such as muscle, are classified as 'deep' cells. Noxious stimuli other than mechanical, which may excite many spinothalamic tract cells, include noxious heating or cooling of the skin, injection of algesic chemicals in the arterial circulation or muscle, injection of hypertonic saline in the muscle, occlusion of a coronary artery, noxious mechanical, chemical or thermal stimulation of the testicle and overdistension of the abdominal or pelvic viscera.

Spinothalamic tract cells that project to the medial thalamus are often located more ventrally than cells that project to the lateral thalamus. They often have very large receptive fields extending over much or all of the surface of the body and face. In addition to excitatory receptive fields, spinothalamic tract cells often have inhibitory receptive fields. This inhibition is often produced by noxious stimuli delivered to areas remote from the excitatory field, and is most often a characteristic of wide dynamic range cells. The responses of spinothalamic tract cells seem appropriate for a contribution by these cells to pain sensation and to the motivational-affective aspect of pain.

Most spinoreticular tract neurons are located in laminae VII and VIII. The spinoreticular projection from the cervical enlargement is both crossed and uncrossed, while this projection from the lumbosacral enlargement is chiefly crossed. The number of spinoreticular neurons in the monkey appears to be similar to the number of spinothalamic neurons. Some spinoreticular neurons have somatosensory receptive fields and these can often be activated by noxious stimuli. It is unclear if reticular neurons can transmit sensory-discriminative information about pain to higher centers, but it seems likely that they participate in the motivational-affective aspects of the pain response.

Spinomesencephalic tract cells appear to be situated in locations similar to the spinothalamic neurons that project to VPL, i.e. they are concentrated in laminae I and V. Some spinomesencephalic cells also appear to be spinothalamic tract cells giving branches to both the midbrain and the thalamus. Many of the cells projecting in the spinomesencephalic tract in the rat respond to noxious stimuli and they could participate in both nociceptive signalling and pain modulation.

The spinocervical tract originates from neurons concentrated in laminae III, IV and V, and relays in the lateral cervical nucleus. Many of the spinocervical tract cells respond to tactile stimuli, but some can also be activated by noxious stimuli. Finally there is a postsynaptic dorsal column pathway that originates from neurons that are concentrated in laminae III and IV and that terminates mostly in bulbar dorsal column nuclei. In addition to the cells of origin in deep layers of the gray matter there are a few in laminae I and II. Some neurons in the postsynaptic dorsal column pathway are low threshold cells and others are wide dynamic range cells. It is possible that the postsynaptic dorsal column pathway contributes to nociception, possibly also to pain modulation. When extrapolating to man from these anatomical and physiological data, nearly all obtained from animals, it is necessary to be well aware of the fact that significant differences exist between the organization of the nociceptive (and all other) pathways between different laboratory animals and man. This is represented in figure 7/3 in some detail for the localization of spinothalamic neurons and in a schematic way in figure 7/4 for the representation of nociceptive pathways in the spinal cord. For instance the very existence of the spinocervical tract in man remains controversial [Kircher and Hongchien, 1968; Truex et al., 1970].

Some physiopathological changes at the level of the dorsal horn which may have a bearing on the genesis of central pain have already been discussed in the section on spinal rhizotomy (chapter 4). The medium-term physiological consequences at the level of the dorsal horn after rhizotomy are, however, not the same as after avulsions. In one study in the cat, it was found that more than 6 weeks after extradural rhizotomy of roots L4–S1, proximal to the ganglion, receptive fields of dorsal horn cells shifted onto the flank and even to the thoracic dermatomes. Often only light stimuli were required to fire these dorsal horn cells. On the other hand, after avulsion injury in the same conditions, the receptive fields were more restricted; general pinch moderate to strong, superficial or deep, was necessary to fire the dorsal horn cells. Moreover, with avulsion injury, there was damage to the medial portion of Lissauer's tract and more gliosis in the substantia gelatinosa. It was suggested

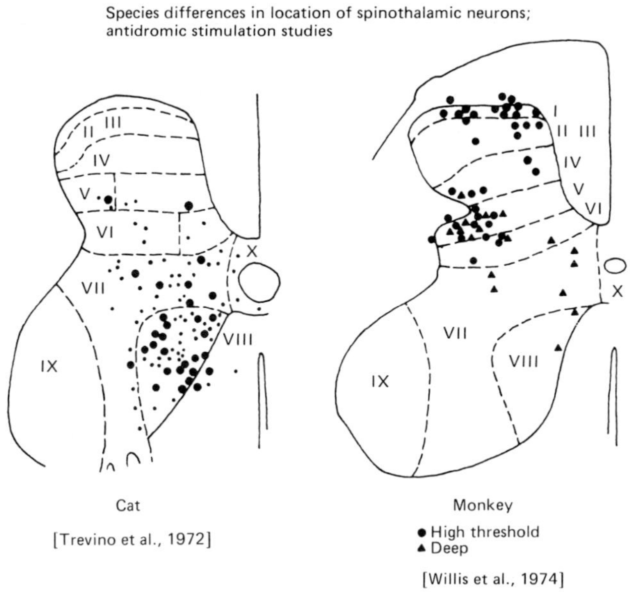

Fig. 7/3. Species differences demonstrated by antidromic activation of neurons in the spinal gray. In the left-side figure, large dots represent cells from which antidromic potentials greater than 100 μV, small dots cells from which maximum potentials less than 100 μV were obtained. From Kerr [1975a].

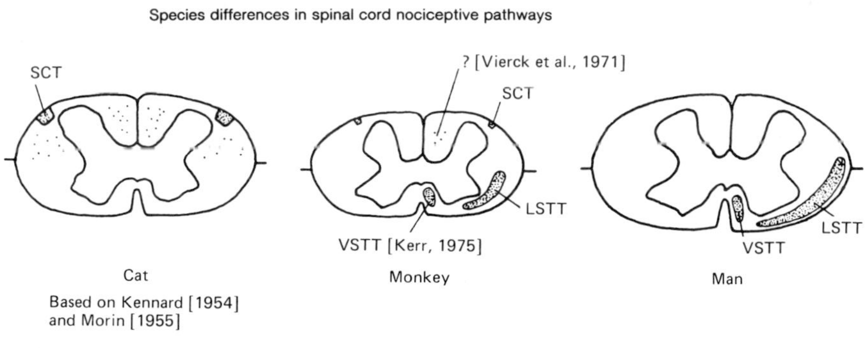

Fig. 7/4. Nociceptive pathways in the spinal cord are located predominantly dorsal to the horizontal plane passing through the dentate ligament in the cat, and almost entirely ventral to this plane in the human; the situation in the macaque appears to be intermediate. The progressive decrease in size and significance of the spinocervical tract (SCT) is indicated. From Kerr [1975a].

that the loss of this propriospinal pathway might explain the lack of receptive field expansion onto the thoracic dermatomes and the stronger natural stimuli that were required [Ovelmen-Levitt et al., 1984] (chapter 8).

To summarize then, according to one hypothesis cells in the dorsal horn, whatever the pathophysiological mechanism, may become hyperactive and send impulses via spinoreticular and spinothalamic pathways to supraspinal structures. DREZ lesions would act by either destroying these hyperactive neurons or by destroying the cells of origin of the spinothalamic and spinoreticular tracts.

According to a second theory [Pagni, 1976], central pain would be due to the conduction of afferent impulses in only one part of the anatomical substrate which in the intact nervous system subserves pain. The paleospinothalamic and nonspecific thalamic projection systems would become of particular importance when other afferent pathways have been damaged. As a consequence of this type of lesion a new permanent pathophysiological equilibrium would be reached, and only an additional lesion or restoration of the lost afferents could alter the situation. DREZ lesions would cause a rebalancing of inhibitory and excitatory pathways within this damaged sensory network [Nashold and Bullitt, 1981]. Some authors suspect that an abnormality involving either neurons in the substantia gelatinosa or the internuncial fibers in Lissauer's tract is responsible for pain in patients with primary sensory deafferentation. This conclusion is based on the results of laser-produced DREZ lesions; these in the cat do not extend into the deeper layers of the dorsal horn but remain limited to the substantia gelatinosa or the associated Lissauer's tract. Such lesions in man yield relief of pain from avulsions of the brachial plexus [Powers et al., 1984]. Although these different theories all have some experimental evidence in their favor, the shortage of physiologic and postmortem data correlated with clinical analysis leaves much to be desired in our understanding of the rationale for DREZ lesions.

Historical Note

In 1979, Nashold and Ostdahl published the methods and results of an operative procedure in which RF heat lesions were placed in the DREZ in 18 patients with partial or complete plexus avulsion. Nashold operated on his first patient in March 1975. The lesions were originally intended to destroy the substantia gelatinosa of Rolando at selected levels [Nashold et al., 1976].

In view of the complex anatomy of the DREZ and the lack of histological confirmation, the thermocoagulation target was referred to as the 'DREZ'. As experience, and particularly that of Nashold [Nashold et al., 1976, 1986; Nashold and Ostdahl, 1979; Nashold and Bullitt, 1981; Friedman et al., 1984] accumulated, results of this intervention in different 'central' pain states were reported, respectively plexus avulsion with phantom pain, pain in paraplegics, in post-herpetic neuralgia, pain after amputation, and finally in varieties of craniofacial pain. It is interesting to note that already in 1961, on the evidence of experimental work, Kerr suggested for atypical facial pain a procedure which he termed spinal V nucleolysis, and in which the entire nuclear column of the subnucleus caudalis was to be destroyed.

Technique

The surgical technique of thermal coagulation for DREZ lesions has been described in detail by Nashold and collaborators in a number of publications [Nashold et al., 1976, 1984; Nashold and Ostdahl, 1979; Nashold, 1981; Friedman et al., 1984; Bronec et al., in press] and for DREZ lesions made with microsurgical lasers by Levy et al. [1983] and Powers et al. [1984].

In the cervical region, the laminectomy is performed one level rostral to the dermatomal localization of the pain, in the thoracic region two to three vertebral segments rostral to the affected dermatomes, and at the conus medullaris a laminectomy of T10, T11, T12 and L1 is carried out for exposure of the lumbar and sacral root entry zones. Radiographic confirmation of appropriate spinal segments is obtained prior to the bone removal. Intraoperative localization of the appropriate segments for thermocoagulation is done by following the nerve root identified by its associated intervertebral foramen to its entry zone. In the case of prior spinal cord injury such as root avulsion and contusion, anatomic abnormalities often correlate with the dermatomal distribution of the pain symptoms. Identification of the root and corresponding cord segment can be confirmed by recording of root and spinal cord potentials evoked by stimulation of a given peripheral nerve [Nashold et al., 1985]. Once segmental localization is satisfactory, the operative microscope aids identification of the DREZ lateral to the dorsal column at the level of the posterolateral sulcus on the dorsal surface of the spinal cord. The more medially lying postero-intermediate sulcus in the cervical region may be more obvious than the scarred line of former entry of the posterior rootlets and should not be confused with that line.

The posterolateral sulcus forms the line along which the posterior roots enter the spinal cord. 'Through the cervical and upper thoracic segments the posterior funiculus is subdivided by another longitudinal groove, the postero-intermediate sulcus' [Gray's Anatomy, 36th ed., 1980, p. 865].

The intact roots on the opposite side of the cord and those above and below the lesion ipsilaterally may serve as a guide for the location of the sulcus. The locus for coagulation should include the abnormal segments as well as two normal cord segments rostral to and one segment caudal to the abnormal segments. Impedance measurements may be helpful to localize the abnormal segments. Normal impedance values in the spinal cord range from 900 to 1,200 Ω, when the measurement is made with a 2-mm bare, 0.25-mm diameter electrode tip. Following avulsion of spinal roots or cord trauma the impedance drops below 1,000 Ω to as low as 600 Ω due to the pathological changes in the spinal cord tissue [Vieira et al., 1988]. Superficial vessels which obscure the region for DREZ thermocoagulation must be dissected free. Since 1982, using a redesigned electrode, Nashold makes a series of RF lesions at 1-mm intervals; for each spinal cord segment 10–15 lesions are necessary. To do this, a thermocouple temperature monitoring needle 0.25 mm in diameter is used [Cosman et al., 1984]. The needle is introduced 2 mm into the cord by transpial penetration at an angle of 30–45° with respect to the sagittal plane into the posterolateral sulcus in order to interrupt the tract of Lissauer and laminae I down possibly to V or VI of Rexed; the needle should avoid penetration of surface blood vessels. The sequential lesions are produced by heating the tip of the electrode to 75–80 °C for a period of 15–30 s. Rapid tissue heating, thermal vaporization of spinal cord parenchyma and tissue scarring at the electrode tip should be avoided. Protein coagulum should regularly be removed from the tip of the needle. Usually steroids are started the day before operation and continued postoperatively for several days. Persistent new postoperative weakness in 11 of the first 21 patients and some new sensory deficit in 15 of the 21 consisted of a proprioceptive loss in the ipsilateral lower limb in most of the 15. These lesions were made at a depth of 3 mm with an electrode of 0.45 mm in diameter. A dramatic reduction in these neurological deficits has been achieved by the use of the new smaller temperature-monitored electrode.

After studying the effects of laser irradiation in the spinal cord of animals, Powers et al. [1984] have used the argon and carbon dioxide microsurgical lasers to produce the lesions in the dorsal root entry zone. The power setting with the Ar laser was 6–7 W for a duration of 1 s at an optical spot size of 150 μm. For the CO_2 laser, lesions were made at 5 W for 1 s at a spot size of 300–400 μm. With the CO_2 laser, it was necessary, in order to avoid thermal disruption that would create diffuse lesions, to keep the spinal cord clear of CSF. While the lesion was being made, ventilation was stopped. Lesions were probed with a microinstrument marked at 1-mm increments to assure that their proposed depth of 1–2 mm has been achieved. Other necessary steps included detailed dissection in order to preserve surrounding vasculature and angulation of the laser beam into the region of the dorsal horn [Powers, 1984]. It has been pointed out [Nashold and Walker, 1984] that the pathological state of the cord, as with scarring of the injured spinal cord in plexus avulsion, may interfere with the effect of laser irradiation and that this irradiation may induce the formation of a syrinx in the central part of the spinal cord.

Results

Nashold and his colleagues [personal communication, 1987] have now operated on over 400 cases without mortality. Their criteria for classifying a result as 'good' are commendably rigorous; the patients must be off all analgesics and have no limitation of activity due to pain. A 'fair' result means that no narcotics are used and the patient has no limitation of activity by pain.

Avulsion of Brachial Plexus

In 39 cases of brachial plexus avulsion, followed for 1–8 years, 54% of the patients meet this stringent requirement to be classified as having a 'good' result. 13% of these avulsion patients had a 'fair' result — a total of 67% then have really eminently satisfactory long-term results. None of the patients even in the originally treated group has had such changes in sensation or strength that he/she could not walk independently. The improved technique used since 1982 has increased the numbers in the good category to 82%.

The next largest reported series, that of Thomas and Jones [1984], is of 34 such patients. At a follow-up 4–44 months later 60% had a good result according to less rigorous criteria — i.e. 20 of the patients had 75–100% pain relief. Relief was graded at 20–70% in 9 of them and 5 had less than 20% relief. Thomas notes that neurological deficits have likewise been reduced by use of the new temperature-monitored electrode. New neurological deficits persist in 12% of his patients although they too are all ambulant. Accounts of 98 cases have been presented by 10 other services. Different grading systems were used for the results, but roughly 67% may be classified as having about 70% or more relief at the last follow-up. This, however, was relatively short in many of the patients.

Central Pain of Paraplegics

The technique has been used by Nashold to treat the pain of paraplegia, i.e. that referred to an anesthetic area below the level of the lesion in the cord or cauda equina. Such pain tends to persist if it lasts for over 6–8 months and occurs in 5–10% of severe injuries to the cord or cauda. The results of DREZ lesions in the treatment of such pain vary markedly depending on the locus and the type of the pain [Bullitt and Friedman, 1987]. One group of patients have pain in the segmental boundary zone or 'end zone', beginning at the dermatomal level of the cord injury and extending a variable distance caudally. This tends to be of two types: (1) paroxysms of one to several minutes of a pain often cramping in character, and (2) a constant aching and burning pain. In this category they have 31 patients of whom 80% had good or fair relief by their stringent criteria. Another group of patients have diffuse pain which often involves the entire body and limbs below the level of the cord lesion. This tends to be worst in the saddle region and in some patients is confined solely to the sacral segments. Their 25 patients in this group had good or fair relief in only 32%. They found that electrical signals recorded from the posterior columns do not become normal until circa two to three segments above the level of the obvious injury. Consequently, they usually made their DREZ lesions from a few segments above to a few segments below this level. They extended the DREZ lesions down through the sacral dermatomes in a number of patients in whom diffuse or sacral pain was present, improving the pain in only one of these patients. Most of the patients have bilateral leg pain; however, a subgroup of 10 with only unilateral pain did much better — 9 had good relief. Another favorable group were those who proved to have nerve root avulsions at operative exposure. When the pain was worsened by distension of bowel or bladder it was also likely to be improved by the operation. Three patients had a complication of new postoperative weakness and 3 more had other neurologic deficits postoperatively, but none had further loss of any useful function. Only 2 patients developed new paresthesias which were referred above or below the level of the old pain, somewhat analogous to the situation which occurs rarely after posterior rhizotomy.

An intramedullary cyst was diagnosed by a combination of myelogram, CT and MR scanning plus ultrasound at operation in 18 cases. There were 2 independent cysts in 7 of these patients, one above and the other below the transverse lesion. It did not suffice merely to drain the cyst, but in the 18 in whom this was combined with DREZ lesions 12 good and 2 fair results were achieved.

Wiegand and Winkelmüller [1985] have carried out this operation in 20 patients who have been followed for 5–34 months. The excellent result of 9 maintaining 100% relief and one with 80% relief was achieved. As occurred with the Duke group, at follow-up of these patients 10 had maintained their early postoperative relief. Actually one moved from 80 to 100% relief. A new paresis developed in only one of the 20. Powers et al. [1984] made lesser lesions with their laser in another series of 7 cases. These were followed for 5–19 months and 'end zone' pain was relieved at a level of 80–100% in 6 of them. In 2 patients with 90–100% relief of this pain, however, their low back and coccygeal pain were not helped at all, again confirming the experience at Duke with respect to this type of pain. Samii and Moringlane [1984] secured 70–100% relief in 2 of 5 patients. Richter and Seitz [1984], Thomas and Jones [1984], and Dieckmann and Veras [1984] all achieved no benefit in any of 5 patients in toto. None of them used the procedure further in this group of patients.

Inasmuch as we have used a slight variation in technique, we shall describe in some detail our results in one case with a traumatic total transverse lesion at T5. His pain was both of upper thoracic 'end zone' location as well as coccygeal and in one foot. Since these patients probably all have a more extensive lesion than one in the dorsal root entry zone and superficial layers in the posterior horn it has seemed rational to us to make a more extensive lesion into the deeper lying nociceptive neurons in the entire dorsal horn and on down into lamina X around the central canal. We have thought that this would be unlikely to increase the serious deficit these patients already have. This we describe as a posterior poliotomy rather than a DREZ lesion. The improved apparatus of Nashold was used to make 48 lesions, half on each side, each at 85 °C for 15 s. They extended for 40 mm from the lower T3 through T5 levels down into abnormal cord. A striking difference in the electrical parameters required was noted. The voltage varied from site to site from 12 to 20 V and the milliamperage from 20 to 50 to maintain 85 °C. Although the patient had complete relief for only 3 months, he said his worst pains were two thirds as bad as those preoperatively by 13 months later and an average of 40% of the original severity. Although this discouraging percentage of pain persists he did stop all of his preoperative narcotics and alcohol. He also says his 'personality is now 10 times better'.

No new neurological deficits appeared despite the higher lesions in the presumed normal cord.

Post-Herpetic Neuralgia

Once such pain becomes well established for a year or more after the acute attack, we find that it is likely to persist indefinitely. The Duke series numbers 32 spinal cases of whom only 2 were less than 60 years old, with some over 80. Postoperative follow-up extends from 6 months to 6 years. Early relief was the happy result in 90% but unlike most of the other categories of pain treated by this operation, recurrence took place in these by 6 months in 50% of them with a present recurrence rate of 66%. Only 3 remain relieved at 25, 36 and 48 months and only 25% continue with excellent pain relief. A new type of pain appeared in 10 of the 24 recurrences; this was not as severe and rated as 20–60% of the original pain. It has been called aching in 6, indescribable in 3 and cold in one. It limited the activity in all 10 patients and they required analgesics. Fortunately the original hyperpathia usually does not reappear. New neurological deficits have been more common in this older age group; one fourth must walk with a cane and 44% have mild unsteadiness along with increased deep tendon reflexes. The surgical lesion failed to denervate a 1.5-cm strip along one margin of the painful area in 3 patients. Consequently the DREZ lesions are now made from one half a spinal segment above to one half below the area of pain — an extension of the original procedure. About 25 lesions have been made at each spinal segment. The only other surgeon to do the DREZ operation for spinal post-herpetic neuralgia, Thomas, records a failure.

Pain in Amputation Stump and/or Phantom Limb

Saris et al. [1985] have noted a difference in the results correlated with the site of the pain in the 22 patients in this category operated on at Duke. He used a less rigorous appraisal system than was used for the other Duke patients, giving a rating of good if there was an overall improvement in the pain as graded by the patient of 3 points on a scale of 1–10. If the pain was confined to the phantom, 'good' improvement of 3 points or more occurred in 6 of 9 patients, whereas in the 7 whose pain was in both stump and phantom there were only 2 'good' results. No good result occurred in those with pain only in the stump. No other report appraises outcomes according to site of pain. The best group were the 6 patients in whom a traumatic amputation was associated with root avulsion, 5 having achieved good results. There are five other publications totalling 17 patients of whom 6 were described as totally relieved and 2 as having greater than 50% relief [Samii and Moringlane, 1984; Powers et al., 1984; Thomas and Jones, 1984; Wiegand and Winkelmüller, 1985; Dieckmann and Veras, 1984]. Although all 5 of Wiegand's lower limb amputees lost any original DREZ relief, full relief persisted in 2 of Power's 3 amputees for over a year, the amputation being below the knee in all 3. In the Duke series the results of lower versus upper limb amputation were about the same. New persistent dysesthesia occurred in 2 of Power's cases. In one the operation was for amputation stump and phantom pain and in the other for dysesthesias after posterior rhizotomy.

Lumbar Arachnoiditis and Failed Back Operations

Powers et al. [1984] and Powers [1987] have given a thorough trial with DREZ lesions in the hope of help in this vexing group of patients. Unfortunately, they record an uninterrupted succession of early or late failures in 20 cases. In 2 of these cases 2 operations were done. Wiegand and Winkelmüller [1985] and Dieckmann and Veras [1984] each describe one case of arachnoiditis with no relief.

Autopsies

Postmortem studies of the RF cord lesions in man have been carried out in 3 cases. In that of Barcia Salorio et al. [1985] the lesions were made without temperature control at 40 mA for 15 s; they extended deeply into Rexed's lamina IV as well as somewhat in the column of Burdach medially and the lateral corticospinal tract laterally. The lesions made by Richter and Schachenmayr [1984] were at 45–50 mA for 5–10 s. The histologic sections following death on the 5th postoperative day revealed that almost the entire posterior horn was replaced by a pseudocyst which was described by the pathologist as due to the original root avulsion. The illustrations reveal a complete absence of any tissue for virtually the entire extent of the posterior horn — a most unlikely result of the DREZ lesion only 5 days earlier (fig. 7/5). Clearly in this patient no irritative process in the posterior horn was causing the pain. This important case strongly suggests that we should be looking elsewhere as well in the CNS for the pathophysiologic process in the disorder. The adjoining posterior and posterolateral white columns were but little involved. In the third case from Duke the lesions were made with the new electrode with thermocouple temperature control at the appropriate 75–

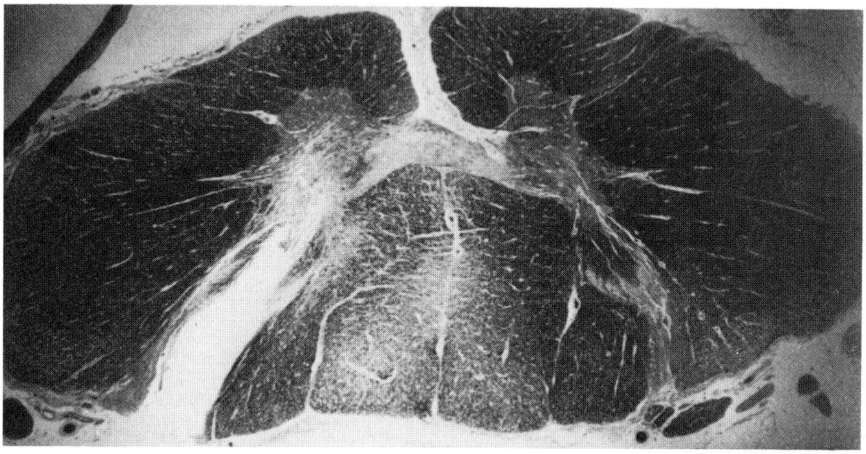

Fig. 7/5. Section through the 8th cervical segment of the spinal cord at the level of the previous attachment of the posterior root. There is a sharply bordered tissue defect reaching from the torn-out entry of the left dorsal root deep into the gray matter of the posterior horn. Beneath the destroyed dorsolateral fascicle (Lissauer's tract), the loss of gray matter comprises the following posterior horn nuclei: nucleus posteromarginalis, substantia gelatinosa, nucleus centrodorsalis, parts of the nucleus reticularis, and parts of Clark's column. Paraffin section, Luxol-Nissl stain. × 16. From Richter and Schachenmayr [1984].

80 °C for 15 s. The patient died on the 28th postoperative day. There had been 48 lesions on one side and 35 on the other in the lumbar cord. These extended halfway into lamina VI with minimal impingement on the white matter, indicating that the current improved technique is indeed accomplishing its objective. The groups of Levy et al. [1983], Campbell and Miles [1984], Powers et al. [1984], Powers [1987], Nashold et al. [1985] are all exploring the evoked potential techniques during operation as an aid to monitoring of lesion size.

Conclusions

The present technique of Nashold and colleagues is of proven efficacy with a low rate of complications for pain related to avulsion of sensory rootlets from the cord, even though the site of generation of the abnormal neural impulses for pain is not entirely clear. For treatment of the neurogenic pains of traumatic paraplegia the rostral 'boundary or end zone' pains are more likely to be relieved than the more diffuse, more caudal pains. However, the low rate of neural complications makes such cases suitable for critical evaluation of the operation. For other types of pain the use of the operation is in the exploratory phase with the exception of the pains related to lumbar arachnoiditis and other causes of failure of lumbosacral surgery for pain. In this group the procedure appears proven to be of no value.

Chapter 8. Section of Lissauer's Tract

Hyndman [1942] confirmed earlier observations in his series of 100 cases after anterolateral cordotomy that the level of skin analgesia and thermanesthesia was nearly always four or five segments lower than that which would correspond to the level of the cord section. Since in a complete transverse section of the cord the level of skin anesthesia more nearly corresponds to the level at which the cord is severed, and since pain and temperature fibers may course upward in Lissauer's tract for a distance of four or five segments before crossing over, he reasoned that this may account for the zone which fails to be made analgesic and thermanesthetic after cordotomy. He therefore added to an anterolateral cordotomy on one side a section of Lissauer's tract on the other side at the same level (fig. 8/1).

On the evidence of 5 cases he found that such a section about 2 mm wide and 1.5–2 mm deep, directly into the line of entry of the posterior rootlets, would bring up the level of analgesia and thermanesthesia to the level of the cordotomy incision. He also noted that sensory modalities other than pain are impaired and assumed that some of this loss might be a result of carrying the incision into the posterior column. Further, he noted that the section did not appear to be of great value in the cervical region.

From the time of the original description of the so-called posterolateral tract of Lissauer in 1885, there has been considerable controversy concerning the origin of fibers which make up this neural pathway. On the one side there have been investigators who considered that these fibers arose exclusively in the posterior root ganglia [Ranson, 1913], while on the other side there were anatomists who believed that the fibers were endogenous in origin, i.e. arising exclusively from nerve cells in the tip of the posterior horn [Earle, 1952; Nathan and Smith, 1959]. Lissauer's tract would then be considered as a portion of the propriospinal system. It is now clear that this tract contains both primary afferents [LaMotte, 1977] of which many are small myelinated and unmyelinated axons [Chung et al., 1979] and axons of propriospinal neurons.

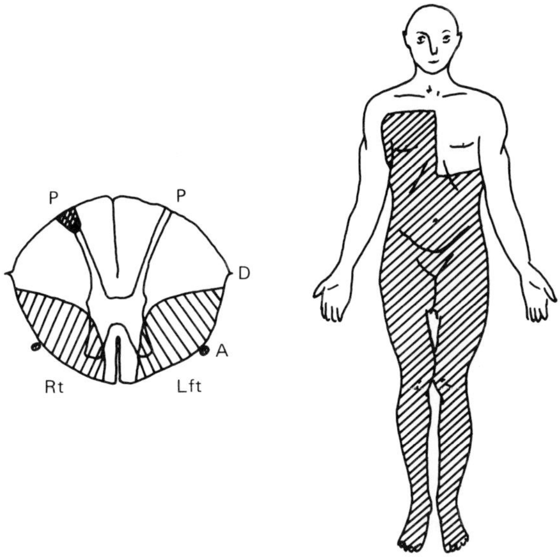

Fig. 8/1. Diagram illustrating sensory losses with lesions of the spinal cord as shown at the left. In the hatched zone the sensibilities were as follows: Touch, normal except for about a 25% reduction in the upper 5 dermatomes on the right; temperature discrimination, 0; pain, 0. The diagram on the left represents the sections made in the cord at D1. D = Dentate ligament; A = anterior root line; P = posterior root line. At P on the right is shown the section through Lissauer's tract. From Hyndman [1942].

Lesions of the medial portion of Lissauer's tract in the macaque, which are followed by some atrophy of the medial portion of the substantia gelatinosa at the level of the incision, cause a contraction of the isolated dermatome. This is related to the fact that the remaining lateral part of Lissauer's tract has a suppressor effect from neighboring segments, whereas the medial portion has a facilitatory effect. Therefore, section of the medial portion results in a predominance of the suppressor effect [Denny-Brown et al., 1973].

There is not much human material available to judge the importance of Lissauer's tract for dispersion of nociceptive inputs over several segments. Today, this tract is destroyed together with the anterolateral part of the dorsal root when a selective posterior root section is performed, and with the dorsal horn when a DREZ operation is done. From the few cases he reported, Hyndman [1942] concluded that a section of Lissauer's tract eliminates pain sensibility in three or four adjacent lower segments. As has been pointed out by Vierck et al. [1986], indirect evidence of rostral excitatory influences on pain via Lissauer's tract can be found in the appearance of pain from a stimulus to an analgesic zone caudal to a cordotomy referred to levels rostral to the anterolateral cordotomy cut. Repetitive, vigorous stimulation with a hot object or pin within the analgesic area can be perceived as touch along with slowly incrementing, burning pain localized above the analgesic level [Nathan, 1956; Nathan and Smith, 1979]. This rostral referral is rare and occurs only locally near the lesion for most forms of pain.

Conclusions

Incisions specifically to destroy Lissauer's tract are not used currently in neurosurgery although the incidental division of fibers entering this tract from the posterior root in the selective posterior rhizotomy of Sindou probably plays a role in the relief afforded by that procedure.

Chapter 9. Open Anterolateral Cordotomy

Historical Note

In 1911, Martin, at the suggestion of Spiller, performed the operation of anterolateral tractotomy for pain, after Spiller correlated clinical with pathological evidence that lesions of the anterior quadrant of the spinal cord were associated with contralateral loss of pain and temperature sensation [Spiller and Martin, 1912]. Foerster [1913] had been thinking along the same lines and reported the same operation the following year. From then until the present time, open anterolateral cordotomy has been performed and its results reported by many surgeons. While the operation has remained in essence the same as that introduced by Spiller and Martin some 76 years ago, much effort has been devoted to produce lesions in the anterolateral quadrant of the cord with minimal morbidity and maximal pain relief. A key role in this effort has been the correlation of anatomically verified lesions at autopsy with the results of detailed clinical observation.

Among the many publications devoted to this effort, special interest attaches to those of Foerster and Gagel [1932], Hyndman and Van Epps [1939], Walker [1940], Hyndman and Wolkin [1943], French and Peyton [1948], Kahn and Peet [1948], White et al. [1950, 1956], Nathan and Smith [1951, 1953, 1958, 1966, 1979], Nathan [1952, 1963a, b], Bowsher [1957], Grant and Wood [1958], Schwartz [1960], Mehler [1962], Hitchcock and Leece [1967], White and Sweet [1969], Cowie and Hitchcock [1982] and Vierck et al. [1986].

General Anatomical and Physiological Considerations

In human studies, the term 'spinothalamic tract' has often been used very loosely and refers to any ascending fibers in the anterolateral part of the cord which have to do with the ability to feel pain and temperature [Nathan and Smith, 1966]. Many of these fibers make synaptic connections at nuclei of the reticular substance in cord or brain stem; some are spinotectal, and only a small part in man are true spinothalamic fibers reaching the thalamus before undergoing synapse.

To characterize these different ascending systems, the terms paleo- and neospinothalamic tracts are often used. These terms were coined by Bishop [1959] to replace older terms such as 'medial spinoreticulothalamic system' and 'classical spinothalamic tract'. These terms stressed the findings of comparative anatomy in which analogies were shown between different species with respect to the relationship of premammalian spinothalamic projections and the fine fibers coursing medially as spinoreticulothalamic systems projecting to the mammalian 'paleothalamic' region. A predominance of the spinoreticulothalamic system was observed in lower 'nonprimates', e.g. in the opossum and the rat, in contrast to the paucity of the coarser, classical spinothalamic fibers projecting to the neothalamic ventral nuclei [Mehler, 1969]. These terms are still used in the clinical literature and the term spinoreticular system has been added [see reviews by Bowsher, 1957; Mehler, 1962; Hassler, 1972; Kerr, 1975a; Vierck et al., 1986].

The neo- and the paleospinothalamic tracts are often viewed as two parts of the lateral spinothalamic tract. The paleospinothalamic tract does not have a precise somatotopic arrangement. It ascends from dorsal horn cells together with the neospinothalamic tract to the level of the midbrain and from there on diverges medially to project to periaqueductal gray and the intralaminar nuclei and centrum medianum of the thalamus, although this last point is not accepted by some [Mehler, 1962, 1969]. The neospinothalamic tract is organized somatotopically; at the level of the upper midbrain it diverges laterally to enter the thalamic specific sensory relay nuclei and the PO region (posterior gray nuclei). Spinoreticular tracts follow a course deep to that of the spinothalamic tract and synapse in various brain stem nuclei; ascending connections from these nuclei reach periaqueductal gray and thalamic periventricular and intralaminar nuclei.

In the clinical literature concepts of the 'pain tract' range from oversimplifications, such as identifying the spinothalamic fibers as the principal pathway, to the hypothesis of Noordenbos [1959] of a 'Multisynaptic Afferent System' in which he proposes an imbalance between slow and fast conducting fibers in neuronal networks. Neuroanatomists have been struggling for years to identify the central 'pain pathway' in man. One account reports a study of 4 cases in which the diencephalon and brain stem were

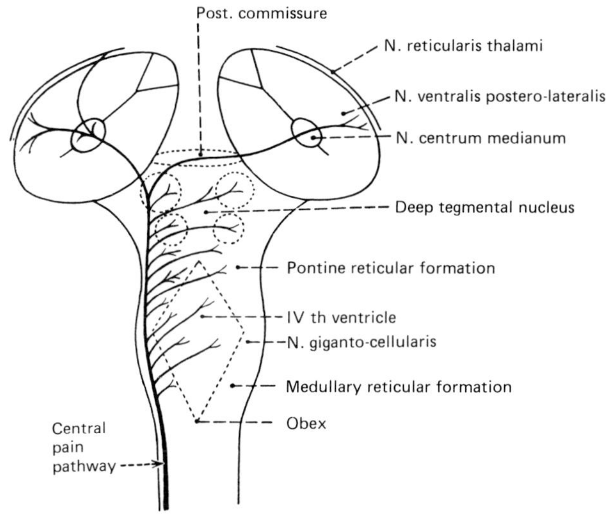

Fig. 9/1. Diagramatic representation of the termination of the central pain pathway, as revealed by silver impregnation techniques in human material following anterolateral cordotomy or medullary tractotomy. From Bowsher [1957].

examined for axonal degeneration following successful anterolateral cordotomy for the relief of pain. The following conclusions were reached: (1) Terminal degeneration was found in the specific sensory ventroposterolateral nucleus of the thalamus of both sides, in the ipsilateral centre médian, and possibly in the anterior part of the ipsilateral thalamic reticular nucleus; in the nuclei of all four quadrigeminal bodies and ipsilaterally in the lateral reticular nucleus of the medulla oblongata. Massive bilateral degeneration was found at the cells of the medial reticular formation of the medulla, and to a lesser extent in these regions of the pons and mesencephalon (fig. 9/1). (2) It was suggested that the direct spinothalamic system is responsible for the type of pain that is immediately felt, sharply localized, and which lasts for only as long as the provoking stimulus is applied, while the spinoreticulothalamic system is responsible for diffuse, poorly localized pain or discomfort with an appreciably slower conduction time to consciousness, and which persists after the withdrawal of the initiating stimulus. (3) It was shown that the two types of pain fibers run together below the level of the inferior olive, and meet again in the centrum medianum thalami [Bowsher, 1957]. As noted earlier, this last point is disputed [Mehler, 1969].

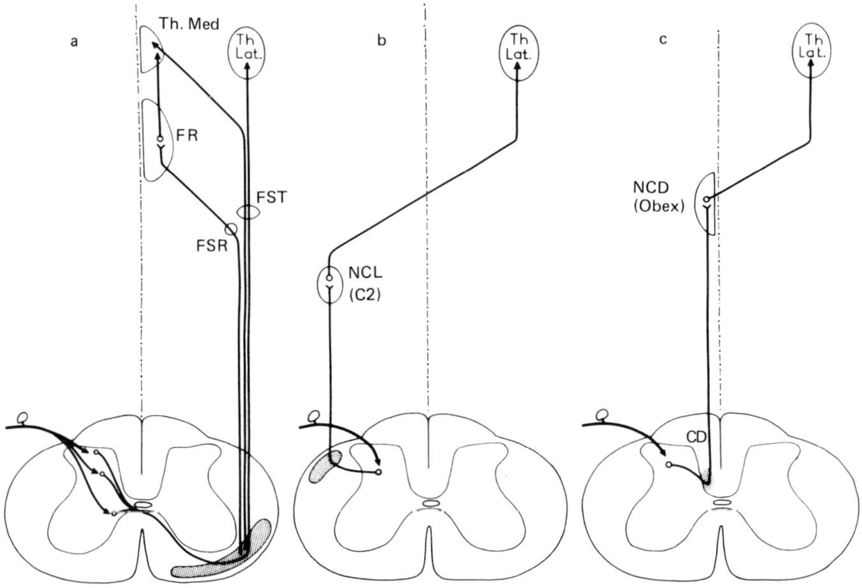

Fig. 9/2. Schematic representation of the principal ascending pathways transmitting nociceptive information. *a* FSR = spinoreticular tract; FST = spinothalamic tract running through the anterolateral quadrant of the spinal cord; FR = reticular formation; Th Med = medial thalamus; Th Lat = lateral thalamus comprising also the nuclei of the PO area. *b* Spinocervicothalamic tract coursing through the dorsolateral spinal cord and making relay in the n. cervicalis lateralis (NCL). *c* Post-synaptic fibers in the dorsal column (CD) projecting towards the dorsal column nuclei (NCD). It is not certain whether the neurons receiving input from the post synaptic fibers project to the thalamus. From Besson et al. [1982].

Neuroanatomical and physiological aspects of nociceptive pathways have been extensively studied in animals and have been the object of recent reviews [Besson et al., 1982; Besson and Chaouch, 1987; Perl, 1984; Willis, 1985; Yaksh, 1986]. Figure 9/2 is a schematic representation of principal ascending pathways which have been identified in rat, cat and monkey as being implicated in nociception. The neurons of origin and the stimuli that activate them, the target nuclei of these tracts and the location of these tracts in the spinal cord, are summarized in table 9/I and table 9/II. Recently, a spinothalamic tract has been described in the cat that courses in the dorsolateral funiculus of the spinal cord, lying thus outside the classical course of the spinothalamic tract. This originates almost exclusively from spinal lamina I neurons [Jones et al., 1985].

Table 9/I. Ascending tracts in spinal cord implicated in nociception

Tract	Location in the spinal cord	Neurons of origin	Input	Destination
Spinothalamic tract	crossed through ventral white commissure to anterolateral quadrant	dorsal horn — lamina I + V intermediate region ventral horn	low threshold wide dynamic range high threshold deep	VPL Pom intralaminar n. n. submedius
Spinoreticular	crossed and uncrossed to anterolateral quadrant	VII + VIII dorsal horn, including I	often nociceptive input	n. in pontomedullary reticular formation see table 9/II
Spinomesencephalic	crossed to anterolateral quadrant	I + V	often nociceptive input	midbrain see table 9/II
Dorsal column postsynaptic elements	uncrossed in dorsal column and dorsal lateral funiculus	III + IV	wide dynamic range	rostral and ventral parts of n. gracilis and n. cuneatus
			proprioception for hindlimb	n. Z.
Spinocervical	uncrossed in dorsal lateral fasciculus	III + IV (+ V)	low threshold hair follicle receptors wide dynamic range	lateral cervical n.

Table 9/II. Nuclei of termination of spinoreticular and spinomesencephalic tracts. From Willis [1985]

Nuclei of termination of spinoreticular tract	Nuclei of termination of spinomesencephalic tract
N. retroambiguous	deep layers of colliculus superior
N. supraspinalis	n. intercollicularis
N. medullae oblongatae centralis (dorsal and ventral parts)	lateral periaqueductal gray
	n. cuneiformis
N. reticularis lateralis	n. of Darkschewitz
N. gigantocellularis	n. of Edinger-Westphal
N. interfascicularis hypoglossi	
N. of Roller	
N. olivaris inferior	
N. paragigantocellularis lateralis and dorsalis	
N. pontis centralis caudalis and oralis	
Subcoerulcus complcx	

Besides these principal ascending pathways which have been implicated in nociception, the possibility that propriospinal systems might play a role in transmission of nociceptive impulses should not be overlooked (fig. 9/3).

This notion is supported by experiments involving lateral hemisections of both the left and right halves of the spinal cord that are spaced more than several segments apart. In such animals thresholds for aversive reactions were elevated but the responses for suprathreshold noxious stimuli were not absent [Basbaum, 1973]. This subject will be discussed again in chapters 11.A and 11.B.

Characteristics of Ascending Pathways for Pain in the Human Anterolateral and Ventral Columns

In figure 9/4 are represented diagramatically lesions that were insufficient to cause adequate analgesia contralaterally below the cord lesions and incisions that caused dense analgesia in a limited region of the body. These diagrams of the data from 14 patients were established from a case material of 80 patients with cancer who had postmortem examinations with histological studies of the spinal cord and who survived more than a month and less than 2 years after cordotomy [Nathan and Smith, 1979].

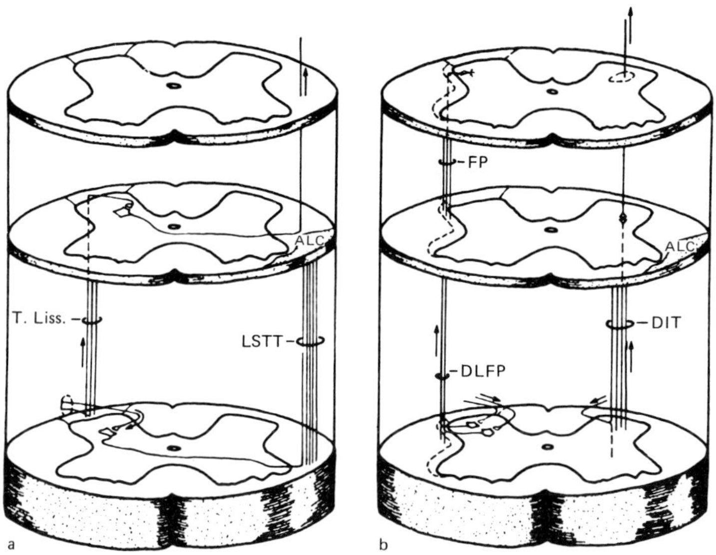

Fig. 9/3. Some potential supplementary pathways for relay of nociceptive input for short distances in the spinal cord. In *a*, according to classical views, primary afferents in the tract of Lissauer would account for 1–2 segments of conduction. In *b*, 2 alternative possibilities are indicated. On the left, secondary relays in the dorsal horn (lamina I or IV) which enter the dorsolateral fasciculus proprius (DLFP); on the right, the longitudinal system of the dorsal horn or dorsal intracornual tract (DIT) composed of primary afferents and secondary relays. From Kerr [1975a].

From this type of evidence, in which a correlation has been established between sensory effects, the location of the spinal lesion and resulting ascending axonal degeneration, different diagrams of the anatomy of the anterolateral and ventral white columns have been proposed.

There is indeed a vast but often controversial clinical literature on the functional anatomy of the anterior quadrant of the spinal cord, but from the point of view of applied anatomy, the important aspect for the operating surgeon, the features described below are particularly relevant.

Somatotopy

The most cranial fibers lie deepest and most anteriorly and the most caudal fibers most posterolaterally and near the surface, but there is overlap between the fibers of the different body segments. In fact reversal of the usual

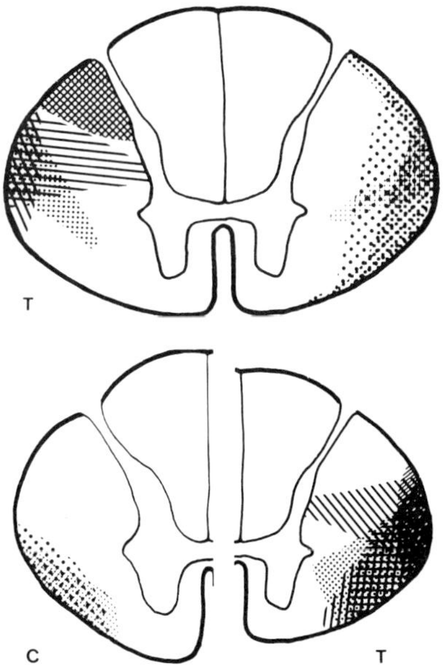

Fig. 9/4. Upper: A diagram of cordotomy lesions that were insufficient to cause adequate or dense sensory loss contralaterally below the lesion. Lower: A diagram of cordotomy incisions that caused dense analgesia in a limited region of the body. Left, cervical cord; right, thoracic cord. Every case of cordotomy in both illustrations has the lesion illustrated by a different form of cross-hatching. From Nathan and Smith [1979].

disposition with a far ventral locus for the sacral dermatomes has been described by Schwartz [1960] in 3 cases and by Voris [1951] in one. The posterior limit of the spinothalamic tract is slightly posterior to the postero-lateral angle of the ventral horn [Nathan and Smith, 1966]. Some authors have favored the concept of an 'onion skin' lamination, with thoracic and cervical fibers lying most medially since they suggest that only incisions reaching a depth of more than 5 mm are effective, while others regard the lamination of the spinothalamic fibers as having a more postero-anterior distribution, and that consequently a superficial incision should be capable of producing high levels of analgesia as readily as a deep incision [Hitchcock, 1971]. Besides a somatotopographical pattern for the different body parts, a modality topography is often described: impulses for 'pain' from the superficial part of the body are transmitted by fibers close to the surface while at progressively deeper levels are, respectively, the fibers transmitting impulses for the senses of temperature, deep pain and visceral pain. Consequently, many authors recommend transection of virtually the whole anterior quadrant of the cord, including the medial and anterior portion of the anterior quadrant [Poletti, 1982].

Cross-Over

Classical teaching is that the axons of the spinothalamic neurons cross the midline at the levels of the anterior commissure, and according to Foerster and Gagel [1932] the cross-over is prompt with analgesia extending to within one or two segments of the level of the incision in the cord. However, as noted by Sweet and Poletti [1984a] the cross-over may be delayed for many segments. For this reason, several authors prefer the high cervical level for all unilateral incisions, because complete cross-over is more likely to have occurred. According to Poletti [1982] fibers arising in the dorsal horn may at times cross through the anterior commissure almost immediately from which they then move laterally while ascending five to eight more segments to take up their final lateral position to move rostrally to the brain. The only evidence for this is that the more medial the incision the higher the analgesic level tends to be. Therefore, a lesion in the lateral anterior quadrant, even deep, may produce analgesia extending rostrally only eight or more segments below the lesion. In contrast, a lesion of the anterior quadrant extending to the midline may in some individuals produce analgesia to within one segment of the lesion. Therefore, Poletti [1982] recommends, especially in cervical cordotomies where the primary goal is a high permanent level of analgesia, to extend the lesion at least 1–2 mm medial to the most medial part of the ventral root, i.e. 1–2.5 mm from the anterior spinal artery. Extreme instances of anatomical variability are represented by those rare cases in whom upper thoracic cordotomies were followed by ipsilateral loss of pain and temperature sensation [French and Peyton, 1948; Voris, 1951; Brenner and Pendl, 1966]. Other gross anatomical variations have been reported by Moossy and Rosomoff [cited by Sweet, 1976a] in 5 postmortem studies on patients after C1–2 percutaneous cordotomies. All 5 had lesions confined to virtually total destruction of the posterolateral column of white matter. This in 3 had produced an analgesic level to pin with corresponding relief of pain and no hemiparesis. The other 2 had no hemiparesis, but also no pain relief.

Ventral Spinothalamic Tract and Sensory Modality

In the clinical literature the existence of a ventral spinothalamic tract is generally accepted and it is thought that this pathway mediates touch and light pressure, as distinct from the lateral spinothalamic tract, which is concerned with the relay of information on pain and temperature, and some light touch. From the anatomical point of view Kerr [1975b] has shown in the monkey that the ventral spinothalamic tract is indeed an entity independent of the lateral spinothalamic tract; its fibers are widely distributed in the ventral funiculus and it establishes connections in the brain stem and the thalamus which are similar but not identical to those of the lateral tract.

From physiological evidence in animals it seems difficult to maintain a separation in the spinothalamic tract between a lateral component, which would be responsible for pain and thermal sensitivity, and a ventral component, participating in tactile sensibility, since there is a total overlapping of axons of the spinothalamic tract which are activated by different cutaneous stimulations, mechanical and thermal, and with low or high thresholds [Besson et al., 1982].

Sensory Effects of Anterolateral Cordotomy

Superficial Sensations

Pain evoked by vigorous mechanical stimulation such as that with a pin is no longer felt contralaterally after anterolateral cordotomy; however, repeated pinprick may provoke pain [Nathan and Smith, 1979]. The sensation of sharpness is lost, whether this sharpness is felt as painful or not [White and Sweet, 1969]. There is a high correlation between the relief of clinical pain when the upper level of pinprick loss is higher than the highest level at which the clinical pain is felt. Warmth and cold are reported as lost contralaterally after cordotomy [Hyndman and Wolkin, 1943; Nathan and Smith, 1966; White and Sweet, 1969] and ice-cold water and noxious heat are not perceived as painful [Hyndman, 1942; Hyndman and Wolkin, 1943]. There are cases in which innocuous and noxious thermal sensations remain intact in the area hypalgesic to pinprick suggesting a more central location for the temperature signaling fibers [Stookey, 1929; Taren et al., 1969]. However, the reverse findings were recorded by White et al. [1950] who, upon late testing in 20 patients, found complete thermanesthesia persisting in 16 whereas complete analgesia persisted in 13.

Itch sensation is almost always lost in the area which becomes analgesic following an anterolateral cordotomy. Indeed intolerable itching and destructive scratching are nearly always eliminated by the analgesia of an effective cordotomy [White and Sweet, 1969, pp. 688–689]. Tickle as tested by light stroking remains intact [Hyndman and Wolkin, 1943; White and Sweet, 1969, p. 688].

In early descriptions Head and Thompson [1906] reported that impulses giving rise to light touch were transmitted via fibers situated in the contralateral anterolateral quadrant of the spinal cord, and in classical textbooks a ventral spinal pathway subserving touch is often described, but we find no report of patients with a selective section of the ventral columns who were tested for tactile thresholds. However, Wall and Noordenbos [1977] have described a case with nearly total transection of the spinal cord sparing only one anterolateral quadrant in whom thresholds for touch were slightly elevated contralaterally. When touch was tested in a quantifiable manner with von Frey hairs, White et al. [1950] reported that the threshold was usually increased on glabrous skin, but remained intact on hairy skin. This made White and Sweet [1969] tell their patients that after anterolateral cordotomy, 'they will be able to detect a mosquito when he alights, although they will not be able to feel him bite nor be annoyed by the subsequent itch'.

Deep Somatic Sensations

Deep somatic pain, as estimated by applying weight to compress tissue over bone, squeezing the Achilles tendon, and pressure measurements, is reduced by anterolateral cordotomy [White and Sweet, 1969] and is the objective test which correlates best with the clinical results [Nathan and Smith, 1979].

Conflicting data have been presented for the localization of fibers transmitting deep somatic pain. Some evidence points to a localization dorsolaterally in the anterior quadrant [Kahn and Rand, 1952], other evidence to a localization medial to the fibers subserving superficial pain [Taren et al., 1969]. Position sense remains intact after anterolateral cordotomy [White and Sweet, 1969]. However, it was preserved in the case of Wall and Noordenbos with an intact cord only at one anterior quadrant, not consonant with the concept that the posterior columns are solely responsible for this function [Wall and Noordenbos, 1977].

Visceral Pain

There are numerous reports of relief of clinical pain of visceral origin by anterolateral cordotomy. In patients in whom visceral sensation has been tested objectively by distension of the ureter or intestinal loops [Nathan and Smith, 1953; White and Sweet, 1969], greatly elevated thresholds have been found after anterolateral cordotomy. According to many surgeons, cordotomies for the control of visceral pain should extend medial to the gray matter [Hyndman and Wolkin, 1943; Taren et al., 1969] and some stress the need for bilateral sections [Taren et al., 1969] but this is denied by others [White and Sweet, 1969] when the pain is referred entirely to one side.

Levels of Pain Relief Following Anterolateral Cordotomy

The clinical literature reports that when the anterolateral column (extending from the dentate ligament to well medial to the ventral roots) is completely cut, pain sensitivity is diminished within two or three levels below the cordotomy [Hyndman and Van Epps, 1939; Kahn and Rand, 1952; White et al., 1956] but as we have noted when discussing the cross-over of spinothalamic fibers, the results may be extremely variable. Comparisons of upper levels for different noxious stimuli show that the rostral level for thermanesthesia can be slightly higher than the level for pinprick analgesia [Taren and Kahn, 1966; White and Sweet, 1969]. More importantly the loss of deep pain may be three or four segments lower than the loss of light cutaneous pinprick [Nathan and Smith, 1979]. These workers find that the relief of cancer pain correlates best with loss of deep pain as determined by the pressure algometer.

Other Tracts of Importance in Cordotomy

The Descending Respiratory Pathway

Knowledge of the location of the descending respiratory pathway is important, not only theoretically but also from a practical point of view for those practicing anterolateral cordotomy. Evidence from animal work has shown that the descending fibers run in the anterior and/or the lateral column of the cord but it was Nathan [1963b] who first worked out the location of the descending respiratory pathway in man. The material of his study consisted of 13 cases in all of whom the operation of cervical anterolateral cordotomy was performed for cancer pain. He showed that fibers subserving respiratory movements do not descend via the corticospinal tract, but that a lesion of the most anterior part of the lateral column of the three cervical segments of the cord causes paralysis or a very great reduction in the ipsilateral respiratory movements. He found these descending respiratory fibers forming either a part of the reticulospinal tract or running with the

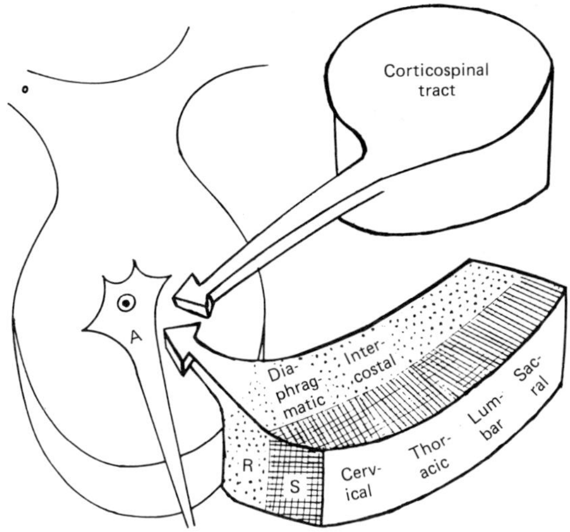

Fig. 9/5. Diagram of the relationship between the spinothalamic (S) and reticulospinal (R) tracts showing the voluntary and involuntary influences on a respiratory neuron (anterior horn cell, A). The diaphragmatic and intercostal components of the reticulospinal system lie adjacent to the cervical and thoracic fibers in the spinothalamic tract. From Hitchcock and Leece [1967].

olivospinal tract. According to Hitchcock and Leece [1967] the more posterior portion of the respiratory tract appears to be closely associated with posterior portions of the spinothalamic pathways; i.e. the area of the respiratory tract having maximal effect on respiration is adjacent to the cervical segments of the spinothalamic tract (fig. 9/5, 9/6). They suggest that the anterior portion of the respiratory tract is largely related to the diaphragmatic function whereas the posterior portion of this tract supplies the rest of the respiratory musculature, namely the intercostal muscles and the abdominal and lumbar musculature used in respiration. They suggest further that the voluntary control is presumably through the corticospinal tract. This concept of voluntary and automatic respiration regulated by two distinct pathways is a possible explanation for the fact that patients have died in their sleep following high cervical cordotomy because of destruction of the system for automatic respiration.

Pathway for Micturition and Defecation

In a series of papers Nathan and Smith [1951, 1953, 1958] have worked out the location of the pathways in human spinal cord implicated in voiding

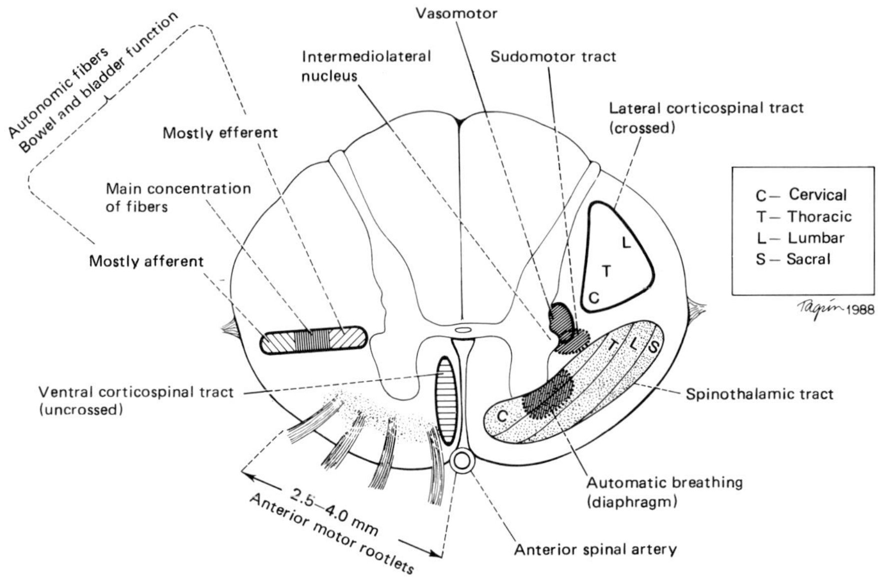

Fig. 9/6. Diagram of spinal cord at circa T2–T3 level to show structures affected by cordotomy of anterior quadrant. Note that although dentate ligament is shown arising from equator of cord that it may arise further posteriorly, leading to inadvertent incision into lateral corticospinal tract if used as an infallible landmark. The ventral rootlets do not emerge from a single sulcus as do the posterior rootlets but are scattered over an extensive mediolateral area as indicated in the diagram. At any one cross-sectional level, however, there is only one emerging rootlet — not a whole row as presented in diagram. Locus of ventro-lateral reticulo-spinal tract for automatic breathing, from Hitchcock and Leece [1967]; locus of sympathetic preganglionic vasomotor and sudomotor centrifugal pathway, from Nathan and Smith [1987]; locus of centrifugal pathway for micturition, from Nathan and Smith [1958]; locus of centrifugal pathway for defecation and sensation from lower bowel, from Nathan and Smith [1953].

and defecation. These fibers are situated within a narrow band extending from the periphery to the lateral horn of the gray matter (fig. 9/6). The lateral part of this band is mainly afferent, and the more medial part mainly efferent. Bilateral cutting through the spinothalamic tract posteriorly to interrupt the fibers from sacral segments will necessarily involve a large proportion of the fibers subserving micturition and defecation, and lead to impairment of these functions, while a unilateral cordotomy itself causes at most only a temporary disturbance of them [Nathan, 1963a].

Descending Fibers to Sympathetic Neurons

A descending vasoconstrictor and sudomotor pathway for the head and neck and for oculosympathetic neurons has been identified in the cervical region of the human spinal cord. It lies close to the posterior angle of the anterior horn and runs entirely unilaterally [Nathan and Smith, 1986]. The pathways from the brain to the thoracic and lumbar autonomic centers have now been well worked out in man by Nathan and Smith [1987] in their recent careful study of 88 human anterolateral cordotomies and correlation with the previous literature. The location of the descending fibers for vasomotor control and for sweating are similarly placed and shown in figure 9/6.

Each descending pathway supplies both sides of the person so that a clear-cut deficit ensues only when both tracts are destroyed. The fibers for vasomotor control appear to leave the cord cranial to the T7 segment but the sudomotor fibers descend at least as far as L2.

Corticospinal Tract

In rare cases, the corticospinal tract descends uncrossed in the anterior medial part of the cord to cross finally near the segment of its termination on the lower motor neuron. Frequently the decussating pyramidal fibers may not be fully crossed and remain in the posterior aspect of the cord until they reach the caudal half of C2 [Yakovlev and Rakic, 1966]. As reported by Sweet [1976a], anatomical studies of Rakic and Yakovlev on 144 specimens of human fetal and neonatal cords and/or brain stems revealed that at the level of C1–C2 25% of the specimens showed bilateral or unilateral absence of the uncrossed ventral corticospinal tract. In 79% of the specimens the pyramidal tracts were 'patently unequal' on the two sides.

Technique

The technique of open anterolateral cordotomy has been described in numerous publications [Kahn and Peet, 1948; White et al., 1950; Grant and Wood, 1958; Schwartz, 1960; Brihaye et al., 1962; Cloward, 1964; White, 1966; White and Sweet, 1969; French, 1974; Tasker, 1977; Poletti, 1982].

Particular points of technique can be summarized as follows. In order to facilitate rotation of the cord over 45°, the dorsal roots are freed from the cord to their point of exit; if the possibility of rotation is limited, a dorsal root is cut. Too much traction on a dorsal root may be followed by girdle pain at that level postoperatively. If necessary the dentate ligament above and below the level of the planned incision is cut to facilitate rotation of the cord in order to identify the anterior median fissure containing the anterior spinal artery. A dental mirror can also help to identify this artery or its fissure and the medial limit of the ventral rootlets. For most surgeons, the goal is then to transect at the least vascular rostro-caudal level of the pia almost the entire anterior quadrant of the cord. The cut should extend from the equator of the cord medial to the most medial of the anterior rootlets as they emerge from the cord. It should be as close to the midline fissure as possible, avoiding injury to the anterior spinal artery. The origin of the dentate ligament from the cord is usually near enough to its equator so that this is a valid landmark for the dorsal extent of the main crossed tract for pain and temperature. Infrequently the origin of this ligament is well posterior to the usual site, a possibility which must be carefully checked by the surgeon lest he make a major cut in the lateral corticospinal tract.

Poletti's [1982] technique has increased both the safety and the reliability of transecting the entire quadrant. He incises the tough pia with a sharp blade, but then divides the nerve fibers with a metal instrument carrying a small round, electrically insulated shaft. At its tip is a tiny, smooth, uninsulated sphere which prevents the instrument from penetrating the medial pial envelope and damaging the anterior spinal artery. Electrical stimulation at 2 Hz activates any lateral or ventral corticospinal motor fibers encountered by the ball tip, thereby enabling the surgeon to extend his incision as far dorsally and medially as necessary and with impunity. Furthermore, the cord need be only minimally rotated.

In the upper thoracic region the cord diameter is about 10 mm and a depth of incision of approximately 5 mm is warranted. In the cervical region the diameter may be as large as 16 mm, allowing for a cord incision up to 8 mm deep. Since the diameter of the cord is variable in different individuals, it is a wise precaution to measure the cord's diameter at the level of the proposed incision. Some surgeons make use of wake-up anesthetics to test the levels of analgesia and motor strength as well as to stimulate within the cord for localizing purposes. When a bilateral cordotomy is indicated, several options are possible, depending on the area to be denervated. These include a high cervical and contralateral thoracic cordotomy, a percutaneous C1–2 cordotomy with a contralateral lower open cordotomy, etc. Most surgeons are reluctant to perform a bilateral high cervical cordotomy because of the major risk of complications, particularly sleep apnea.

Results

For decades, unilateral or bilateral cordotomy has been one of the most successful operations for pain control in the neurosurgical armamentarium. In many of the published series, it is difficult to evaluate fully the precise results of these cordotomies, but a few representative examples of big series allow one to trace general trends. Patients with cancer pain comprise by far the largest group and we shall discuss them first. According to the 1963 study of Nathan on the results of the procedure for cancer pain, roughly half of the 114 operations gave complete relief of pain; a quarter gave partial relief, and a quarter failed to give adequate relief [Nathan, 1963a]. White in 1966, when describing the effectiveness of high thoracic cordotomy in 271 cases of malignant disease, reported an initial success rate of 86%, dropping to 77% by the time the patients left the hospital. Similarly, Piscol [1975] in his review gives in cases of malignant processes a success rate from 72 to 88%. The series of Mansuy et al. [1976], based on 124 patients, quotes 60% good results in perineo-pelvic cancers when a bilateral low cervical cordotomy was performed. However, when such cancers presented with unilateral pain, relief occurred in only 36% because in 39% pain soon appeared on the other side. A 62% success rate was obtained after a unilateral C2 cordotomy in hemithoracic or cervicothoracic cancers such as those of the breast. Cowie and Hitchcock [1982], using a well-defined grading system, described their late as well as early results. In a series of 33 patients with pain of malignancy, they noted in 95% a satisfactory postoperative outcome which was well sustained for the first 3 months after operation, but they observed a gradual reduction in effectiveness over the ensuing 6 months so that at the end of one year only approximately 55% of the patients were still relieved of their pain.

As can be learned from other series as well, there is a marked tendency as time passes for recurrence of pain; this often reappears within months to a year or so after the operation. For this reason one often hears in the neurosurgical milieu that anterolateral cordotomy is not indicated in chronic pain of noncancerous origin. In their review, Sweet and Poletti [1984b] observed that the data regarding long-term relief of individual types of noncancerous pain are too sparse to allow valid comment by type with the exception of the pains related to spinal trauma from the mid-thoracic canal down and to those related to amputation stumps and phantom limbs.

For the pains related to lesions of spinal cord or cauda equina, Botterell et al. [1954] secured long-lasting relief in 4 patients out of 7, and Sweet and

Poletti [1984b] in 10 out of 17 patients. In the large series of Porter et al. [1966], all 34 with injuries of the cauda equina, 62% maintained relief for 8–20 years. Their pains continued to be insignificant or relieved by non-narcotic drugs. Less troublesome burning pain in legs, when present, persisted. For the painful phantoms, Falconer [1966] and Perneczky et al. [1975] report 67% long-term relief in 12 patients each, while Sweet and Poletti [1984b] had 12 early or late failures and 10 with continuing relief. In 3 of the late failures recurrence did not take place until 5, 5 and 8 years. In the 13 patients of Cowie and Hitchcock [1982] including, besides painful phantoms, postlaminectomy sciatica, causalgia, joint disease, etc., just over 60% were pain-free at 6 months, but at the end of one year only 50% had satisfactory analgesia to pin, and even in these pain relief was not sustained. The largest series of long-term follow-up results of anterolateral cordotomy in patients with nonmalignant pain has been published by White and Sweet [1969]. In 70 patients, with a high thoracic cordotomy, 56% had continuing relief, in 30 patients with a high cervical cordotomy 30% had prolonged pain relief.

Complications

Mortality

Obviously, making a cut in the spinal cord can produce many complications. The mortality in many of the reported series varies from 3 to 21% [Poletti, 1982]. The deaths depend of course on several factors, of which the general health of the patient undergoing major surgery is an important one. White and Sweet [1969] report an 8% mortality after open high thoracic cordotomy for pain in malignant disease and no mortality for nonmalignant disease after the same procedure. The mortality is higher for cordotomies in the cervical region than in the thoracic region and higher for bilateral than for unilateral incisions.

Respiratory Failure

Respiratory hazards during high cervical cordotomy are well documented [Belmusto et al., 1963; Nathan, 1963b; White, 1966; Hitchcock and Leece, 1967]. They are due to a lesion of the descending respiratory pathways, described earlier, the automatic components of which are responsible for the involuntary control of breathing, such as occurs during sleep. Unilateral destruction of this pathway results in little functional respiratory loss unless contralateral pulmonary function is itself poor, but bilateral C1–2 lesions produce a high incidence of sleep apnea and death. Rosomoff et al. [1969] measured several parameters, such as vital capacity, maximal breathing capacity, maximal thoracic pressure, tidal volume and movement of the diaphragms, and came to the conclusion that even this screening is not always prognostic. Although this dangerous state of sleep-induced apnea tends not to persist, most neurosurgeons have abandoned bilateral high cervical incisions. It is also good practice to monitor respiration continuously for one week after unilateral percutaneous high cervical cordotomy, lest an intended unilateral lesion be actually bilateral.

Motor Impairment

Transitory motor weakness, particularly of the ipsilateral lower limb, is very commonly observed after anterolateral cordotomy and is of the order of 13% [White and Sweet, 1979]; it is due to damaging the lateral pyramidal tract. It has been shown that each lower limb runs a greater risk from a bilateral cordotomy than does the one limb from a unilateral cordotomy, indicating that the incision in each side of the cord affects the motility of both lower limbs. Bilateral operation done in two stages was not less dangerous than the one-stage bilateral procedure in the series of Nathan and Smith [1973].

Bladder, Bowel and Sexual Dysfunction

As was mentioned earlier, the afferent fibers for micturition and defecation run with the spinothalamic fibers from the sacral segments of the body [Nathan, 1963a]. A bilateral lesion cutting through the spinothalamic tract in the sacral fibers proves to convert the voluntary functioning of the bladder and rectum to one of automaticity. A unilateral cordotomy causes at most only a temporary disturbance of function. Urinary tract dysfunction and fecal incontinence are often accompanied in the male by the inability to develop erections or to ejaculate. A review of the literature [Sweet and Poletti, 1984b] shows that there are wide differences between different authors as to the frequency of bladder, bowel and sexual dysfunction after cordotomy.

Hypotension

Already in 1936 Foerster reported his observations on vasomotor alterations following bilateral cordotomies. He concluded that vasoconstrictor pathways to both sides of the body were represented in each anterolateral quadrant of the cord. Following bilateral lesions postural hypotension may be marked but in most cases gradually the vasomotor tone will adjust to postural changes even after bilateral C1–C2 incisions [Nathan, 1963a, b; Sweet and Poletti, 1984b].

Dysesthesias

Either early or even many months after anterolateral cordotomy, subjective sensory phenomena can appear in which usually a distinction can be made between new dysesthesias and the original clinical pain. As pointed out by Noordenbos [1959], terminology of these sensory phenomena consequent upon lesions of the CNS in general, and cordotomy in particular, is confusing. But from the practical point of view, the dysesthesias are often of major clinical importance, because of their severity. They arise in the areas rendered analgesic to pin. No cases have been described in whom a unilateral lesion of the spinal cord produces bilateral pain and hyperpathia [Cassinari and Pagni, 1969]. At times these pains do not appear in the absence of tonic or intermittent stimuli. Thus, they may disappear during a spinal anesthesia [Nathan and Smith, 1984], and contrariwise they are increased when the analgesic area is strongly stimulated. Often the dysesthesias are most pronounced in the original painful area for which the cordotomy was performed. Happily they occur infrequently; for example, Nathan and Smith [1984] mention 3 cases in a series of 114 cordotomies, White and Sweet [1969] had 12 in 276 cases. These complaints usually appear only when analgesia has given way to hypalgesia and therefore they are more likely to affect patients who live longer. They are clearly a form of central pain and are appropriately discussed in the framework of the classical neurosurgical survey of central pain by Cassinari and Pagni [1969]. The following points in the pathogenesis of this type of pain seem to be reasonably well established: (a) for such pain to arise, a lesion of the neurons or axons of the paucisynaptic 'pain' system, the spinothalamocortical fibers proper, seems to be necessary; (b) inside the neuraxis it does not seem to matter whether the first, second, or third order neuron is affected; (c) central pain may occur in association with a partial or total lesion of the spinothalamic tract; (d) isolated lesions of the spinoreticulothalamic polysynaptic system do not seem to be sufficient to give rise to central pain, and (e) pure lesions of the first order neuron of the pathways for touch and kinesthesias do not seem to give rise to central pain but only to paresthesias. It has also been suggested that dysesthesias arise from lesions of the spinothalamic tract sparing the spinoreticular fibers, or when an interruption of the spinothalamic pathways is combined with that of the medial lemniscus.

It is interesting to add to these clinical interpretations, based on lesions in the nervous system of patients, two other sets of data. (1) Monkeys, after spinal lesions, may develop a syndrome in which the animal severely attacks a hypalgesic area of the body; the release of this syndrome is dependent on the integrity of a widespread bilateral spinal pathway for peripheral nociception, but is independent of the integrity of specific sensory tracts [Levitt and Levitt, 1981; Levitt, 1985]. (2) Data from stimulation of the human thalamus suggest that the paleospinothalamic pathways have a role in the appreciation of sensation of a burning quality, and this role is much more pronounced in patients with neurogenic pain than in patients without such pain [Tasker et al., 1982].

Postoperative Girdle Pain at the Level of Incision

This is a rather frequent complication [White and Sweet, 1969]. It usually disappears in a few weeks, is due to trauma to the exposed spinal roots, and can be avoided by care when rotating the spinal cord so that minimal tension is placed on the roots in question [Sweet and Poletti, 1984b]. According to Cassinari and Pagni [1969], however, some authors think that in some cases ipsilateral girdle pains may be due to lesions of the primary afferent neuron within the spinal cord.

Horner's Syndrome

This syndrome is almost the rule following high cervical cordotomy. The location of the fibers descending toward the sympathetic neurons in the intermediolateral cell column explains the frequency of this side effect.

Referred Pain

By this, one means that the pain is no longer felt at the site of the original stimulus but seems to be elsewhere. This phenomenon has been termed allachesthesia [Nathan, 1963a; White and Sweet, 1969]. Noxious stimuli, cold or certain other sorts of stimuli applied to the part of the body rendered analgesic, are referred to parts of the body that still have a normal or almost normal innervation, suggesting that such impulses giving rise to pain reach the neurological substratum of consciousness by other pathways than those sectioned [Nagaro et al., 1987]. Common patterns of the reference of sensation after unilateral cordotomy are rostrally and ipsilaterally to the corresponding general area on the opposite side. This contralateral reference occurs most often in patients with bilateral malignant disease in the torso and is likely soon to be followed by spontaneous pain on that contralateral side for which a cordotomy to denervate that side may be needed [White and Sweet, 1969, pp. 692, 748]. A further cordotomy on the opposite side will abolish this referred pain. Another reference pattern is to the level immediately cranial to the region of total loss of pain sensibility.

Causes for Failure

According to general neurosurgical experience and well-documented observations [Nathan, 1963a; Nathan and Smith, 1979] total division of the spinothalamic tract by anterolateral cordotomy stops pain from cancer. This means that the section should include the medial and anterior portion of the anterior quadrant, extending 1–2 mm medial to the most medial fibers of the ventral root. An incomplete anterolateral cordotomy may give rise to hypalgesia over an extensive region, with total analgesia and cessation of pain over a much smaller region. As the cancer spreads, pain may appear or reappear in the hypalgesic region. It is also a common observation that the area of total analgesia will shrink in both a cranial and caudal direction as time passes; this may take weeks or months to occur. However, when this happens in a few days, it is logical to conclude that some fibers have not been severed but only temporarily put out of action. But when the area of analgesia decreases a long time after the section of the spinothalamic tract, there is no simple and satisfying explanation. Several unproven hypotheses have been proposed, such as collateral sprouting and unmasking of existing synapses in alternative nociceptive pathways.

Conclusions

Although cordotomy is now carried out far less often than formerly, its capability of producing a completely pain-free state in the appropriately selected and fortunate case should not be forgotten — the more unilateral the pain the more likely is a gratifying success.

Chapter 10. Percutaneous Anterolateral Cordotomy

Historical Note

Mullan et al. introduced in 1963 a percutaneous method to perform an anterolateral cordotomy. They chose to introduce the needle at the C1–C2 interspace, the site of the largest intervertebral interval; this makes insertion lateral to the cord simple and the anterior migration of the interarticular joints at C1 and C2 allows percutaneous access to the anterior as well as to the lateral aspect of the cord. The vertebral artery is well out of the way at this level, entering the dura mater at the atlanto-occipital space one level higher. To make a lesion they used a strontium needle placed so that the radioactive source lay in the subarachnoid space against the anterolateral quadrant of the spinal cord. The problems of precise dosimetry to determine lesion size and the latency in the development of the lesion proved to be such gross disadvantages that the tactic was soon abandoned.

Rosomoff et al. [1965] therefore developed a technique by which an RF electrode permitted the lesion to be made promptly in a fractional manner with the patient awake so that the development of analgesia could be monitored and the size and the localization of the lesion could be adjusted. Since respiratory failure is a possible complication of cordotomy at the C2 level, Lin et al. [1966] modified the Rosomoff technique, devising an anterior approach in which the needle was inserted through an intervertebral disc in the lower cervical area, below the emergence of the phrenic nerve fibers. The introduction of the needle through the disc makes it difficult, however, to redirect the needle in the event that it does not hit the target in the spinal cord [Gildenberg et al., 1968]. With the development of stereotactic apparatus for spinal procedures, a posterior approach to the anterolateral tract has also been proposed [Crue et al., 1968; Hitchcock, 1969].

Surgical Technique

The technique for percutaneous anterolateral cordotomy has been described in detail by several authors [Mullan et al., 1963, 1965; Rosomoff et al., 1965; Lin et al., 1966; Rosomoff, 1968; Gildenberg et al., 1968; Crue et al., 1968; Hekmatpanah, 1968; Taren et al., 1969; Lorenz, 1976; Tasker, 1976/77; Gildenberg, 1976/77, 1982; Ganz and Mullan, 1977; Lipton and McLennan, 1980; Tasker, 1982b; Ischia et al., 1983].

Whatever approach is used, percutaneous methods offer with respect to an open operation a lower risk and the advantage of constant checking that the lesion is beginning and evolving properly. Most authors use the lateral approach and attention will be focused on this inasmuch as the posterior and anterior approaches have several disadvantages.

Target Localization in the Lateral Approach (at C1–C2 Level)

Radiological Localization

The dentate ligament in front of which lies the dorsal margin of the lateral spinothalamic tract is situated approximately in the antero-posterior center of the spinal canal at the C1–C2 interspace. This ligament can usually be visualized by injecting a small amount of emulsified insoluble positive contrast medium. The position of the point of the needle with respect to bony landmarks is an unsatisfactory way to judge its position outside of or within the spinal cord because of anatomic variation, toughness of the pia mater and mobility of the whole cord.

Impedance Measurement

Usually when the needle penetrates the cord, the patient feels pain referred to the ipsilateral side of the neck. As the tip impales the cord, the impedance shows a sudden shift from low to high (of the order of 200 Ω in spinal fluid to 500 Ω in spinal cord when a 3-mm-long, 0.5-mm diameter electrode tip is used [Taren et al., 1969; Gildenberg et al., 1969].

Stimulation: A physiological puzzle; Difference in threshold between primary and secondary afferent neurons for pain.

A remarkable difference in stimulus thresholds for the subjective response to pain distinguishes the behavior of axons of the primary afferent neurons in the posterior rootlets from that of the axons of the secondary afferent neurons in the anterior half of the white matter of the spinal cord. Gentle mechanical stroking of a posterior rootlet may suffice to evoke pain. In an effort to provide a minimal quantifiable electrical stimulus which would at low levels elicit a nonpainful sensation localizable by the patient, one of us decades ago asked the Grass Instrument Company to supply a stimulator with incremental increases of 0.01 V. The increase in voltage required to convert a nonpainful to a painful stimulus at the normal rootlet is at the most 2-fold or a fewfold higher. In sharp contrast are the extreme increases in both mechanical and electrical thresholds for pain within the cord's anterolateral columns. Thus, one can usually transect in the fully awake patient the entire anterior quadrant containing nearly all the fibers for pain from the opposite side without producing contralateral pain in any of the zone which becomes analgesic. Any pain during the maneuver is usually related to tension in the posterior rootlets ipsilaterally at the level of the incision. This difference between the primary and secondary afferent neurons is dramatically brought out by manipulations where they lie in juxtaposition in the lower medulla oblongata. When one deliberately heats with RF current the pain tract from the opposite limbs and torso lying just ventral to the descending cephalic (trigeminal) tract, there is no clue from the patient's sensation at this time that a lesion has been made. This determination requires subsequent examination, as with a pin. However, as soon as a knife blade or heating current affects the primary afferent ipsilateral fibers, the patient typically emits an agonizing cry because of severe pain in the face, and a lesion here is best made with the patient unconscious under general anesthesia. Likewise in the anterior quadrant of the cord the thresholds for any sensory response tend to run of the order of 1 to a few volts [White and Sweet, 1955, p.45; 1969, pp. 756–757; Tasker, [1982b].

Possibly some of the basis for the difference lies in the electrical and mechanical excitability of the primary afferent large myelinated fibers for touch and kinesthesis comprising most of the large fibers in the posterior columns of the cord and lower medulla oblongata. Touch or very low-voltage electrical stimulation to the pia over the posterior column may elicit an intolerable electric shock-like sensation. It is conceivable but surprising that elimination of these fibers from the anterior white columns may be the basis for the increased thresholds here. If so this would be the more puzzling because deliberate electrical stimulation of the posterior columns tends to relieve rather than provoke pain.

During stimulation at percutaneous cordotomy, spread of current to the more responsive posterior roots, with pain therefrom as well as highly variablc types of response from the secondary afferent neurons themselves makes the stimulation less precisely applicable during this operation than that of posterior rootlets for rhizotomy. Some neurosurgeons have abandoned its use during cordotomy; we however strongly recommend it as a major adjunct to improving the accuracy of the procedure.

Table 10/I lists the criteria, as summarized by Tasker [1982b] for the identification by threshold electrical stimulation of cord structures at C1–C2. We have found his observations so complete and helpful that we are reprinting them in full.

Table 10/II lists the responses this same author noted in 244 procedures when the spinothalamic tract was being stimulated at threshold at, respectively, 2 and 100 Hz.

He states that provided radiologic and impedance criteria have been met, it can be assumed with confidence that the electrode lies in the main ascending pain tract at a site where a lesion will be effective and safe when threshold stimulation at 2 Hz and at about 3 V induces 2-Hz contractions in the ipsilateral neck muscles, and at 100 Hz and at about 0.5–1 V contralateral sensory effects, usually of warmth. An ipsilateral motor effect induced at 2 Hz involving other than cervical myotomes or any tetanization induced at 100 Hz contraindicates lesion making.

Mayer et al. [1975b] also concluded that determination of the electrical threshold for pain sensation is a sensitive quantitative index for predicting optimal electrode position in percutaneous anterolateral cordotomy. In their experience if the threshold for pain elicited by the stimulating electrode was less than 300 μA (1-second trains of 0.2-ms pulses, monophasic, rectangular wave cathodal pulses delivered at 50/s) a 5-second RF lesion of 50 mA would produce complete contralateral analgesia with no weakness. They also note that the results further suggested that the fibers in the anterolateral quadrant that transmit pain are discretely rather than diffusely localized. Mayer et al. [1975a] in an elegant study used threshold, frequency, and refractory period characteristics to define a neural population in the anterolateral quadrant of the spinal cord of man, stimulation of which produces pain. They found these characteristics to be similar to those found for wide dynamic range neurons in the ventral half of the dorsal horn in the monkey, suggesting that activation of these cells is a sufficient condition to produce pain in man. Occasionally other sensations are evoked by stimulation in the spinal cord, but the pathway stimulation of which elicits them is not clearly identified.

Table 10/I. Identification of cord structures at C1 by threshold electrical stimulation. From Tasker [1982b]

Structure stimulated	Effect of electrical stimulation	
	2 Hz	100 Hz
Anterior horn	2–Hz twitches in C1–2 myotomes, ipsilaterally	tetanization of C1–2 myotomes
Corticospinal tract	2-Hz twitches of any ipsilateral musculature from C1 to sacral myotomes	tetanization of C1–sacral myotomes sometimes preceded by tingling, shock, or vibration in the same area as that from which the motor response arises
Descending tract or spinal nucleus of V	usually none; occasionally ipsilateral facial throbbing or bumping	ipsilateral facial tingling, electric shock, or vibration
Dorsal column	usually none; occasionally ipsilateral bumping or throbbing anywhere below face	ipsilateral tingling, vibration, or electric shock anywhere below face
Lateral spinothalamic tract	nearly always ipsilateral 2-Hz twitches of muscles innervated by cervical roots including upper extremity; usually no sensory effect occcasionally contralatcral bumping or throbbing below neck	no motor effect; contralateral warmth, coolness, or burning; rarely pain or tingling

These sensations include: nausea [Taren et al., 1969], abdominal burning [Taren et al., 1969], vegetative phenomena such as awareness of heart beating and discomfort during heating [Lorenz, 1976]. Bilateral sensations, especially hand sensation, occur if the electrode is too far forward [Mullan, 1971]. Superficial stimulation close to and especially behind the dentate ligament tends to be painful in the neck [Mullan, 1971].

Evoked Potentials

Taren et al. [1969] proposed that the most precise identification in the spinothalamic tract would probably result from recording spontaneous and evoked potentials from the cord. However, even today this method has not been applied clinically on a wide basis. In one study [Campbell and Lipton, 1983], recording from the anterolateral quadrant of the spinal cord was made

Table 10/II. Responses elicited in 244 procedures with threshold at 2 Hz in lateral spinothalamic tract at C1–2. From Tasker [1982b]

Response	Percentage
2-Hz contractions in ipsilateral cervical myotomes	72.2
2-Hz contractions in ipsilateral cervical myotomes plus contralateral sensation	20.1
Contralateral sensory only	0.9
Contralateral motor only (significance unknown)	5.1
Ipsilateral sensory only (probably subthreshold motor)	0.9
Not specified	0.9

Contralateral sensory effects produced by 100 Hz threshold stimulation of the lateral spinothalamic tract at C1–2 in 244 procedures

Effect	Percentage
Warmth or heat	70
Cold or cool	24
Burning or pain	5
Tingling or vibration	1

in 53 patients. One positive wave, appearing with a latency of about 24 ms after stimulation of the median nerve at the contralateral wrist, and only appearing after stimulus intensities which gave rise to an unpleasant sensation, was thought to be a true crossed-pathway response, originating within the anterolateral quadrant.

Lesion Making

The lesion is made in successive steps and between or even during each step a check is made on the strength in the ipsilateral limb and on the analgesic level if any, in the contralateral limb and torso. For making the lesion an RF generator is usually used. Parameters for making a lesion may be expressed in current and time; typical electrodes are insulated wires with a bare tip of 2–3 mm. Different authors give current intensity values ranging between 30 and 100 mA, delivered in increments of 5–10 s, for a variable total time (30–60 s) depending on the degree of analgesia obtained and preservation of other neurological functions. More logical parameters for lesion making are temperature and time, since an RF current destroys neural tissue by local heating. This can be done by using a thermocouple-monitored electrode [Levin and Cosman, 1980]. Temperature values used range between 75 and 90 °C up to 30 s in increments of 5–10 s.

Since the size of the lesions produced depends not only on time, current and temperature, but also on tip diameter and other factors [Organ, 1976/77] it is necessary for a given electrode and a given RF generator prior to clinical use to make experimental lesions with different parameters in order to know the geometry of the lesion produced with a given set of parameters.

Results

Open versus Closed Anterolateral Cordotomy

Results and complications of percutaneous cordotomy do not differ in quality from those of the open operation. It is pertinent though to compare quantitatively end results of the two procedures.

In 1979, White and Sweet pursued this objective and we shall summarize the results of their detailed study. To do this comparison, they collected through the efforts and courtesy of many neurosurgical colleagues a total of 3,357 cases, treated by percutaneous cordotomy and 691 cases of open cordotomy. The study showed conclusively that the percutaneous method is effective, at least for pain of malignant origin, and that it carries a small risk of mortality and serious complications. In these respects, it is superior to open cordotomy. There is not enough evidence yet to make sure that this is equally true for victims of chronic pain of nonmalignant origin. It is not known yet whether (a) the initial analgesia will persist as frequently, and (b) whether the incidence of postcordotomy dysesthesia will be as low after percutaneous as after open cordotomy. In special circumstances there is still an indication for the open operation, especially when several attempts with the percutaneous method have failed. In the past several years some neurosurgeons are reverting to open cordotomy principally related to the greatly reduced use of both operations. In the experience of many of us the percutaneous approach to the cord requires continuing practice in order to maintain consistently good results.

Conclusions

This is not an easy procedure. For the neurosurgeon experienced in its use percutaneous cordotomy is a significant improvement over the open operation.

Chapter 11.A. Commissural Myelotomy

Historical Note and Surgical Variants in Location and Technique

Commissural myelotomy for the treatment of pain was conceived as an alternative to bilateral anterolateral cordotomy in patients in whom a restricted and bilateral area of analgesia was sought. Since the pain and temperature fibers were all presumed to decussate in the cord, it offered the attraction of interrupting all these bilateral fibers by a single cut. This was advantageous for the relief of bilateral shoulder, girdle and visceral pain, and especially in the typically bilateral pain of luetic crises. Moreover, the touch sensory and most of the motor fibers decussate only in the brain stem or uppermost cord, respectively, so are of necessity spared. Consequently, inspired by Greenfield, Armour [1927] in 1926 performed the first commissural myelotomy of the thoracolumbar segments on a patient suffering from tabetic gastric crises. Taking the anatomy of the spinothalamic decussation into account, his intention was to perform a complete sagittal section of the commissure while avoiding damage to the anterior spinal artery by the use of a ball-pointed knife in the deepest stage of the section. This feature of the technique continues to be emulated today.

Leriche [1936] cut only the posterior commissure, whereas Putnam [1934] inserted a needle — and later a needle-shaped 'myelotome' — between the posterior columns at intervals of a few millimeters and maneuvered it up and down in such a way as to pass completely through the commissure (as proven by autopsy).

In the 1940s, commissural myelotomy became quite popular among French neurosurgeons. The level of myelotomy was always attuned to the presumed metameric 'pain' input, taking into account a slight cephalic shift of the fibers as they ascended a variable number of segments before crossing

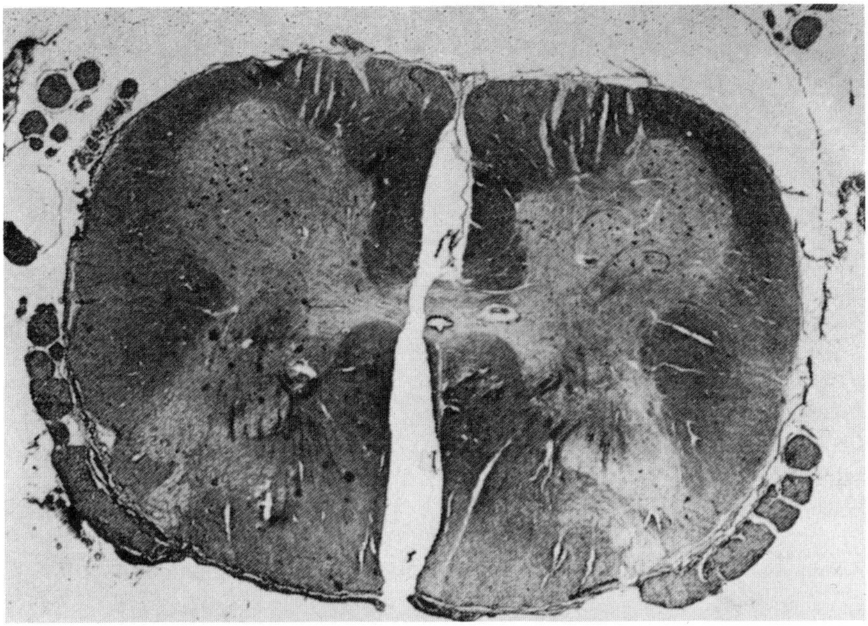

Fig. 11/1. Specimen of spinal cord 2 days after commissural myelotomy at D12–L2. From Sourek [1969].

in the midline. Controversy seemed to reign as to the depth of the cut. Some authors limited the incision to a depth of 2–3 mm, just reaching the gray substance [Mansuy et al., 1944]; some took care not to exceed 4 mm, thereby seeking to limit the incision to the posterior commissure [Wertheimer and Lecuire, 1953] while some cut deeper ventral to the central canal [Guillaume et al., 1945] (fig. 11/1).

As experience has accumulated, it has become clear that it is advisable to maximize the extent of analgesia by dividing the commissures completely. Dargent et al. [1963], reviewing the patients of Wertheimer and Lecuire 10 years later, concluded that the operation was effective only for the treatment of vaginal and visceral pain. It is useful to recognize that the posterior median sulcus is shallow and soon gives way to a posterior median septum of neuroglia. Hence even with the microscope two layers of medial pia cannot be separated from each other because they are not there. Lack of awareness of this fact may account for some surgical deviations from the midline.

Table 11/I. Late results of commissural myelotomy. From Van Roost [1988]

Author, year	Operation level	Late success		Malignant		Benign	
		%	n	%	n	%	n
Arutjunov, 1952	compl. C–T/T–L	87	15	87	15		
Wertheimer and Lecuire, 1953	post. T4–6	65	80				
Lembcke, 1964	compl. C2–5–T1	86	7	0	1	100	6
Sourek, 1969 1977	compl. C4–7/T7–L1	84	38				
Grunert et al., 1970	compl. C3-T1/T-L	55	11	56	9	50	2
Broager, 1974	compl. T9-11	58	33				
Cook and Kawakami, 1977	compl. C4-T1/5-L1	20	10	67	3	0	7
King, 1977	compl. T9-11-S1	70	10	86	7	33	3
Fascendini et al., 1979	compl. T6-8-L1			17	6		
Adams et al., 1982b	compl. T2-4/low T-L-S	63	24	62	21	67	3
Goedhart et al., 1984	compl. S2-5	37.5	8	37.5	8		
Sweet and Poletti, 1984a	compl. conus	33	9	33	9		

Results

Table 11/I, taken from Van Roost [1988], summarizes late successes of commissural myelotomies, with a follow-up ranging from one month to 12 years.

Since many of the patients had cancer pain, most of these lived only a few months. In table 11/I success means: (a) total disappearance of the pain syndrome or such an improvement that the patient no longer requests narcotic drugs; and (b) troublesome postoperative dysesthesia must also subside. In eight articles reporting on 175 cases [Lembcke, 1964; Sourek, 1969, 1977; Grunert et al., 1970; Broager, 1974; Cook and Kawakami, 1977; King, 1977; Adams et al., 1982; Sweet and Poletti, 1984a] of complete commissural myelotomy early complete relief of pain was achieved in an average of 92% of the cases, but with time the outcome decays. In the cases where follow-up was longer and up to 11 years, 59% of 63 patients with malignant tumors and 48% of 21 with other than malignant causes of their pain showed a good outcome at the latest follow-up by the less rigorous criteria than complete relief mentioned above. Since the 'benign' group live longer, they have more time for spinal pathways to recover. In three articles reporting 151 cases [Arutjunov, 1952; Wertheimer and Lecuire, 1953; Broager, 1974] the cause of the pain was not specified. The deficits in bowel, bladder and sexual function, so prominent after bilateral anterolateral cordotomy of the lumbosacral segments, have been largely avoided.

Side Effects and Their Implications Related to the Anatomy of 'Pain Pathways'

Table 11/II summarizes the changes in neurological status reported after commissural myelotomy. Among these the variability in the sensory changes is particularly striking. In the literature, the terms 'hypesthesia or hypo-esthesia' and 'hypalgesia or hypo-algesia' are often used in an ill-defined fashion. In table 11/II we have tried to ascertain whether the authors meant a sensory loss for tactile or for noxious stimuli and to tabulate the data accordingly. A girdle-shaped hypalgesia is usually seen in cases of complete commissural myelotomy, while a less consistent configuration of the hypalgesia is often reported in posterior commissural myelotomy. Paresthesias and dysesthesias in the legs, usually transient, and girdle pains are frequently seen with commissurotomies. At times gross asymmetry in the sensory loss on the two sides occurs, apparently due to surgical incision off the midline. These problems have been largely eliminated by the use of the operating microscope which enables the surgeon to avoid the trauma to the fasciculi gracili which was causing the dysesthesias.

It is especially noteworthy that the clinical pain is often relieved even when there is slight or no hypalgesia. Less often the opposite occurs; i.e. even when there is loss of pinprick sensation, the clinical pain may not be relieved. Moreover, there may be loss of pain and temperature sensibility far caudal or more cranial than would be expected from the level and length of the commissurotomy, a helpful but puzzling finding [Cook et al., 1984; King, 1977; Sourek, 1977; Wertheimer and Lecuire, 1953; Sweet and Poletti, 1984a]. These results, especially the good ones, are inexplicable on the basis of present understanding of pathways for pain and how they function, and will be discussed in the next chapter.

Table 11/II. Side effects of commissural myelotomy. From Van Roost [1988]

Authors, year	Tactile hypes-thesia	Palles-thesia dimin-ished	Proprio-ception dimin-ished	Girdle-shaped hypal-gesia	Hypal-gesia other type	Thermo-hypes-thesia	Pares-thesias legs	Dyses-thesias	'Radi-cular' pain	Paresis transient	Paresis perma-nent	Gait incoor-dina-tion	Mortality within 10 days of op., %
Putnam, 1934		1/3		1/3 t		1/3							3
Guillaume et al., 1945			+	+ t	+	+ t	+ t	+t	+t				0
Lembcke, 1964				(+)						2/12		1/12	0
Grunert et al., 1970				+++	(+)	+++				5/24			8
Broager, 1974			+++				+++ t	2/33 p		3/33	3/33	+++	3
Lippert et al., 1974	4/16			9/16		1/16	4/16 t	1/16 t		1/16	1/16	1/16	0
Cook and Kawakami, 1977			13/24 (2 p)	18/24t		18/24t		12/24t					0
King, 1977	+++ t	+++ t	+++		9/10		3/10t				2/10	+	0
Sourek, 1977	+++ p	+++	+++ p	+++ t	+	++ t	+++ t	+++ t				+	3
Sweet and Poletti, 1984a			4/9					++ t	+ t	4/9	2/9		0
Mansuy et al., 1944					6/20t	6/20	++ t	++ t	++ t				7
Wertheimer and Lecuire, 1953	13/80*	6/80	6/80		24/80	24/80		28/80 (1 p)	27/80 (1 p)	15/80			7

* = Sharp-blunt discrimination spared; + = few patients affected (± 10%); (+) = imprecise designation; ++ = moderate number of patients affected (± 30%); +++ = great number of patients affected (± 75%); t = transient; p = permanent. Complete myelotomy upper and posterior commissurotomy lower part of table.

Conclusions

Current enthusiasm for the lower stress and lower risk epidural or intrathecal morphine and other pain suppressor agents has for the present greatly reduced the use of this operation. However, if as experience accumulates, the incidence of the development of major tolerance to these agents frequently leaves the patient dying in painful misery, it may prove advisable to resort to commissural myelotomy once tolerance looms on the horizon, and well before the patient's state has deteriorated to a level at which the procedure would be too risky.

Chapter 11.B. Stereotactic C1 Central Myelotomy (Central Cord Lesion)

Although the term extralemniscal myelotomy has also been used to designate this procedure, we and Hitchcock prefer the term indicated in the title because of its greater specificity. Hitchcock developed a stereotactic frame enabling him to introduce an electrode via a posterior approach to the atlanto-occipital membrane above C1 or one interspace below [Hitchcock, 1974]. With the patient seated so as to keep the midline of the cord near the skeletal midline and with the head flexed to keep the cord taut, he used bony landmarks and positive contrast myelography, with the later addition of impedance monitoring, to determine the site of penetration of the cord by his 1-mm bare electrode. With this he made lesions in one area in each patient in the C1 segment of the cord. The final location and extent of the lesion were decided occasionally by evoked potentials recorded at the electrode tip, but chiefly by the patient's reactions during electrical stimulation and clinical testing as the lesion was enlarged. A burning sensation in chest or abdomen was found to be characteristic of central cord stimulation at 50 Hz.

This type of 'central myelotomy' differs from commissural myelotomy in three important respects: (1) the larger spatial and especially lateral extension of the lesion; (2) its location limited to a single level in the spinal cord not determined by the metameric distribution of the pain, and (3) by the minimal injury to the dorsal columns.

The early extent and severity of the loss to pinprick usually produced by such a lesion is so astonishing that it compels a major revision in our thinking anent the pathways for pain in the spinal cord of man. The deficit in the appreciation of pin as determined by Hitchcock [1970b] was of two types: (1) a complete inability to distinguish sharp from blunt as, for example, after anterolateral cordotomy, and (2) ability to distinguish sharp from blunt, but appraisal of the point as painless. Figure 11/2 shows the loss 24 days after operation in the first of Hitchcock's 8 patients reported in 1970. Early after operation there was the 'spinothalamic' type of analgesia on both sides,

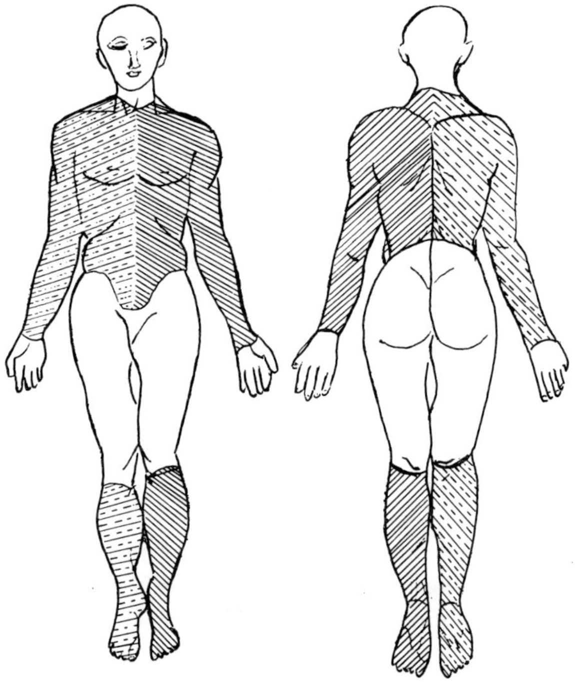

Fig. 11/2. Stereotactic C1 midline myelotomy (Hitchcock's case 1). Early after operation there was symmetrical loss of discrimination between sharp and blunt — the same on right side as persisted 24 days later in the left diagram slightly modified by authors. From Hitchcock [1970b].

which soon faded on the right, as illustrated, to feeling the stimulus as a point but painless. However, the patient remained free of pain in the neck and both arms caused by cervical vertebral cancer until his death on the 26th postoperative day. The postmortem study revealed an electrode track the full dorsoventral extent of the cord 1–2 mm to one side of the midline without clear-cut depiction of an obvious electrolytic lesion. The unexpected analgesia in both legs led Hitchcock to the logical trial of the method for lower midline pain. This in his case 2 was perineal from extensive cancer and was stopped by a lesion which preserved the patient's ability to distinguish sharp

Table 11/III. Late results of stereotactic C1 central myelotomy. From Van Roost [1988]

Author	Year	Operation level	Late success		Malignant	
			%	n	%	n
Hitchcock	1970b	centr. C0–1	43	7	43	7
Papo and Luongo	1976	centr. C2–4	40	10	33	9
Hitchcock	1977	centr. C0-1	80	25		
Schvarcz	1978	centr. C0-1	78	75	79	61
Eiras et al.	1980	centr. C0-1	58	12	58	12
Gildenberg and Hirschberg	1984	compl. + centr. T9/10	66	12		
Sourek	1985 1987	centr. C0-1	57	30	minority	

from blunt but rendered cutaneous pinprick painless everywhere below D12. Moreover, literally everywhere above this she had analgesia except for the medial parts of her face. Even though completely normal sensation was recovered in the sacral area by 6 weeks, the relief of pain was persisting at last follow-up 4 months later (table 11/III). By 1977 Hitchcock could report on over 30 patients with C1 operations at and near the midline — mainly for cancer pain. The procedure was not completed in 5 patients due to technical problems, but there was no mortality at all. Of 25 patients who were followed until death or for over 5 years, 55% had complete relief or required only weak nonnarcotic drugs and a further 24% required only strong but nonnarcotic drugs. In these two groups there was well marked sensory loss in 75 and 85%, respectively. Poor or no relief occurred in 20% of the patients who also had no sensory loss.

Hitchcock's pupil, Schvarcz [1977a, 1978] has an even larger experience reporting on 75 patients. His target was the same, i.e. in the midline 5 mm deep to the dorsal surface of the cord. The lesion was usually made at the site at the base of the dorsal funiculi at which threshold stimulation — 0.5–1.0 V at 50–75 Hz — evoked tingling or electrical feeling starting in one or both feet, spreading with increased stimulus intensity to the dorsums of the legs to any combination of all limbs or trunk, or amazingly enough to the whole trigeminal area. His lesions averaged 2.5–3 mm in diameter. In 61 of the patients the pain was related to tumor; of these, 42 had lower dorsal midline and/or bilateral pain; 19 had unilateral upper body pain. Satisfactory relief persisted in 78% at follow-up at 0.5–2 years, 81% of these patients having died, however, in the first 6 months. Of the group with a nonmalignant cause of pain 4 had causalgia, 4 post-herpetic neuralgia and 6 had other painful central lesions in the cord. In these neurogenic types of pain abolition of hyperpathia and elimination or marked reduction of background pain was achieved at follow-up times ranging from 0.5 to 4 years. The only deficit in most of Schvarcz's cases was the description of a pinprick as sharp but not painful. In only a few was there inability to distinguish sharp from blunt stimuli, e.g. conventional analgesia. This might be in one or both arms or the face; more rarely it occurred below the waist. These deficits could be correlated neither with the responses to stimulation induced at operation nor with the areas of relieved pain. There were no lasting neurological disturbances of any kind, including no postoperative dysesthesias.

Papo and Luongo [1976] tried a more extensive operation in 9 cancer patients of whom 5 had pain in the lumbosacral segments; another had a brachial plexus avulsion. They exposed the cord in the upper C1 to the C3 segments and made six or seven RF lesions in this region with the electrode tip at the usual site of the central canal 6 mm deep to the posterior surface of the cord. They then split between the two posterior columns to a depth of 5 mm for the full length of upper C2 through lower C4 segments. All 10 patients were completely relieved of their pain for from 2 weeks to 3 months, which was until death in 4 of them. The relatively prompt recurrences in the other 6 discouraged these surgeons from continuing the procedure. In only 3 patients was there a band of mild hypalgesia from C2–T10 dermatomes lasting about 3 weeks. Special interest attaches to 2 of these patients. The one with the central pain of a brachial plexus avulsion was completely relieved of pain for the remaining 9 weeks of his life. In the second patient the surgical lesion damaged the right posterior column producing hypesthesia to touch and very distressing dysesthesia in the right half of the body. But the original bilateral sacral, testicular and lower limb pain was abolished on the right side, persisting unchanged on the left, pointing to ipsilateral conduction of the impulses for pain.

Eiras et al. [1980] have carried out this operation in 12 cancer patients with total relief in 7 for from 3 to 14 months. In only 3 patients were 'nondermatomal' areas of hypalgesia detected. As was described also in the reports from the previous three services, postoperative gait disturbances were common, but limited at worst to a few weeks.

By 1985 Sourek [1985, 1987] could report on 34 such thermocoagulations at the C1–2 level on 30 patients whose chronic pain was predominantly of nonmalignant cause. There was no intraoperative stimulation, the circa 2 × 3 mm lesion being performed under general anesthesia. The loss of pain in various parts of the body was accomplished 'without any sensory deficits', and with no side effects including no sphincter disturbances. In only 8 of the 30 was the operation unsuccessful and 4 of the 8 were relieved by repeating the procedure. In 16 patients the completely new observation was made that in 11 of the 12 with pain relief the plasma levels of metenkephalin (ENK) rose immediately after operation, whereas in the 4 without relief these levels fell or remained the same. The preoperative skin temperatures were 'very low' in 10 of these patients. Relief of the pain in all 10 was accompanied by a rise in skin temperature of up to 5 °C. Despite recurrence of the pain in 3–6 months, in about 30% of the patients Sourek recommends the procedure even for nonmalignant pain in the upper limbs and thorax. We need more details.

These operations led Gildenberg and Hirschberg [1984] to carry out open lower one level lesions near the central canal in 16 cancer patients. These were at T9 or T10 vertebral levels in 14 patients but were made mechanically with a blunt dissection in 12 patients with 8 good or excellent relief. The same tactic used at C1 in 2 cases failed in both. Less trauma to the posterior columns from a central RF lesion made in 2 patients at the low thoracic level gave one good and one excellent result with no demonstrable sensory loss, motor weakness or sphincter disturbance. The heat lesion with a diameter of 2–4 mm is more likely to have the necessary bilateral extent.

Significance of the Sensory Findings

The relief of pain unaccompanied by analgesia to pin after commissural myelotomy led a number of workers to join the ranks of those who hypothesize that in addition to long tracts there is a chain of short tracts in the cord used for pain conduction. This had been conceptualized as a multisynaptic afferent network by Noordenbos [1959] in an extensive cogent exposition. An excellent review of the relevant animal studies has been published by Cook et al. [1984], but the crucial species for us is man. Of the many papers on the differences between the CNS of primates and that of lower animals the 1914 work of Karplus and Kreidl germane to this area may be cited. They based their conclusions that there are short multisynaptic pain pathways on the persistence of pain following their bilateral cord hemisections at different

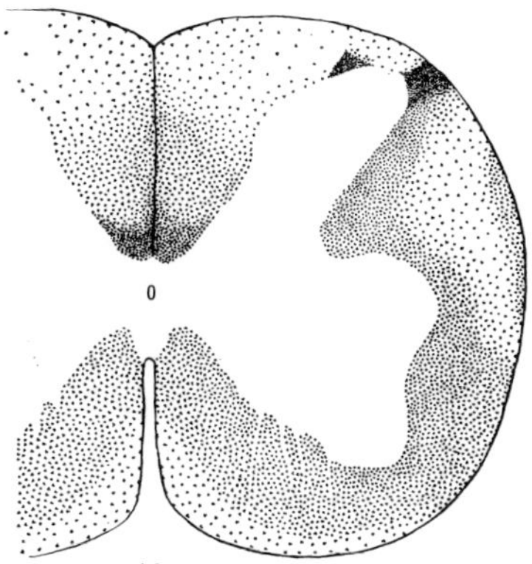

Fig. 11/3. Silver-stained section of lumbosacral cord of monkey 14 days after isolation of this segment of the cord by T12–L1 transection rostrally and at S5 caudally as well as by cutting all posterior roots to these segments. This caused degeneration of all fibers arising from neurons outside this segment of cord. The vast majority of the surviving fibers are small and unmyelinated. The densest bundles of such fibers are medial and lateral to the apex of the posterior horns. The next densest bundles are at the ventral tips of the posterior columns. These presumably largely ascending fibers are destroyed by the C1–2 myelotomy of Hitchcock. From Tower et al. [1941].

spatial intervals in cats. They were able, though, to find no trace of pain conduction after similar operations in monkeys. However, the sensory findings regarding pain, both subjective and objective, following high cervical central lesions in the majority of over 100 patients just summarized, leave no doubt that somewhere in the central gray or nearby perigriseal white matter lies an ascending pathway for pain whose destruction produces at least temporary relief of clinical pain along with patchy total loss of appreciation of a pin as painful. In at least one patient of Papo and Luongo the pathway was ipsilateral rather than crossed. Davis et al. [1929] have found both crossed and uncrossed pain pathways in the cat close to the gray matter and ascending into high cervical and lower bulbar areas before crossing. Richards et al. [1966] have evidence for small fibers ascending uncrossed. The locus of this pathway is suggested by the work of Tower et al. [1941] in monkeys (fig. 11/3). They isolated the lumbosacral cord by total transverse incisions and by cutting posterior roots to this segment. Two weeks later one of the densest collections of surviving unmyclinated fibers lay bilaterally as two tiny bundles at the base of the posterior columns in exactly the position to be destroyed by the Hitchcock type lesion. Hitchcock's [1970b] and Schvarcz' [1978] proposal of an entirely separate pain pathway ascending in the spinal cord, possibly multisynaptically, close to the midline, seems inescapable. This pathway shares the feature of pain relief without analgesia to pin characteristic of the medially lying paleospinothalamic tract in the brain stem which appears to be simply an upward extension thereof. Schvarcz has also relieved intense pruritus up to the C1 level by this operation [Hitchcock, 1974].

These observations in man as to the existence of a pain pathway are buttressed by experimental evidence that the gray matter around the central canal of the spinal cord is implicated in nociception. From the anatomical point of view there are connections between this area and brain stem structures [Martin et al., 1981; Kevetter et al., 1982; Light, 1983; Menétry et al., 1983; Nahin et al., 1983, 1984] that have to do with stimulation-produced analgesia [Akaike et al., 1978; Takagi et al., 1978; Zorman et al., 1981]. From the physiological point of view in this area neurons can be activated by noxious stimuli [Honda and Perl, 1985; Nahin et al., 1983]. From the biochemical point of view substances which are implicated in nociception or its modulation are present in the same area [Hökfelt et al., 1977; Oliveras et al., 1977; Barber et al., 1979; Gibson et al., 1981; Steinbusch, 1981; LaMotte et al., 1982; Schoenen et al., 1985]. These include substance P, CCK, neurotensin and ENK. Even more helpful is the study of Lauterborn et al. [1987] who have demonstrated cells lateral to the central canal in the lumbar region of rats which localize simultaneously ENK and CCK and which project directly to the periaqueductal gray at the mesodiencephalic junction. Another long central pathway has been found by Bernard et al. [1987b] who, following a lesion in the spinal tract ascending from lamina X in rats, find degenerating fibers which are contacting cells in the pontine parabrachial nucleus (PB) that project to the central nucleus of the amygdala. That many PB neurons are concerned with nociception is indicated by: (1) the response to noxious inputs in their extracellular records in 24 of 30 such cells; (2) PB receives a large input from (the largely nociceptive) lamina I neurons of the cord and trigeminal nucleus caudalis as shown by retrograde labeling, and (3) electrical stimulation of PB suppresses pain in the cat.

Among the continuing mysteries is the explanation for the often long-lasting relief from anterolateral cordotomy and the shorter relief of pain after upper cervical central myelotomy in the presence of an apparently completely functional alternative pathway for pain. These facts have led Cook et al. [1984] to suggest that the pain-relieving effect of a commissural or central myelotomy is due to the blocking of impulses entering into, or in, or leaving the spinothalamic and spinoreticular tracts.

Conclusions

The extent to which both commissural myelotomy and central myelotomy should be utilized at present is unclear. What is clear is that we have learned from the lessons of precise surgical therapy in man that there is a central pathway for pain in the human spinal cord whose destruction diminishes or eliminates the conscious awareness of clinical persistent pain with modest, if any, loss of pain from discrete noxious stimuli. These conclusions could be reached only by studies in man.

Chapter 12. Cordectomy

Historical Note

The first cordectomy for pain of which we are aware was carried out by Armour [1927] in 1916. In a post-traumatic paraplegic he totally excised 'from above the lesion' a mass of scar tissue including cord and cauda equina from the upper border of T12 to the L2 vertebral levels. Intense pain in the lower abdomen and in the legs, especially the thighs, was completely eliminated. Later the same year Cushing [cited by Armour, 1927] had transected the entire cord cephalad to spinal metastases which were causing excruciating pain 'with an entirely satisfactory result'.

Clinical Data

Patients with complete lesions of the thoracic or lumbar cord may have at least 3 types of pain: (1) 'segmental', 'root', or 'girdle' related to the dermatomal level of the lesion; (2) visceral, usually referred to lower bowel or bladder, and (3) focal or diffuse pains referred to one or more insentient areas below the level of sensory loss. As already noted in earlier chapters on cordotomy and DREZ lesions, the first of these types of pain tends to be somewhat more readily relieved than those in the other two categories.

Results of A. Jefferson

A new and far more encouraging light has been cast on limitations and value of this procedure by the report of Jefferson [1983] on 19 cases — nearly as many as have been reported altogether in the rest of the world. These cases are all from the Sheffield Spinal Injuries Unit where 'low overall incidence of intractable pain is a tribute to the quality of pain management by the staff of the unit', says Jefferson. Indeed, many patients did not develop major pain until years later, the mean elapsed time after injury being 5.8 years. This also indicates that those submitted to cordectomy had really bad pain despite excellent care. One patient thought at one point to be a candidate for cordectomy was cured of his pain by clonazepam and carbamazepine and had remained pain-free for 4 years. All operated patients had no useful function below the hips and had as well extended conservative management with a mean time from the onset of severe pain to operation of 3.4 years.

Striking features of the Jeffersonian series are: (1) the main pain was referred below the hips, i.e. was of the diffuse or caudal type in all 15 of the patients whose cordectomy (and injury) were at, and/or below D11 vertebra. Whether their pain was predominantly in thighs, knees or legs it was 70–100% relieved in 14 of the 15, and in 7 of the 14 the relief was 100% complete. The 15th patient (whose leg pain disappeared) graded himself as having only 50% relief because of continuing pain in lower abdomen, genitals and buttocks. In sharp contrast were the results in 3 patients with cordectomies one level higher opposite T10 or T10–11. The 2 with pains referred to tops of thighs, lower abdomen, buttocks and rectum secured no benefit and the unsatisfactory level of 25% relief was the lot of the third patient with pain throughout the legs. The one patient with a higher lesion had his cordectomy from the body of D3 to the upper border of D7; he too obtained no relief. In a subsequent letter Jefferson [1987] tells us that almost none of the patients in the Sheffield Unit had severe pain when their lesion was above D10 vertebra. Episodic pains were the ones most likely to respond to operation.

In 4 other patients pain in the legs was triggered by touch on the abdomen. In them, one or two posterior roots above the level of the cord section were divided bilaterally; none of them had satisfactory pain relief. In contrast with some other neurosurgeons Jefferson did not insist that the excision extend rostrally into normal cord. Nevertheless, in some who were cured of their pain 'there was still severe widespread cord damage at the level of the upper incision into it'.

Results of Others

The report of Durward et al. [1982] includes 6 patients, in 5 of whom a post-traumatic syringomyelia was present in addition to pain. In the 3 in whom the progressive syringomyelic deficit was accompanied by a new pain in the arm, the syndrome had appeared 2, 2 and 15 years, respectively, after injury, but cordectomy was not done until another 4, 4 and 1 year, respectively, had elapsed. The upper surgical transection in each case extended somewhat above the area of trauma at T6, T7 and T8, respectively. Although the syrinx continued upward for many segments above the level of cordectomy and the upper ends of the specimens of cord showed pathological changes in all 3 patients, they were all relieved of their arm pain. In these 3 patients the upper level of surgical transection was far below the upper level of the syrinx, indicating that this type of abnormality may not be a generator of pain. However, in 3 other patients who developed neurogenic buttock and leg pain, 13, 1 and 5 years, respectively, after injury, cordectomies at T10–12, T2 and T4–5, yielded no change in the pain. The levels of excision were at T10–12 for an injury at that level, at T2 for a C6 lesion, and at T4–5 for a major injury at T7. In this last case the operative specimen confirmed the presence of a syrinx lined by gliosis. In none of these 3 cases was the rostral incision into histologically normal cord. In 2 of them with a post-traumatic syringomyelia, earlier drainage of the cyst had improved the syndrome with the exception of the continuing pain. It is noteworthy that the pain in these latter 3 failures was all referred well below the level of the lesion in the cord, and especially that these lesions were all at levels at which Jefferson's cordectomies had also failed.

Further successes have been described in 6 earlier reports, each in one or 2 cases [Botterell et al., 1954; Druckman and Lende, 1965; Melzack and Loeser, 1978; Smolik et al., 1960; Tasker, 1984; White and Sweet, 1969]. In Botterell's case excision carried up into grossly normal cord at T5 was supplemented by bilateral posterior rhizotomy at T4 and T5. At last follow-up root pain remained relieved and burning pain in the feet was less severe. The result was considered 'good'. This is the only case report in which additional posterior rhizotomy may have contributed to the good result. In Druckman and Lende's instructive report the upper transection of the removed cord was through tough gliotic tissue at the junction of the T10–11 vertebral bodies and did not help the pain. A second transection 3.5 weeks later and 3 cm higher was through histologically normal cord. This was followed by a complete cessation of the original main bilateral lower abdominal and groin pain; relief continued 40 months later. The patient was aware of slight burning in the legs when he concentrated on it. This success led Druckman to do cordectomy in a second patient through normal cord at the upper end, again with persisting relief of the pain at over 12 months. Similar experiences are recorded by White and Sweet [1969, p. 400], namely failure of a resection at T2–3 to relieve when gliosis extended rostrally several segments above this, whereas in a second patient resection through normal cord at the T11 vertebral level gave relief, lasting at 4 years, of severe burning pain in both legs. This good result ensued despite gliosis at the rostral end of the cord specimen. Melzack and Loeser's case 3 operated on by Collin MacCarty of the Mayo Clinic had his resection at the T10–11 level with complete relief of pain in the low back, hips, posterior thighs and calves, lasting for 11.5 years when it recurred. In agreement with the prognosis given by Jefferson for episodic pains, these favorably affected pains were spontaneous, shooting, lasting 3–4 s and occurring up to 60 times an hour. The pain in the late recurrence was of exactly the same type. An unusual distribution of pain in relation to the site of cord injury occurred in Melzack and Loeser's case 5. The traumatic total transverse lesion at the T10–11 level was accompanied by a much higher severe pain around the right lower chest and abdomen. Cordectomy at the T8–9 levels yielded the partial success of initial disappearance of the pain with gradual return to its original severity by 5 years.

Failures dominate the reports described in this paragraph. In Tasker's two-sentence summary of his 6 cases of cordectomy he notes cure of another case of episodic, severe sharp pain with ability of the patient to return to work. However, in none of the 6 cases was pain in the anesthetic lower limbs relieved. A complete failure to relieve diffuse burning pain in the legs was also recorded in one case of Davis and Martin [1947]. Similarly, Freeman and Heimburger [1947] failed to relieve pain in a leg by removal of a 2.3-cm segment of cord at the T3–4 level. Major abnormality of the whole operative specimen was the microscopic appearance. Melzack and Loeser's cases 1, 2 and 4 were also not benefitted. In the first case a T6 cordectomy did not help the principal pain in the abdomen and legs. In the second case a T11 cordectomy did not alter burning pain in distal legs, perirectal or buttock areas — the only reported case in the literature of total failure of a cordectomy at this low level. Case 4, a complex case with intrinsic cord disease, did not get lasting help for unilateral abdominal and leg pain by three extensive unilateral operations plus two cordectomies, the first from T9 to T12, the second at T4–5. However, the extensive removal of spinal cord segments T9–12 stopped the pain completely for 2 years with only gradual worsening during a third year. A second cordectomy estimated to be at T4 and T5 unfortunately failed utterly to help pain extending from the right chest to the right toes. In none of these 5 cases were there descriptions of the histology at the upper end of the transection of the cords. These authors determined in their cases by appropriate sympathetic blocks that impulses causing the pain were not traveling over these autonomic routes, leaving no other source of pain than the CNS somewhere above the cord transection.

MacCarty [1954], a pioneer in the field, who has carried out the most extensive total cordectomies for spasticity or intramedullary tumor, treated the pain at the T5–6 segments and the severely spastic legs in a patient with a traumatic T7 total transverse lesion by removing the lower 21 cm of the cord from T5 down to the conus. Despite 'persistent annoying girdle sensation and occasional root pain at the T5 segment' narcotics could be stopped and effective rehabilitation begun. The good result was continuing 6 months later. Smolik et al. [1960] have also used cordectomy to treat spastic paraplegia in 4 cases, in 3 of whom the spasms were severely painful. In all 4 cases the cord was removed from the T10 level down through conus medullaris and upper cauda equina, producing the expected flaccid paralysis of legs. The pain was stopped with cessation of the muscle spasms in 2 of the patients but continued diffusely in both legs despite flaccidity throughout them in a third patient. Her diagnosis was thrombosis of the anterior spinal artery. The poor result in this case, and in case 5 of Melzack and Loeser in whom the diagnosis was likewise not one of focal trauma to the cord, suggest that the operation should be reserved for a severe focal injury to the cord. The current successes with intrathecal baclofen, if borne out in long-term follow-up, will render obsolete the use of cordectomy for treatment of spasticity.

Conclusions

The outstanding success of Jefferson [1983] in controlling pain by cord resections at and below the T11 vertebra, the mysterious abrupt decline (but not total disappearance) of good results when lesions are above this, and the 3 successes of Durward et al. [1982] in dealing with the post-traumatic syringomyelia syndrome when it includes a painful upper limb encourage us all to take a new and perhaps much more optimistic look at this operation.

Section V. Lesions in the Brain Stem

Chapter 13. Bulbar Trigeminal Tractotomy and Nucleotomy

In 1938 Sjöqvist published his studies on pain conduction in the trigeminal nerve. These started with the distribution of pain-conducting fibers of the sensory trigeminal root, were gradually widened and finally led to a bulbar procedure for the relief of facial pain which he termed trigeminal tractotomy. He was led to do this by a description of Hun [1897] of a patient who developed complete trigeminal analgesia with preservation of touch ipsilateral to an 8-mm softening dorsal to the inferior olive at the rostro-caudal level of its middle third. This indicated to him that all of the pain fibers descended to at least this level before terminating in the nucleus of the descending tract, and that a surgical section here might eliminate post-rhizotomy dysesthesias. Accordingly he selected for his incision a point immediately caudal to the lowest vagus filaments and a few millimeters dorsal thereto at which point the spinal tract is overlain to some extent by the restiform body. This level generally corresponds to the border between the middle and inferior thirds of the eminentia olivaris, 8–10 mm cranial to the inferior end of the fourth ventricle. The depth of his incision was 3–3.5 mm. The central connections of the afferent trigeminal fibers to their central sensory nuclei differ from those of any other posterior roots in that they consist of five different components extending continuously through the brain stem from the second cervical segment of the cord upward through the mesencephalon. In a caudorostral direction these are the three nuclei of the spinal tract, the main, or principal sensory nucleus, and the mesencephalic sensory nucleus (fig. 13/1). The fibers of the sensory root upon entering the pons traverse its basilar portion, and cross dorsomedially in the direction of the main sensory nucleus. Many of the fibers then bifurcate into ascending and descending branches. Many of the latter are very long, desending as a distinct bundle, the spinal tract of the trigeminal nerve, to below the caudal end of the medulla oblongata where it merges with the dorsolateral tract of Lissauer in the spinal cord. As the fibers descend each gives off many

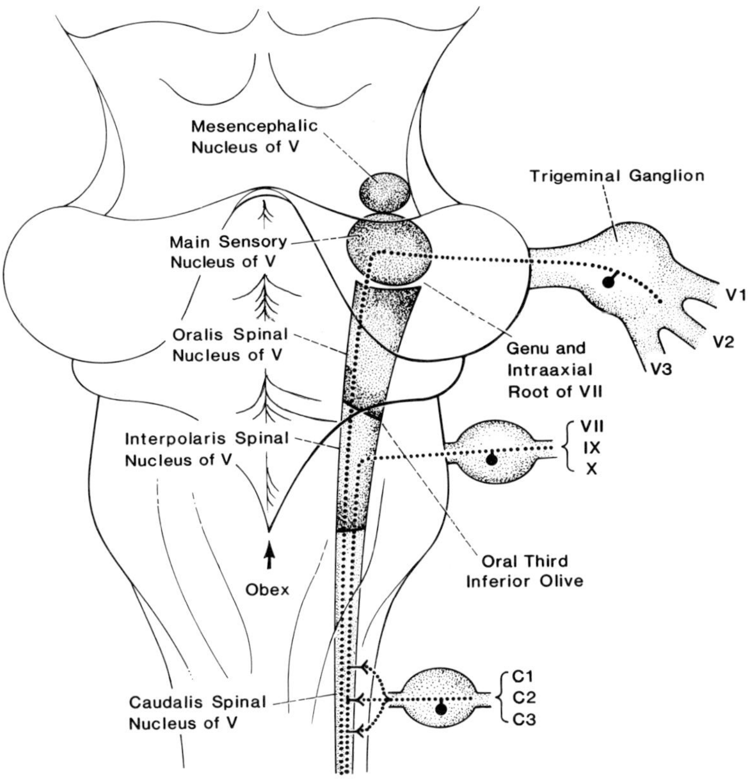

Fig. 13/1. Topography of brain stem trigeminal nuclei. Levels of boundary zones of subnuclei are indicated.

collaterals and finally terminals to a long small-celled nucleus, lying immediately medial to the tract, the nucleus of the spinal tract which is continuous with the gelatinous substance of the dorsal horn of the cord. In the medulla oblongata below the cross-sectional level of the obex the tract and its nucleus are situated almost at the surface covered only by a thin layer of external arcuate and dorsal spinal cerebellar fibers. The rostral parts of the tract are covered by the fibers of the brachium pontis. It is plausible to regard the main sensory nucleus as being partially homologous to the nuclei of the dorsal funiculi of the cord, concerned with tactile sensibility. The mesencephalic nucleus has been assumed to mediate proprioceptive impulses from the muscles of the jaw.

Winkler [1921] was the first to note that one caudal group of cells was the only part of the spinal trigeminal nucleus whose cells resembled those of the substantia gelatinosa Rolandi of the spinal cord, so he called this the nucleus gelatinosa tractus spinalis. This nucleus is well developed at levels below the obex, and he finds only scattered clumps of cells from the obex to the bulbopontine junction. No such cells are seen above this point. Olszewski [1950] subdivides the nucleus of the spinal tract into three architectonically different portions, called the n. caudalis, interpolaris and oralis, respectively. His nucleus caudalis includes the subnucleus gelatinosus, homologous to the cord's nucleus of similar name, and he finds that it extends in man only up to 1–2 mm below the obex. N. caudalis also includes two other subnuclei. As will become apparent we think the clinical observations may be more in accord with Winkler's description. Olszewski's n. interpolaris extends from just below the obex to the rostral third of the inferior olive and n. oralis lies between here and the level of the genu and intra-axial root of the facial nerve where the main sensory nucleus starts.

During the last decade much work has been devoted to the central organization of the trigeminal nerve. With respect to bulbar trigeminal tractotomy and nucleotomy in man a useful account can be found in Kruger and Young [1981]. Stated succinctly, the functional role of the subnucleus oralis remains undetermined. The subnucleus interpolaris has substantial projection to the cerebellum, and its role also remains enigmatic; cornea and dental pulp are represented in it rostral to n. caudalis. The intranuclear organization of the sensory V complex is poorly understood but an anatomical substrate for intranuclear interactions within the spinal trigeminal complex has been clearly demonstrated [Stewart and King, 1963].

As is often the case with new operations, Sjöqvist's level of tractotomy was adopted by several neurosurgeons but soon abandoned because of erratic postoperative analgesia and the serious lasting side effects of ataxia of the ipsilateral upper limb, ipsilateral lateropulsion and paralysis of the recurrent laryngeal nerve. On the favorable side was nearly complete preservation of touch, as hoped for. Inasmuch as the descending trigeminal tract in the closed medulla, i.e. below the obex, lies almost at the surface, Grant and Weinberger [1941a, b] placed the incision 4–5 mm below the obex, and the overwhelming majority of neurosurgeons followed this lead because the three major complications were greatly reduced and more consistent analgesia was achieved. However failure to secure initially or to maintain over the longer term the necessary sensory loss remained a problem. Although focal stimulation of the suspected site of the tract enabled one to delimit its boundaries, there seemed to be no certain way to assure that the relevant fibers were fully divided and not just contused by the incision. This problem was largely solved for trigeminal neuralgia by Sweet who noted that there was no contraindication to producing some analgesia in the opposite leg by extending the incision ventral to the descending trigeminal tract. Moreover, at the level of the obex most of the secondary afferent neurons arising in the nucleus giganto-cellularis of von Monakow (external nucleus of the fasciculus cuneatus) have already crossed in the medial lemniscus to the opposite side. Hence one would expect deficits provoked by injury here to be fairly short-lived — and so they proved to be. In 15 of Sweet's patients with chronic facial pain syndromes, nearly all trigeminal neuralgia, reexaminations at intervals of 16 months to 11 years after such operations revealed ataxia of the upper limb lasting as long as 2–5 months in only 2, and lateropulsion to the side of the lesion lasting beyond 4 months in only one.

Sweet had also noted an illustration and description by Cajal of afferent glossopharyngeal fibers joining the descending trigeminal tract [White and Sweet, 1955]. This led him to check sensation in the zones innervated by nervus intermedius of VII as well as by glossopharyngeal and vagus nerves, i.e. on the oral pharynx, tonsillar fossa, external auditory canal and tympanic membrane. In his 24 extensively and rostrally tractotomized patients, the great majority operated on in World War II, nearly all had initially complete analgesia not only of the trigeminal, but as well of the cephalic domain of VII, IX and X nerves, although dental sensation was not tested. This complete analgesia required an incision at a rostro-caudal level no lower then 3 mm below the obex. In 21 of the patients it lay between 2 mm below and 6 mm above that level. In the 15 chronic pain patients reexamined at intervals up to 15 years only one had 8 years later by 1950 an extensive recovery of pain on pinprick everywhere but the V1 area. In 3 others only small areas of oral mucosa or external auditory canal showed such recovery to pinprick. The hope that this operation would relieve the cephalic pain of cancers was not borne out, although the chronic nonmalignant pain patients were relieved. Similar extensive bulbar incisions no lower than 1 mm below the obex in 5 patients with malignant tumors were followed in 4 of them within a few months by areas of recovered sensation and return of the clinical pain. In one case with pin felt as pain on tongue and both front and back walls of the ear canal, postmortem examination showed complete degeneration of the spinal trigeminal tract caudal to his incision 3.5 mm deep at the obex. This suggests that V3 and VII, IX and X fibers for pain undergo synapse at higher levels than the obex. It is possible that these may occur at the substantia gelatinosa cells opposite the level of the open medulla as described by Winkler [1921]. It seems reasonably clear that if all primary afferent cephalic pain fibers are to be destroyed the lesion must be well rostral to the obex. Kunc [1970] though, after doing 216 bulbar tractotomies, concluded that all trigeminal pain and temperature fibers terminate 6–10 mm caudal to the obex. In addition to our own evidence to the contrary a number of newer animal observations indicate that not only n. interpolaris but also nuclei oralis and principalis may be directly concerned with nociception. Sessle and Greenwood [1976] and Vyklický et al. [1977] all found that the cat's rostral spinal trigeminal nuclei respond directly to nociceptive stimulation of the tooth pulp. Young and Perryman [1984] extended these observations to the monkey finding that electrical stimulation of the dental pulp relayed via the nuclei principalis, oralis and interpolaris while the afferents for cutaneous facial pain relayed mainly via nucleus caudalis. Hayashi [1985] has found in cats some high threshold mechanoreceptors (nociceptive) A-delta fibers from the skin sending a few collaterals to n. interpolaris with more passing to n. caudalis. Hu et al. [1987] raise a question as to the significance of electrical excitation of tooth pulp afferents eliciting responses in cells of n. oralis because the natural stimulus of noxious heat did not excite these cells, whereas both types of stimulation excited cells in n. caudalis. The results of Young [1982] in 2 cancer patients with bulbar tractotomies at the level of the obex extended dorsally and ventrally as we have recommended would appear to settle the question with respect to dental and probably oral mucosal sensation as well. The dental thresholds for noxious heat, cold and electrical stimulation were unchanged and the oral mucosa was rendered only hypalgesic by lesions which at first produced total cutaneous trigeminal analgesia. Later this faded to hypalgesia over the medial upper lip, nose and eye. These studies do not answer the important question as to how far rostrally in man one may need to extend trigeminal tractotomy and nucleotomy in order to destroy the all important substantia gelatinosa of n. caudalis.

However the uppermost pain fibers from V1 terminate at a lower level than those of V2 which are in turn lower than from V3, VII, IX and X. Hence the usual V1–2 post-herpetic pain is in a more accessible part of the medulla oblongata. For a clinical pain which does not require full analgesia for control but for which high-grade extensive hypalgesia in conjunction with good medical treatment may suffice, this operation is in our view indicated. The situation which meets these specifications is chronic migrainous neuralgia (chronic persistent cluster headache) resistant to the many effective drugs and unrelieved by trigeminal analgesia.

Crue et al. [1970] developed a stereotactic apparatus for carrying out a percutaneous RF bulbar trigeminal tractotomy. The lesions in their 6 reported patients were usually inadequate, and they have given us no further account. Hitchcock, however, has had better results with the apparatus he has developed for carrying out this operation [Hitchcock, 1969]. In 1970 he reported pain relief in 5 of 7 patients with lesions made into the descending tract as it lies at the C1–C2 levels of the cord [Hitchcock, 1970a].

Bulbar Trigeminal Nucleotomy

Having demonstrated that the spinal trigeminal tract descends well into the middle of the second cervical segment of the cat Kerr went on with Olafson [1961] to show that volleys from both trigeminal and cervical posterior roots converged on the same cells in the cat's posterior gray matter at the C1–C2 level. He subsequently [Kerr, 1966] showed that he could carry out electrolytic destruction of the nucleus of the spinal tract of V at this level without causing ataxia or weakness. He suggested that such lesions be tried for intractable forms of cranial facial pain. The report by Stewart et al. [1964] of an ascending polysynaptic intranuclear pathway in the nucleus of the descending V tract further set the stage for the human work of Hitchcock and Schvarcz [1972]. These neurosurgeons first described in man the making of RF lesions in the secondary afferent neurons of the descending cephalic pain pathway in nucleus caudalis, and carried this out for post-herpetic facial pain. A further 115 such operations were reported by Schvarcz [1975, 1979] under the rubric of trigeminal nucleotomy. Fifty-three of these were carried out on 52 patients with syndromes of central pain. Using stereotactic instrumentation he sought, by enlarging a lesion at one site toward the rostral pole of nucleus caudalis, to induce hypalgesia rather than dense analgesia in those with preoperative preserved sensation. Facial touch was preserved as expected; contralateral lumbosacral hypalgesia was also produced at times. No new dysesthesias either in face or limbs ensued. In the 16 patients with anesthesia dolorosa he eliminated hyperpathia when present and markedly reduced or abolished deep burning pain in 9 of them or 56%. In another 27 patients with dysesthesia plus additional superimposed tic pain he had a similar type of success in 20 of them or 74%. The patients were followed from 0.55 to 6.5 years. Schvarcz's [1985a] report describes 21 patients with post-herpetic neuralgia in 16 of whom he was able to reduce significantly or eliminate both hyperpathia and constant pain. The neuralgia involved V1 in

19 cases, V3 in one, VII, IX and X in 4, and C2–3 in 5. One patient who recurred at 5 years was operated on again and remained relieved until death 3 years later. These follow-ups were from 1 to 12 years. In another 31 patients with cancer pain satisfactory relief was obtained in 84% who were followed from 2 to 30 months. The pain was exclusively trigeminal in 14 and included lower cranial nerves as well in the other 17.

Multiple Lesions of Descending Cephalic Pain Tract and Nucleus Caudalis – 'DREZ' Lesions

Nashold has extended Kerr's concept of making a lesion in the lowest part of the nucleus of the descending tract to the making of a row of lesions in the axis of the spinal gray column and Lissauer's tract extending from the uppermost C2 dorsal root up to or slightly above the level of the obex. Bernard et al. in 1987 added 9 more cases at the April 1987 Duke Symposium to the 18 reported by them earlier [Bernard et al., 1987a]. Thermocouple-controlled temperatures of a 0.25-mm diameter electrode were kept at 75–80 °C for 15s. The line of spinal and bulbar lesions runs 'along the dorsolateral sulcus'; the lesions are 2 mm deep and about 1 mm apart. Although the dorsolateral sulcus in the cord is distinct, this groove is much less conspicuous in the bulb, moves ventrally, and has emerging from it at the level of the closed medulla the largely motor tiny filaments of the cranial portion of XI and the lower ones of X. The spinal tract and nucleus of V lie completely dorsal to this line and the electrode should penetrate the brain stem 1–2 mm dorsal to it. Placing a lesion a little too ventral will have the relatively innocuous effect of analgesia in the contralateral lower limb. Of course the lesions are distant from the entry zones of the roots of V, VII, IX and X and referring to them as DREZ lesions perhaps obscures the substantial difference between them and the truly DREZ lesions in the cord. The highly variable distance of 10–20 mm from obex to uppermost spinal posterior rootlet means that the number of lesions 1 mm apart will be similarly variable. Nashold points out that unless his lesions extended 1–2 mm above the level of the obex there might be medial sparing — i.e. of nose and medial mouth. These multiple lesions differ from the single lesion of Hitchcock and of Schvarcz not only in this fact but also in their more superficial position at the higher level, i.e. at the obex the tip of a 2-mm electrode is 0.5–2 mm away from the nucleus of the descending tract, so it is not at this level a nucleotomy — only a tractotomy.

The largest group of patients, 9 with post-herpetic pain, includes 6 who maintain good to excellent relief at 4–39 months. The remaining 18 patients fell into 7 diagnostic categories. Tic douloureux which had become atypical after treatment was present in 5; the pain was due to neoplasm in 4 and to anesthesia dolorosa in 3. In each of these 3 groups there was only one good result. Although the mean age of the patients was 58 years major complications occurred in only 2 and there were no deaths from the extensive procedure. Hypalgesia of all 3 trigeminal divisions was produced. A mild transient dysmetria was the only neurological deficit; none developed secondary dysesthesias. The factors associated with a favorable prognosis included a lesser preoperative sensory deficit, confinement of the pain to the trigeminal zone and a burning, lancinating or penetrating quality to the pain in contrast to a dull pain. If only one trigeminal division was involved, a good result ensued in 75%; only 50% were in this category if 2 divisions were involved and when all three divisions were affected only 38% had a good result.

Ishijima [1987] used a shorter electrode only 1.2 mm long and extended his lesions up to only 5 mm below the obex. Otherwise his procedure in 4 patients was similar to Nashold's. Relief graded 100% was achieved in the 2 with post-herpetic neuralgia; however, of the 2 with anesthesia dolorosa, one had some residual pain and the other was a complete failure. Slight truncal ataxia in 2 and a slight paresis in the upper limb in one were the neurological complications. Inasmuch as these RF lesions in these 4 patients were monitored only with milliamperage measurement this may explain the complications not experienced by Nashold.

Although Nashold points out the lesions in the post-herpetic patients at this level may suffer the increasing number of recurrences with time noted for the spinal post-herpetic patients, the present results in this category of patients, extremely difficult to treat effectively, are most encouraging.

Conclusions

Trigeminal nucleotractotomy either at one or many levels needs further critical evaluation before its place can be decided. Intractable facial post-herpetic neuralgia is one of the most promising disorders to explore.

Chapter 14. Bulbar and Pontine Spinothalamic Tractotomy

Schwartz and O'Leary in 1941 described the first section of the spinothalamic tract in the medulla oblongata at the junction of the middle and lower third of the inferior olive and were soon followed by White [1941] who did the first such operation with lasting pain relief. The indications for this operation were cases of intractable pain so high in the shoulder and neck that it cannot be alleviated by spinal anterolateral cordotomy.

In the medulla oblongata the spinothalamic tract runs relatively superficially between the dorsolateral surface of the inferior olive ventrally and the descending or trigeminal cephalic pain tract dorsally (fig. 14/1a). It courses more deeply in the pons until the anterior border of the brachium pontis is reached; at this point it runs dorsally to occupy a more superficial position in the mesencephalon (fig. 14/1b).

Only a limited number of open bulbar spinothalamic tractotomies have been reported [White and Sweet, 1969]. Cassinari and Pagni collected in 1969 about 60 cases in the literature mostly cancer cases with a short life expectancy and commented that it was rare for central pain to occur after bulbar spinothalamic tractotomy. They suggested this low incidence of central pain might be due to the fact that the surgical incision interrupts the spinoreticular fibers which run intermingled with the spinothalamic fibers before the spinoreticular fibers reach the nucleus gigantocellularis of Olszewski in the bulbar reticular formation.

Hitchcock in 1973 introduced spinothalamic tractotomy at the pontine level. He chose this level reasoning that a lesion of the spinothalamic tract here should provide a high level of analgesia without too great a risk to respiration, micturition and upward gaze. To destroy the tract he described a stereotactic technique, and developed a coordinate system for the human brain stem with as vertical axis the floor of the fourth ventricle and as horizontal axis a line at right angles to it and passing through the fastigium (fig. 14/2).

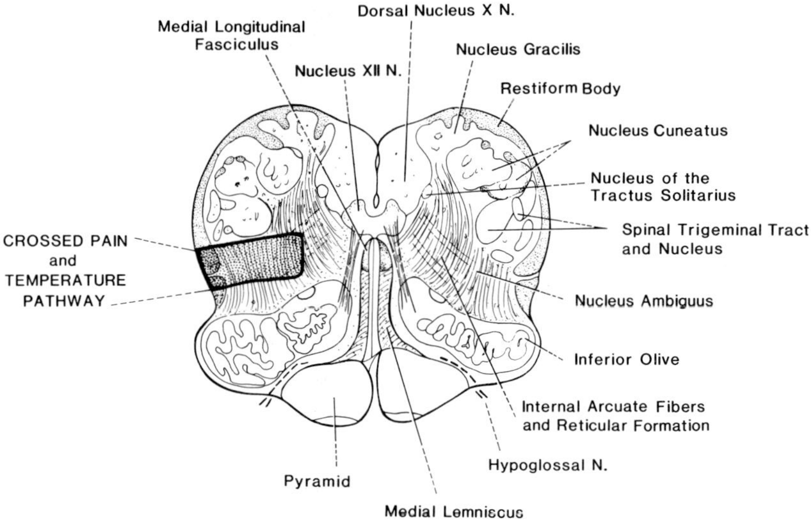

a

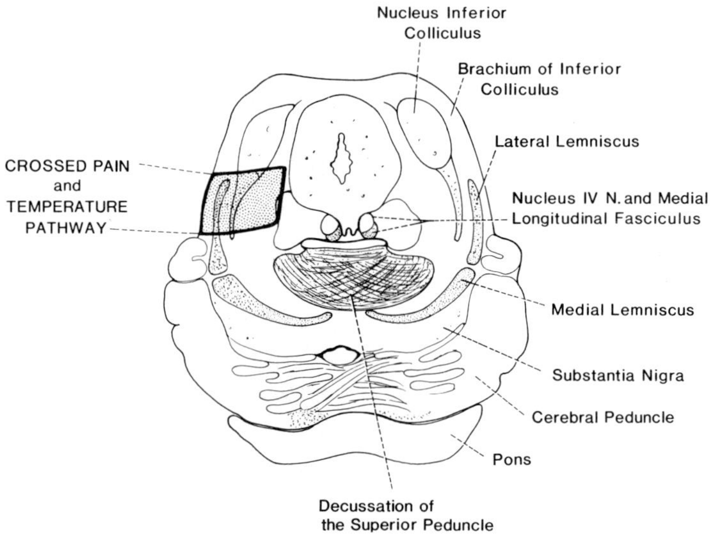

b

Fig. 14/1. a Cross-section of medulla oblongata just below obex through lower third of inferior olives to show locus of crossed pain and temperature pathway from limbs and torso. From Villiger [1931]. *b* Cross-section of midbrain through inferior colliculus to show locus of crossed pain and temperature fibers from entire opposite side. From Villiger [1931].

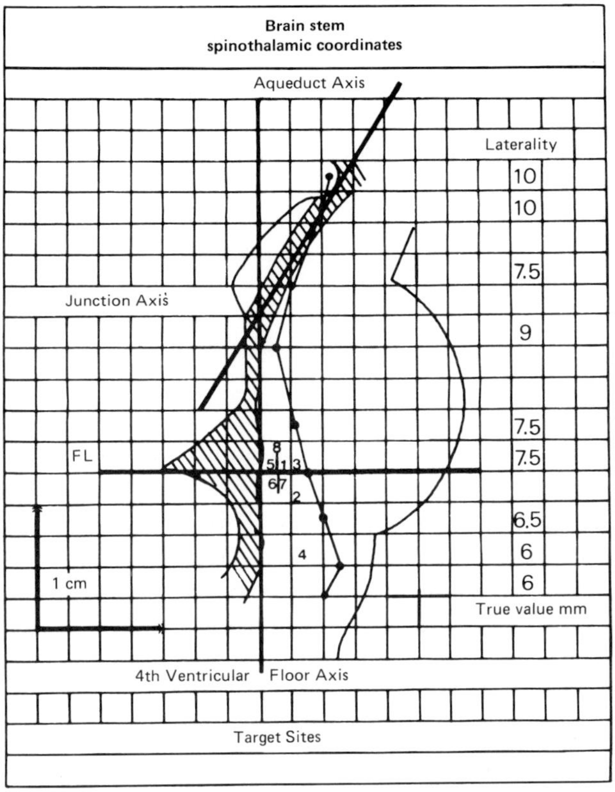

Fig. 14/2. Brain stem coordinates for spinothalamic tract. FL=Line perpendicular to fourth ventricular floor axis and passing through the fastigium. From Hitchcock et al. [1985b].

Conclusions

Published experience with this procedure is limited [Hitchcock, 1973; Barbera et al., 1979; Hitchcock et al., 1985a, b] but according to Hitchcock et al. [1985b] it may offer deep sustained high-level analgesia at lesser risk than many other procedures.

Chapter 15. Stereotactic Mesencephalotomy

Historical Note

In the pons the secondary trigeminal tract or quintothalamic tract joins the spinothalamic tract and therefore it is possible from that level to section nociceptive pathways from one half of the body. This was done in 1938 by Dogliotti in the upper part of the pons and by Walker [1942a] in the mesencephalon (fig. 15/1a). These are major operations and White and Sweet [1955] commented on the three cardinal difficulties with them; the occurrence of severe dysesthesias, the high postoperative mortality, and the tendency of the analgesia to diminish with time. They led Wycis and Spiegel [1962] in 1947 to develop a stereotactic method to interrupt spinothalamic and quintothalamic tracts with adjoining areas of the tegmentum dorsal to the red nucleus (fig. 15/1b).

Stereotactic Coordinates and Target Structures

The stereotactic coordinates, which different authors have used to perform mesencephalotomy, are summarized in table 15/I as well as the anatomical structures the different authors aim for.

It seems then that most surgeons performing stereotactic mesencephalotomy aim at either the spinothalamic and quintothalamic pathways or the spinoreticular pathways or both, and try to avoid the medial lemniscus [Iacono, 1982; Frank et al., 1982]. The spinothalamic and trigeminothalamic fiber tracts mediating pain and temperature in the mesencephalon are situated in the dorsolateral angle of the dorsal tegmentum. There is somatotopic organization with the lower parts of the body represented more laterally than the upper parts, the trigeminothalamic pathway lying medial to the spinothalamic tract [Walker, 1942b; Mazars, 1976]. The trigeminal mandibular division seems to lie more laterally than the ophthalmic division, and there is an intermingling with fibers from the VII, IX and X cranial nerves [Nashold, 1982]. The medial lemniscus lies medially and anteriorly with respect to the spinothalamic tract (fig. 14/1b, 15/2).

The lateral spinothalamic tract as seen in Marchi preparations reveals only myelinated fibers. The bundle at the level of the superior colliculus, after all spinotectal fibers have left, is tiny — only 0.05 mm^2 — with about 1,500 fibers varying from 2 to 6 mm in diameter. There are about 15,000 myelinated fibers in this tract at the cervical level [Glees and Bailey, 1951]. These anatomical facts agree well with the modest role of the lateral spinothalamic tract in the midbrain and the importance of spinoreticular system in pain mechanisms. It has been suggested that at the level of the mesencephalon the ascending extralemniscal fiber system is divided into two different projections, one taking a limbic route terminating in the posterior hypothalamus, and one taking a thalamic route to reach the centromedian-parafascicular nuclear complex. It is postulated that the limbic route subserves motivational aspects of pain and suffering, while the thalamic route is involved in the discriminative aspects of pain [Amano et al. 1978].

From a neurosurgical point of view, not only are the pathways concerned with pain of importance, but in this small region of the brain care must be taken not to damage adjacent structures whose destruction could provoke severe sequelae, such as disturbances of eye motility or worse. Before making the lesion, the final target is determined by physiological means, usually electrical stimulation but recording of evoked potentials [Liberson et al., 1970] and unit activity [Amano et al., 1978] have also been used.

Responses Obtained by Stimulation in the Mesencephalon

In a series of papers Nashold and collaborators have described most extensively the results of stimulation in the midbrain of man [Nashold and Wilson, 1966; Nashold et al., 1969 a, b; 1974, 1977; Nashold, 1982]. These authors recognized two separate zones in the dorsolateral tegmentum (fig. 15/3).

The 'medial' zone was the area just lateral to the aqueduct extending from the midline to a point 5 mm lateral thereto. This zone included the periaqueductal gray (PAG) and the tegmentum surrounding it. The 'lateral' zone was situated between 5 and 12 mm from the midsagittal plane and

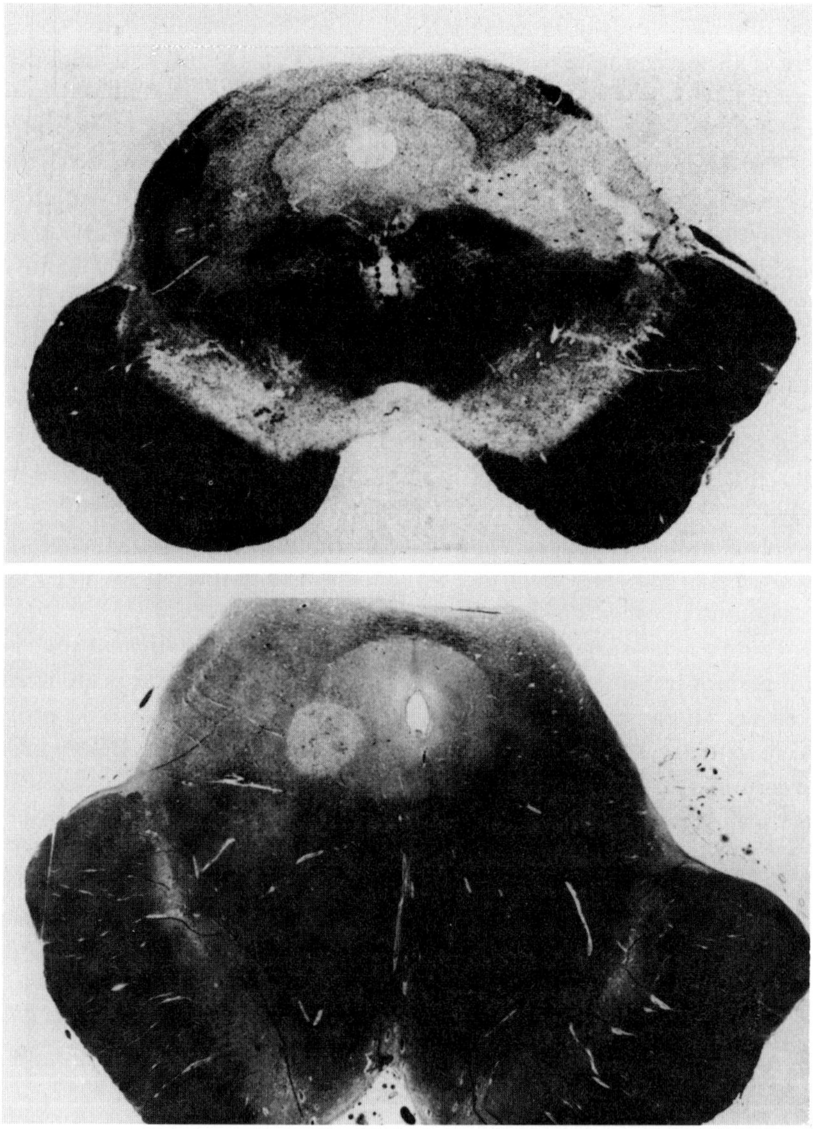

a

b

Fig. 15/1. a Mesencephalic tractotomy: photomicrograph of mesencephalon. 'An untouched photograph of a section at the point of maximum damage to the mesencephalon (immediately caudal to the superior colliculus'). From Walker [1942a]. *b* Cross-section of mesencephalon of patient dying from cancer after mesencephalotomy. Lesion probe produced by Radionics (probe data: 1.6 mm diameter, tip 3.5 mm, 16-gauge tube; 70 °C, 30 s). From Nashold [1982].

Table 15/I. Pathways aimed at in stereotactic mesencephalotomy and coordinates of target used by different authors

Authors, year	Pathways aimed at			Coordinates of target		
	spino-thal.	quinto-thal.	spino-reticul.	PC X	depth Y	lat. Z
Mazars et al., 1960, 1976	+	+		−4	−3	8
Roeder and Orthner, 1961	+	+	+	−1,2	?	7,3
Wycis and Spiegel, 1962	+	+	+ D.M.th.+	0	−1/−5(?)	7,5
Helfant et al., 1965	+	+		−3,3/5	−2/−2,5	5/7
Nashold et al., 1969b	+			−3/−5	−1/−5	5/10
Liberson et al., 1970			N. lat.mes.+	−4	−2	10
Nashold, 1972		+	+	0?	−5	5
Whisler and Voris, 1978			+	−5	−3,5/−5	4/5
Amano et al., 1978			+	−13/−16 from midp. AC-PC	−5/−8	5/8
Frank et al., 1982	+	+		−5,5	−4,5	8/9
Colombo, 1984	+	+		−5	−1/−2	7/8

included the region of the quintothalamic tract, its adjacent lateral tegmentum and the lateral spinothalamic tract. Stimulation of the lateral area evoked feelings of pain, burning, numbness and cold which were referred to the contralateral face, arm and chest. They were often accompanied by contralateral piloerection and sweating and a moderate emotional reaction. There seemed to be a difference between the quality of the sensations from stimulation of the sites in the region of the lateral spinothalamic tract as compared with sites in the region of the medial lemniscus ventral thereto. The feelings evoked from the lateral spinothalamic region were described as 'brighter' or 'sharper' and a painful feeling was more easily evoked. On the other hand, the sensations evoked from the region of the medial lemniscus were less intense and they were described in terms such as a 'numbness' or a

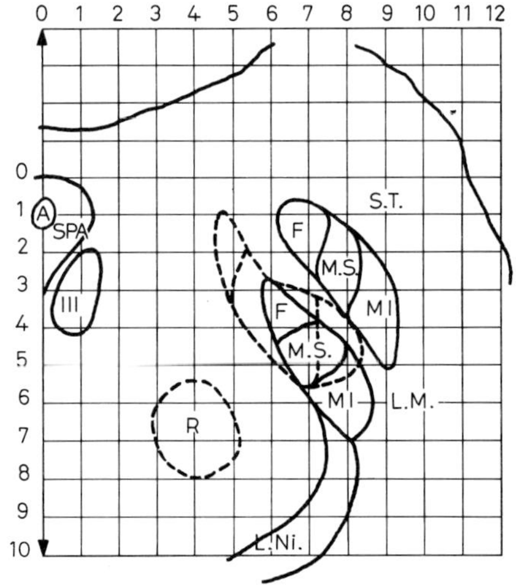

Fig. 15/2. Section situated in a plane perpendicular to the aqueduct of Sylvius, 5 mm behind the center of the posterior commissure. Location as established by electrical stimulation of the spinothalamic tract and lemniscal pathways in the plane, in which the electrode trajectory lies. S.T. = Spinothalamic tract with fibers from the head (F) upper (MS) and lower (MI) limb; LM = medial lemniscus and its topography in a plane 2 mm more anteriorly; A and SPA = aqueduct and periaqueductal gray; R = n. ruber. From Mazars [1976].

'tingling'. Although a painful feeling could also be evoked from this region, higher intensities of stimulation were required and the painful feeling was never as severe. In contrast, stimulation of the more medial zone again evoked feelings of pain, burning, vibration and cold, which were referred to the center of the body, face, nasal and oral cavity, neck and center of the chest, and were accompanied by a blush in the face and neck, contralateral piloerection, hyperventilation or arrest of breathing and pulse increase, and a strong emotional reaction, usually of fear. Moreover, stimulation of this medial area was often accompanied by oculomotor changes, such as conjugate deviations of the eyes, convergence, adduction, lid elevation and nystagmus. There were a few isolated instances when the sensation was referred to the leg alone, but most of the time it was in combination with feelings in the chest or abdomen.

Changes in the frequency of stimulation resulted in differences in the kinds of feelings and the appearance of autonomic responses and facial expressions. Stimulation of the tegmental region near the medial lemniscus at lower frequencies (2–10 cps) resulted in a tremor in the contralateral arm;

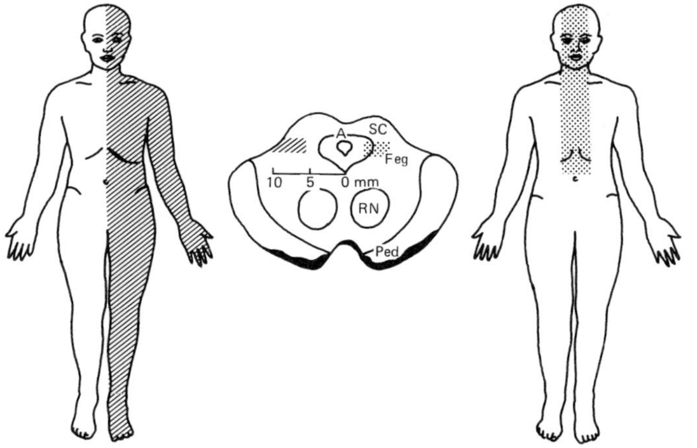

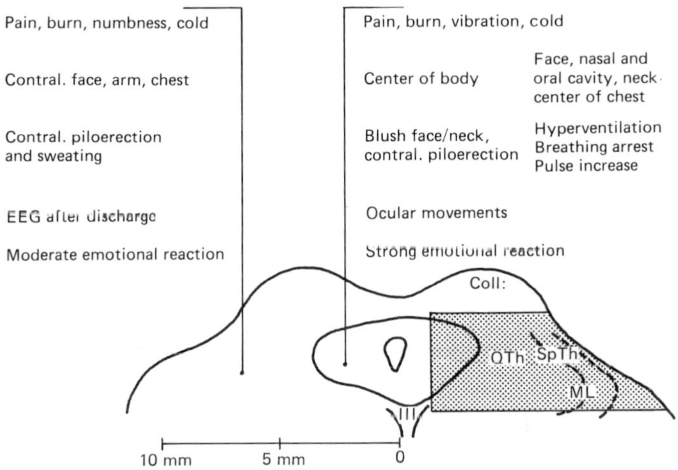

Fig. 15/3. a The figure on left shows area of referred sensation upon stimulation of lateral region of mesencephalon (cross-hatched). The right figure shows midline reference of sensations from the central gray zone 0–5 mm Sylvian aqueduct (dotted area). *b* A coronal section of the dorsal mesencephalon at the level of the superior colliculus. The physiological responses elicited by stimulation of the dorsolateral and dorsomedial mesencephalon. From Nashold et al. [1969a].

with an increase in the frequency above 10 cps, the patient experienced a sensation of movement in the arm. At higher frequencies (60–120cps) the sensation of motion was replaced by a paresthesia which with frequencies of 120–300 cps changed to a hot and painful sensation.

Somatosensory Evoked Potentials Recorded during Mesencephalotomy

Very few data are available. Liberson et al. [1970] recorded in 6 patients the somatosensory responses evoked during peripheral nerve stimulation when the tip of the electrode was located 5 mm below, 10 mm lateral and 5 mm posterior to the posterior commissure; usually their maximal amplitude was observed 2 mm below the intercommissural line, presumably in the vicinity of the nucleus lateralis mesencephali. (This large nucleus lies medial to the lateral spinothalamic tract and extends the full length of the midbrain as the rostral extension of the spinoreticular nucleus of the pons.) The potentials appeared after a latency of 10–16 ms. They state however as well that the recorded potentials, because of their very short latency, obviously do not correspond to the transmission of pain perception. They stated that the improvement in pathological pain was directly related to the amplitude of the potential recorded prior to the making of the lesion. They believed that their therapeutic lesion was located between the lateral and medial lemniscus in the nucleus lateralis mesencephali.

Unit Activity Recorded during Mesencephalotomy

Amano et al. [1978] recorded unit activity in 4 patients during mesencephalotomy. They examined an area 5–8 mm lateral to the midline, 5–8 mm below the AC-PC line and 13–16 mm posterior to the midpoint of this same line. The response of neurons to various sensory stimuli was studied, while the patients were kept in a drowsy state by intravenous administration of diazepam and pentazocine. They could demonstrate in this area, which they term the midbrain reticular formation, neurons which did not respond to touch, joint movement, photic or auditory stimulation, but were activated specifically by pinprick stimulation. Heat pain was not tested. The latencies of responses of neurons ranged from less than 250 to more than 1,000 ms. These units had bilateral, wide receptive fields, and no somatotopic arrangement was noted for them in the midbrain reticular formation.

Indications and Results

Wycis and Spiegel [1962], who carried out stereotactic mesencephalotomy as early as 1947, reported in 1962 on the long-range results of 54 patients. In a relatively recent review Nashold [1982] stated that pain in the head, neck, trunk and arm due to carcinoma, i.e. largely somatic pain, and central pain due to pathological involvement of the ascending pathways, such as the syndrome of Wallenberg of the lateral fossa of the medulla and thalamic syndrome, facial dysesthesia following trigeminal surgery producing anesthesia, post-herpetic facial pain and pain of brachial plexus avulsion, could often be satisfactorily relieved by a stereotactic midbrain lesion. Table 15/II summarizes the results of individual series.

The opinion of the limited number of neurosurgeons who perform this operation is that it is particularly worthwhile for intractable unilateral or bilateral pain caused by carcinoma of the head, neck and brachial region. It is thought that relief of bilateral pain is in all probability due to the interruption of contralateral and ipsilateral pain pathways in the dorsomedial midbrain as well as to a modification of the emotional and affective responses of the patient to his pain.

Adverse Effects

In order to avoid such effects, patient cooperation during localization of the target, particularly by electrical stimulation, and during the production of the lesion, is of primary importance. Even in the most favorable conditions, adverse effects do arise. Mortality is between 0 and 8%. Morbidity includes changes in ocular motility, weakness of the contralateral leg, and contralateral dysesthesias [Nashold, 1972]. A certain degree of malfunction of eye movements occurs with many lesions in the rostro-dorsal mesencephalon (fig. 15/3). This is usually of two kinds: a transitory malfunction, such as myotic pupils, convergence defects, divergence paralysis and skew deviation, which clear in a few days, and a more permanent paralysis of vertical or horizontal gaze. This last condition does not cause a serious disability since most of the time the patient is not aware of it. Weakness of the contralateral leg was observed in the earlier interventions [Torvik, 1959] in which a posterior approach was used, but changing the electrode trajectory to an anterior approach, avoiding injury to the cortical leg area, has practically eliminated this complication. Postoperative painful dysesthesia was a very

Table 15/II. Results of stereotactic mesencephalotomy

Authors year	Benign			Malignant		
	Number of cases	short-term relief	long-term relief	Number of cases	short-term relief	long-term relief
Wycis and Spiegel, 1962	42	33	12	12	6	4
Helfant et al., 1965	3	2	1 60 months	8	6	
Nashold et al., 1969b	15	11 9–30 months	>8 10 years			
Nashold, 1972				8	8 (av. 9.5 months)	
Mazars, 1976	1		0	152	131	
Schvarcz, 1977b	5	4 6–24 months				
Voris and Whisler, 1975	23	8 1–12 months	5 1–3 years			
Whisler and Voris, 1978				38	35 relief to death	1
Colombo, 1984				8	6 1–9 months	
Frank et al., 1985b				38	33 1–7 months	
Amano et al., 1986	34		28 6–70 months (av. 42 months)	6	6 1–18 months (av. 5 months)	
Shieff and Nashold, 1987	27		12 of 24 3 months to 5 years			

serious side effect which occurred so frequently with the open mesencephalotomy that it led neurosurgeons to abandon the procedure [Drake and McKenzie, 1953], but with the smaller stereotactic lesions this complication has become rare. Why this complication occurs remains in fact unknown. This has been discussed in detail in chapter 9 on open anterolateral cordotomy. Two recent reports of long-term follow-ups on large series with rigorous criteria for success warrant more detailed summaries. Amano et al. [1986] did 34 'rostral mesencephaloreticulotomies"; 28 were in patients with central pain of whom 26 had the thalamic syndrome and 6 had pain associated with carcinoma. In the category of patients requiring no medication for pain were 64% of the group with central pain and 83% of the cancer patients. There were no postoperative deaths and no lasting neurological deficits. The pain in all 27 patients of Shieff and Nashold [1987] was due to strokes; 20 of the infarcts were supratentorial and 7 were in the brain stem. The surgical lesion was classified as superior collicular in the first 14; in the second group of 13 the inferior collicular target was about 2 mm posterior and 5 mm ventral to the primary aiming point for the first group. The objective in the second group of reducing orthoptic sequelae was largely achieved in that only 2 in this group as compared with 10 in the first group had such symptoms persisting through follow-up. Pain relief to the extent of no narcotic requirement was the long-term result in 9 of 12 of the superior collicular and 7 of 12 of the inferior collicular group. There were 2 postoperative deaths or about 8%.

Conclusions

From Tokyo and from Duke University two recent long-term follow-ups describe satisfactory relief of central neurogenic pain by mesencephalotomies in about two thirds of 55 patients. The most widespread use of the procedure is pain of malignancies involving the head and neck. It competes with deep brain stimulation and intraventricular morphine.

Section VI. Lesions in the Diencephalon

Chapter 16. Thalamotomy

Historical Note

In 1947, Wycis and Spiegel [1962] added a stereotactic lesion in the nucleus dorsomedialis thalami to a mesencephalotomy in order to influence the psychic components of a patient's pain. Since this first thalamotomy for pain, a number of targets have been selected as anatomical, physiological and clinical knowledge about pain pathways and pain mechanisms was gathered. Earlier, such operations were rather frequently performed by stereotactic neurosurgeons. However, the unpredictability of the results, the poor long-term success rate, and the advent of stimulating techniques and infusion of drugs in different compartments of the CSF, have all greatly decreased the number of thalamotomies.

Some Introductory Remarks Concerning Diencephalic Mechanisms of Pain Sensation

Knowledge about these mechanisms has in part derived from clinical data obtained from stereotactic interventions. Before discussing these data it is helpful to stress a few highlights of the general outline of these mechanisms, as they are understood and questioned today, and have been extensively discussed in a scholarly book [Jones, 1985] and in recent reviews [Albe-Fessard et al., 1985; Willis, 1985].

The clinical syndromes seen with spinal cord lesions and characterized by a dissociation of tactile from pain and temperature sensory deficits have led to the neurological notion of 'epicritic' and 'protopathic' systems with as anatomical corollary 'lemniscal' and 'anterolateral' systems. These terms have now become confusing because they imply a stricter anatomo-functional correlation than experimental data have disclosed. Fibers coursing through the anterolateral system have multiple termination sites in the thalamus but four input sites can be distinguished. It is important to recognize that species differences exist. One termination is in the n. ventralis posterior and the immediately surrounding area. It is thought that this area has something to do with localizing the nociceptive stimulus and sensory discriminative aspects of pain. A second area involves the medial thalamus, either directly or via pathways relayed in the bulbomesencephalic reticular formation. There is, however, very little known about the relationship between spinoreticular and reticulothalamic pathways. Nucleus parafascicularis and centralis lateralis, and the medial part of the centrum medianum are the principal thalamic relays for this second input. It is often assumed that the intralaminar nuclei have something to do with the elaboration of the affective and motivational aspects of pain, as well as arousal and possibly motor reactions in response to nociceptive input. A third area concerns the PO region or the magnocellular part of the medial geniculate body. This posterior group of nuclei receives input from the dorsal column nuclei, the lateral cervical nucleus and the spinal cord gray matter. This area may play some role in pain but not much more can be said; at one time it was thought it had something to do with defining a nociceptive stimulus as painful but this role has now been tentatively taken over by a fourth domain, the nucleus submedius which recently has been described as constituting a separable portion of the medial group of thalamic nuclei. This concept is on the basis of its input from lamina I neurons in the spinal cord and its projection to the orbitofrontal cortex. These thalamic sites, which are thought to be involved in pain sensation, are all associated with spinothalamic, and spinoreticulothalamic pathways, but as pointed out by Berkley [Albe-Fessard et al., 1985] there is concern about placing too much emphasis on the function of these pathways while neglecting the potential involvement of the other somatic 'nonnociceptive' sensory pathways in pain. The many reasons for this include these points: (a) a significant number of neurons in these pathways respond to innocuous stimuli; (b) a significant number of neurons in other ascending pathways respond to noxious stimuli; (c) activation of descending pathways can change the response characteristics of neurons whose axons ascend in all of the purely nociceptive and polymodal nociceptive pathways; (d) the same stimulus can, under some circumstances, produce pain sensation and, under other circumstances, produce a different nonpainful sensation, this is particularly the case in clinical conditions; (e) although apparent complete transection of the spinothalamic and spinoreticular tracts can reduce both normal and pathological pain, often the pathological pain returns, and sometimes painful dysesthesia is produced.

Ventrocaudal Thalamotomy

Originally it was thought that the ventrocaudal nuclei (VPL–VPM) are relay nuclei for the neospinothalamic tract and therefore lesions were aimed at the appropriate parts of their medially to laterally arranged somatosensory homunculus [Hécaen et al., 1949; Monnier and Fischer, 1951; Monnier, 1955; Hassler and Riechert, 1959; Mark et al., 1960, 1961; Ervin and Mark, 1960; Bettag and Yoshida, 1960; Orthner and Roeder, 1966; Richardson, 1967; Uematsu et al., 1974a].

However, very soon after the first interventions, it was realized that 'pain' pathways project to the medial thalamic nuclei, and therefore most authors combined lesions of the ventrocaudal nuclei with lesions of the medial thalamic nuclei (centre médian, parafascicular nucleus and ventrolateral nucleus) a point which will be elaborated later. Hassler and Riechert [1959] presented evidence that the parvicellular portion of the ventrocaudal nucleus, which lies posteriorly and inferiorly, was the specific relay for the neospinothalamic tract. They based their argument: (1) on the observation that its stimulation provoked sensations, not of paresthesias but of cramp-like, burning pain, the responses being arranged from medial to lateral for rostral to caudal body parts, and (2) that lesions in the parvicellular ventrocaudal nucleus induced contralateral dissociated sensory loss with only mild loss of 'lemniscal' modalities for touch and kinesthesis. A further important argument for this view came from the observations of Halliday and Loque [1972]. These authors found in 5 otherwise pain-free patients undergoing stereotactic thalamotomy for Parkinsonism, a small area at the lower end of the specific relay nucleus (ventrocaudalis) in which electrical stimulation produced unpleasant dysesthesias which were described by the patients either as a sharp pain, or an ache or burning sensation. These responses were produced with low current strengths (10–30 μAmp), and the same stimulus evoked only a sensation of tingling without painful quality when the electrode was moved a few millimeters away (fig. 16/1).

These observations are particularly important, since it was generally believed that painful paresthesias are not produced by electrical stimulation within the thalamus except in patients who are already complaining of pain and that, even here, pain is only encountered following the use of strong stimuli well above threshold.

This dual representation in the somatosensory complex has been extensively studied by Tasker and collaborators yielding what they call stimulation mapping of the human thalamus [Tasker et al., 1972, 1977; Tasker and

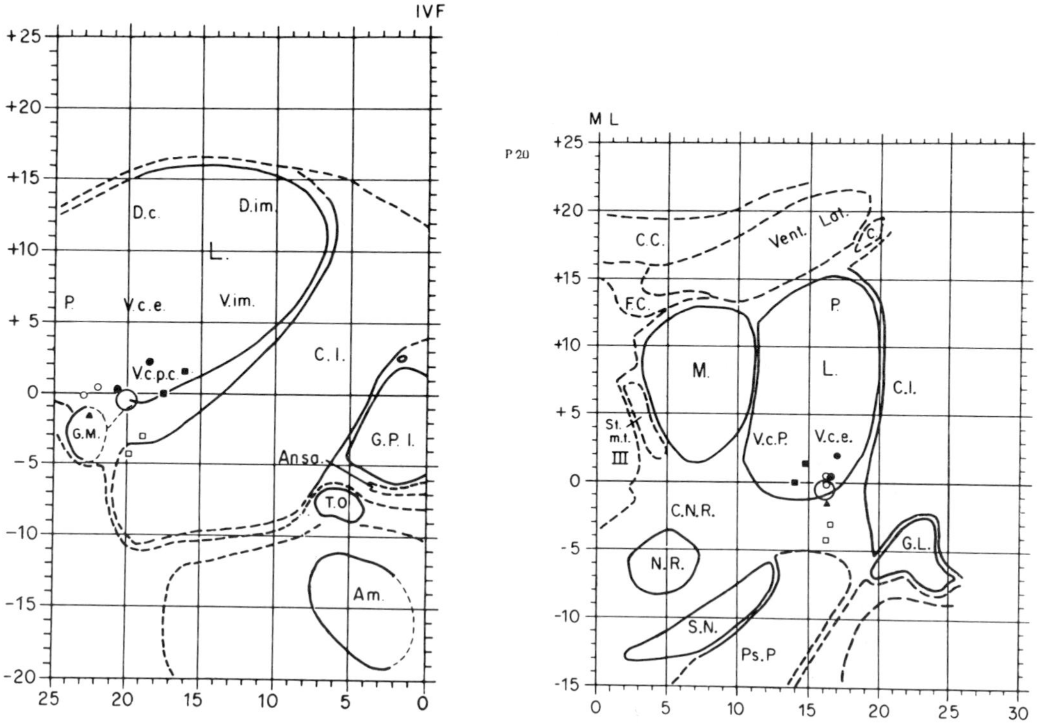

Fig. 16/1. Left: Location in the sagittal plane of the point from which painful paresthesias could be evoked on electrical stimulation at threshold strengths (10–30 μAmp). The mean position for the whole group is indicated by the large circle. The points have been projected onto the sagittal section from the stereotactic atlas of Andrew and Watkins [1969], 16 mm lateral to the midline, which most nearly corresponds to the mean mediolateral position of the group. ■ = Patient 1; ▲ = patient 2; □ = patient 3; ● = patient 4; ○ = patient 5. Right: Location in the coronal plane of the points from which painful paresthesias could be evoked on electrical stimulation at threshold strengths (10–30 μAmp). The mean position of the whole group is indicated by the large circle. The points have been projected onto the coronal section from Andrew and Watkins [1969], 20 mm behind the interventricular foramen, which most nearly corresponds to the mean anterior-posterior position of the group. Symbols as in left figure. From Halliday and Loque [1972].

Organ, 1972; Emmers and Tasker, 1975]. According to these workers stimulation of the anterior portion of the ventrocaudal nucleus, the lemniscal relay, elicits tingling, vibration, electric shock, and these strictly contralateral discrete responses are organized somatotopically from medial to lateral. The lemniscal area for the mouth lies about 8 mm from the midline against the centrum medianum, that for the foot about 18 mm from the midline against the internal capsule. In addition to this anatomical topography of the body's representation in the lemniscal system from head medial to leg lateral, microelectrode analysis of the human thalamus has indicated a spatial arrangement of the different somatosensory modalities of the lemniscal system. Touch-evoked thalamic cellular activity is clustered in the region of the n. ventralis caudalis in a plane 6–15 mm posterior to the mid-commissural plane [Hardy et al., 1981] while activity evoked by kinesthesis of joint and muscle is found in a fairly distinct zone anterior to the 'touch' unit responses 2–11 mm posterior to the mid-commissural plane [Hardy et al., 1980]. Stimulation of the more posterior portions of the ventrocaudal nucleus and of the posterior adjacent structures as far caudally as the anterior portion of the medial geniculate body elicits a sensation of warm or cool tingling, sometimes of burning pain, chiefly but not exclusively in the contralateral half of the body. This changeover from 'lemniscal' responses is abrupt, occurring within 2 mm. The orientation of this second bilaterally represented homunculus is more or less vertical, 'standing' (term used by Tasker) as it were in the posterior thalamus between about 12 and 16 mm from the midline, and immediately posterior to the contralateral horizontally oriented lemniscal homunculus, with its feet in the medial geniculate body. It occupies the posterior and ventral portion of the ventrobasal complex and part of the posterior group of nuclei [Tasker, 1969]. Lesions in the thalamic relay for the spinothalamic tract, this is to say Hassler's ventrocaudalis parvicellularis (V.c.pc) or Tasker's spinothalamic homunculus, cause an initial massive sensory loss affecting all modalities of a large part of the contralateral body. There gradually results a dissociated analgesia and thermanalgesia in an area of the body determined by the location of the lesions in the spinothalamic homunculus, while lesions in the lemniscal part of the ventrocaudal nucleus gradually result in a localized loss in the contralateral body of the modalities of light touch and position sense. Albe-Fessard et al. [1970] have observed that coagulations centered on the V.c.pc of Hassler produce a sensory deficit restricted to the area of the preoperation pain. They propose to explain their observations by the partial and simultaneous destruction of two somesthetic 'pain' pathways adjoining at this level: (a) the neospinothalamic tract (part of the lemniscal system), and (b) the extralemniscal system (paleospinothalamic and reticulospinothalamic tracts), suggesting some kind of collaborating sensory mechanisms inside the lemniscal system. The results of ventrocaudal thalamotomy with respect to pain relief have been reviewed by Tasker [1982a]. He examined the published and his own experience while making a distinction between somatic (nociceptive) and neurogenic pain. According to this review, the results of ventrocaudal thalamotomy show for somatic pain in 22 patients an 82% success rate while in 56 patients with neurogenic pain only 36% were classified as enjoying striking relief. It should be of course kept in mind that patients with somatic pain usually were cancer patients with very short survival times. In both groups of patients, the incidence of complications is high (of the order of 30%), consisting particularly of postoperative sensory ataxia and dysesthesia. By 1972, Siegfried and Krayenbühl had abandoned destruction of the parvicellular part of the ventrocaudal nucleus, since only one procedure out of nine was successful in relieving pain of unspecified type and one resulted in a thalamic syndrome. In this respect, it is not without interest to recall that Hassler and Riechert [1959] described an autopsy specimen in a patient with thalamic pain which showed a softening limited to V.c.pc. Today very few thalamotomies are performed with V.c.pc as the target.

Thalamolaminotomy

Synonym: Medial Thalamotomy

As early as 1949 Hécaen et al. [1949] suggested for the treatment of pain a lesion which interrupts, in addition to the ventrobasal complex, part of the diffuse thalamic projection system. They therefore added to a lesion in the VPL VPM nuclei another of the centrum medianum. As more evidence became available that the intralaminar nuclei including the centrum medianum and parafascicular nucleus receive input from so-called 'pain tracts', a number of surgeons have destroyed this area, either alone or in combination with other thalamic areas [Mark and Hackett, 1959; Mark et al., 1960, 1961; Ervin and Mark, 1960; Bettag and Yoshida, 1960; Urabe and Tsubokawa, 1965; Sano et al., 1966, 1970; Fairman, 1967; Sugita et al., 1972 (fig. 16/2); Fairman and Llavallol, 1973; Richardson, 1974; Tsubokawa and Moriyasu, 1975; Voris and Whisler, 1975; Bouchard et al., 1977; Sano, 1977, 1979; Niizuma et al., 1980; Yoshimasu et al., 1982; Hitchcock and Teixeira, 1981].

The evidence for the involvement of the intralaminar nuclei in pain mechanisms has come primarily from anatomical and physiological considerations (for the evidence, see chapter 9).

We shall now examine the data obtained during thalamotomies relevant to the involvement of these nuclei in pain mechanisms.

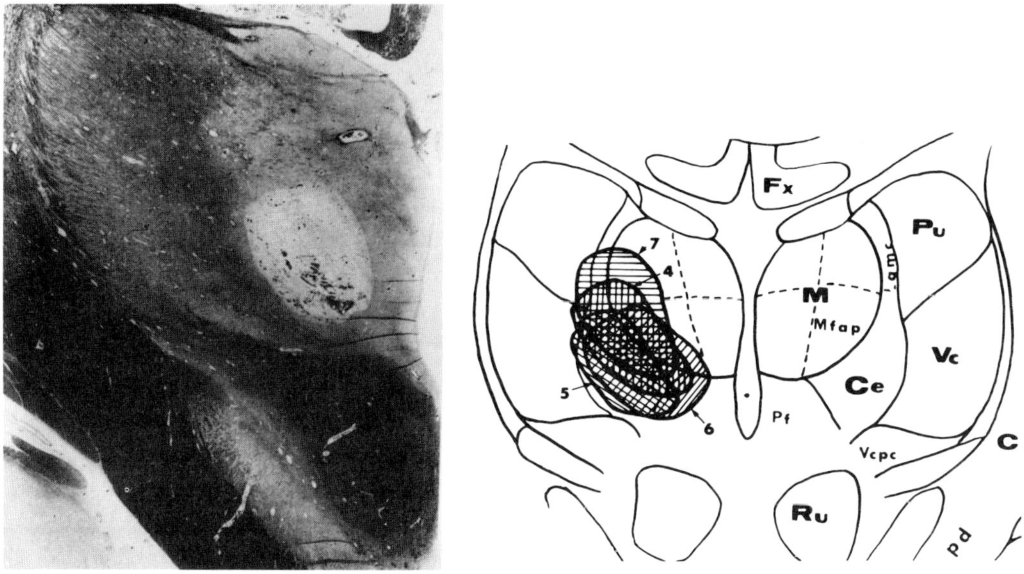

Fig. 16/2. Target for medial thalamotomy (centre médian and n. medialis fasciculosus posterior, which is part of n. medialis dorsalis). Stereotactic coordinates: 3 mm anterior to commissura posterior on the line Foramen of Monro — commissura posterior, and 3 mm above that point, laterality 7–8 mm. In *a,* location of lesion in 1 case, in *b* representation of lesions with same stereotactic coordinates in 4 cases. From Sugita et al. [1972].

Stimulation Data

According to certain authors [Tasker, 1982a; Richardson, 1974] stimulation of the intralaminar nuclei does not evoke sensation within the range of parameters that excite other sensory structures. When responses do occur the high intensity of the stimulating current suggests conduction to adjacent ventrocaudal nucleus and medial lemniscus. Other authors have reported a variety of responses, usually unpleasant sensations in the contralateral half of the body together with an aggravation of existing pain ipsilateral and contralateral to the stimulation [Cassinari et al., 1963; Mark and Ervin, 1965; Sano et al., 1966; Sano, 1977]. Other described effects are dizziness and dyspnea [Richardson and Akil, 1977b], motor and paresthetic effects [Adams and Rutkin, 1965] pain, heat and motor effects [Hassler, 1972;

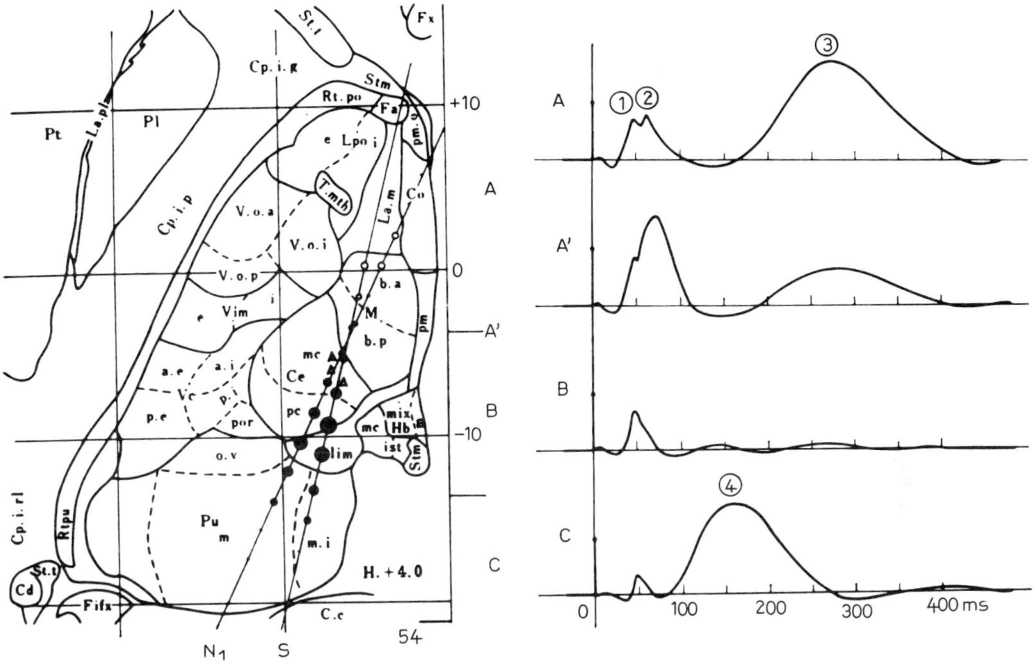

Fig. 16/3. Left: Needle tracks represented on horizontal plane of thalamus. Black circles represent pain evoked by stimulation, the size of the circle is proportional to the magnitude of the effect. White circles: Unpleasant sensation. Triangles: Motor effect. Right: A + A′ = Potentials in frontal and cingulate regions evoked by stimulation in anterior portion of internal medullary lamina. B – Potentials in central regions, evoked by stimulation of posterior portion of internal medullary lamina. C – Scalp potentials evoked by stimulation of pulvinar. From Sano et al. [1970].

Hassler and Riechert, 1959]. Sano et al. [1970] and Sano [1977] have observed that stimulation in the anterior part of the intralaminar nuclei produces an 'unpleasant' sensation which could not be localized anywhere in the body (fig. 16/3), while stimulation in the posterior part of the internal medullary lamina, in an area which ranges from about 4 to 14 mm posterior to the midpoint of the intercommissural line gives rise to a diffuse burning pain in the contralateral half of the body.

Not infrequently the spontaneous pain of the patient was exaggerated at a lower intensity than the threshold for diffuse burning pain, irrespective of the side of stimulation. According to these authors, the n. parafascicularis

(Pf), the parvicellular portion of the centrum medianum (CM) and the n. limitans are especially sensitive to stimulation. In this respect, the work of Tasker et al. [1983] is of great interest since these workers in a careful quantitative analysis of an extensive patient material pointed out that in patients with 'deafferentation pain' there is a peculiar sensitivity to electrical stimulation of the medial mesencephalic tegmentum and medial thalamus, such that stimulation induces contralateral perception of ill-localized burning or pain that frequently resembles the pain from which the patient suffers, but not 'natural' sensations (fig. 16/4).

From these stimulation data in man, it seems that the paleospinothalamic system has a role in the appreciation of a sensation of burning quality, but that this role becomes more important in patients in whom a pain syndrome develops after a neural lesion. It is not known what causes this peculiar sensitivity of these intralaminar nuclei in patients with neurogenic pain, but if the observation is confirmed, the search for the mechanism responsible for this change might be rewarding indeed. Because of Tasker's ultracomprehensive definition of 'deafferentation' pain, we should perhaps be helped in a further analysis of pain mechanisms if Tasker would supplement his brilliant efforts by an attempt to correlate descriptions of pain with specific pathological processes within his 'deafferentation' pain category.

Evoked Potentials

A number of authors have recorded evoked potentials from the medial part of the human thalamus [Ervin and Mark, 1960; Cooper, 1965; Sano et al., 1970; Tsubokawa et al., 1976/77; Sano, 1977] and the cortical-evoked potentials following stimulation of the same thalamic area [Sano et al., 1970; Sano, 1977; Nakamura and Tsubokawa, 1985]. The somatosensory potentials evoked in the intralaminar area showed a long latency, and a rhythmic post-stimulus discharge; they also showed a convergence of different modalities and could be evoked by a flash or a click; their amplitude decreased during distraction and upon the administration of barbiturates. Stimulation of the anterior part of the intralaminar nuclei, from which diffuse unpleasant sensations are produced, evokes potentials predominantly in the frontal and cingulate cortex, more pronounced on the ipsilateral side, while stimulation of the posterior part of the intralaminar nuclei, from which burning pain is elicited, evokes potentials from the ipsilateral second somatosensory cortex suggesting connections between the two areas [Sano, 1977; Yoshimasu et al., 1982] (fig. 16/3).

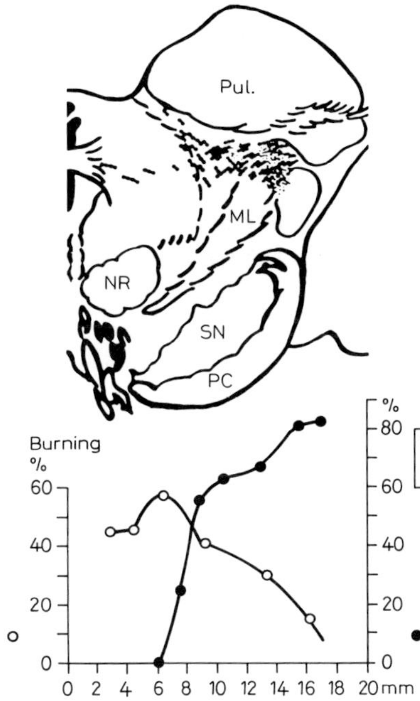

Fig. 16/4. The dimensions of a mesencephalic section of a monkey brain are enlarged to give an idea of the relative position of structures in man at the upper mesencephalic level. The fibers, degenerated after a lesion of the anterolateral cord are represented by small dots. From Mehler et al. [1960]. Below on the same scale are shown the sensations provoked by stimulation applied at different points lateral to the midline in a group of patients of Tasker et al. [1982]. On the left percentages of burning sensation (open circles); on the right percentages of cold, hot or warm sensations (dots). Note that only the burning sensation is provoked in the medial area (between 0 and 6), and that this sensation is progressively less frequent when the electrode is more lateral. On the contrary, discriminative temperature sensations are the most frequent responses between 6 and 18 mm, which is the area through which the spinothalamic bundle passes. From Albe-Fessard et al. [1985].

Unit Activity

According to Sano [1977, 1979] an increase of unit discharges is observed in Pf and CM when the skin is stimulated with a pin. Such discharges are elicited from wide areas of the trunk and extremities on the contra- and ipsilateral sides. Some units in the same nuclei respond to heating the skin, while they are not activated by tactile stimulation. Two types of units can be distinguished: fast-responding ones with a latency of

30–40 ms and short discharges, and slowly responding units with a latency of several hundred milliseconds and long-lasting discharges. The fast responding units cluster in the postero-medio-ventral portion of Pf while the slow responding units are observed in the CM and the dorsolateral part of Pf.

Effect of Lesions

After a lesion in the intralaminar nuclei pinprick sensation is perceived normally [Mark et al., 1960; 1961; Sano, 1977]. Sensory measurements of heat-evoked pain before and after surgery revealed no difference in the pain threshold [Richardson, 1974]. After thalamolaminotomy, slight clouding of consciousness, confusion and hallucinations have been observed, usually after a bilateral operation; but these disturbances seem to be temporary [Sano, 1977]. This absence of severe complications made laminotomy at one time a popular intervention for the treatment of 'intractable' pain.

According to Tasker's [1982a] review of the effects of laminotomy on clinical pain there is a 46–70% (?) expectation for the relief of somatic pain, less than that achieved with lesions of the ventrocaudal nucleus, but with a distinctly lower complication rate. In 'neurogenic' pain only 29% of the patients enjoyed satisfactory and 38% fair results; the making of additional lesions in a wide variety of other thalamic structures did not modify the results.

It is difficult to compare the results of thalamotomies for pain reported in the literature, because information about patient selection and follow-up, target and lesion size vary so much between different authors. Series from one group with a sufficient number of cases studied in sufficient detail are particularly helpful. Hitchcock and Teixeira [1981] published such a series of 43 patients, in which 23 had a basal thalamotomy involving V.c.pc and nucleus limitans portae and 19 a CM thalamotomy. Lesions were made with an 18-gauge electrode bare for 5 mm at a tip temperature of 75 °C for 0.5–1 min. Eight patients had bilateral CM thalamotomies. Basal thalamotomy produced immediate and complete relief in 83% of the patients with malignant disease that fell to 66% during a 6-month follow-up; in patients suffering from neurogenic pain due to a variety of causes, 78% had excellent results during a postoperative period between 2 months and 8 years. With CM thalamotomy good results were obtained immediately in 100% of the patients. Recurrence rate was only 5% during a follow-up period of between 3 weeks and 10 years. The best results occurred in patients with malignancy, in whom none developed recurrent pain during a follow-up period of 3 weeks to 42 months, while in pain of nonmalignant origin, there was a recurrence in

8%. The general conclusion of this series was that the best results occurred in patients with pain in the upper part of the body and in patients who had bilateral CM thalamotomy; this operation was superior to basal thalamotomy both regarding better pain relief and fewer side effects. The authors concluded that despite adverse reports, thalamotomy remains a useful analgesic procedure. Tasker et al. [1982a] were less optimistic and emphasized that patients with symptoms of an organic brain syndrome and those over the age of 65–70 face a high risk of mental decompensation.

Pulvinarotomy

Kudo et al. [1968] chose the pulvinar as their target for treatment of pain. They write: 'We have studied in animal experiments and clinical cases about the invasion to the pulvinar nucleus of the thalamus for several years. Some of the thalamic pulvinar neurons in cats responded to nociceptive stimuli, and clinically we have obtained good effects in relieving intractable and chronic pain by invasion to the pulvinar nucleus. A preliminary report of some of these works has already been published (in 1966).' They suggest that the human medial pulvinar nucleus might correspond to the region of the posterior group as described in animals. An evoked potential study in the cat has shown that cells in the pulvinar can be activated by sensory input, a large part of this via the dorsal column and a smaller part over the ventrolateral column. The ventrolateral column component reaches the pulvinar by way of the mesencephalic reticular formation; this probably represents the pathway for the nociceptive input [Richardson and Zorub, 1970]. However, as stressed by Siegfried [1977a] there is no evidence from fiber degeneration studies after human cordotomies that fibers passing through the anterolateral part of the spinal cord project directly to the pulvinar. However, Kudo et al. [1968] found that 22% of cells in the pulvinar responded to the clear cut noxious stimulation of a toothed forceps or pin to the skin.

Independently in 1967, Richardson reported that stereotactic lesions of the medial pulvinar caused reduction in pain in 12 patients. He [1974] writes that he came to this target for the following reason: 'Patients who have had lesions extending from the CM into the medial portion of the VPM may report loss of both proprioception and touch and complain of upsetting numbness. In an attempt to reduce the incidence of objectionable sensory loss, the lesions were gradually moved posteriorly with similar results. It became obvious that lesions in the medial portion of the pulvinar caused a reduction of painful phenomenon similar to lesions in the CM, that is, abolition of chronic pain without changes in acute pain perception.' He carried out this operation in 20 patients. Stimulation of the pulvinar in man has also been followed by the disappearance of clinical pain and drowsiness [Yoshii and Fukuda, 1976/77] and by the appearance of anomia (from stimulation of the pulvinar in the dominant hemisphere) [Ojemann et al., 1968], and by eye movements [Trachtenberg and Siegfried, 1973].

Following a lesion of the pulvinar, there is usually no clinically detectable sensory loss [Kudo et al., 1968; Cooper et al., 1973]. Visual acuity remains intact and visual fields complete [Yoshii and Fukuda, 1976/77]; there is no deficit on auditory testing [Cooper et al., 1973; Yoshii and Fukuda, 1976/77]. There is no verbal impairment [Vilkki, 1977] but on face matching tests showed slight impairment, suggesting a contribution of the pulvinar in visual association functions or in the regulation of voluntary eye movements in visual searching [Vilkki, 1977]. According to Tasker's [1982a] review, 81% of the patients with somatic pain had pain relief after pulvinar lesions; the number was 22% for patients with 'dysesthetic' pain; unfortunately the relief was usually short lasting.

Dorsomedian Nucleus Thalamotomy

Stereotaxic dorsomedial thalamotomy can be viewed as a prefrontal lobotomy at the thalamic level. According to Hassler [1948] two anterior parts of the medial nucleus (M.fi.a. and M.fa.a.) project to the gyrus rectus (area 11) and the lateral orbital gyri (area 47); the two middle parts (M.fi.p. and M.fa.p.) to prefrontal areas 10 and 46; and the two caudal parts (M.c.i. and M.c.e.) to the large areas 9 and 44 and 45 (fig. 16/5).

It is interesting to note that the first stereotactic operation for pain was a dorsomedial thalamotomy carried out by Wycis and Spiegel [1962] in 1947, in addition to a mesencephalotomy, in the hope of relieving psychic aspects of pain. As in this first case, dorsomedial thalamotomy has usually been performed with other lesions and therefore it is difficult to assess the effects of dorsomedial thalamotomy alone. According to Tasker's [1982a] review, only one case has been recorded in which an isolated lesion was made in this nucleus for somatic pain, apparently with a successful outcome. In 19 patients with deafferentation pain, the success score was 36%. Martinez et al. [1975], rather than making lesions in the dorsomedian nucleus itself, sectioned the thalamofrontal projection in the anterior limb of the internal

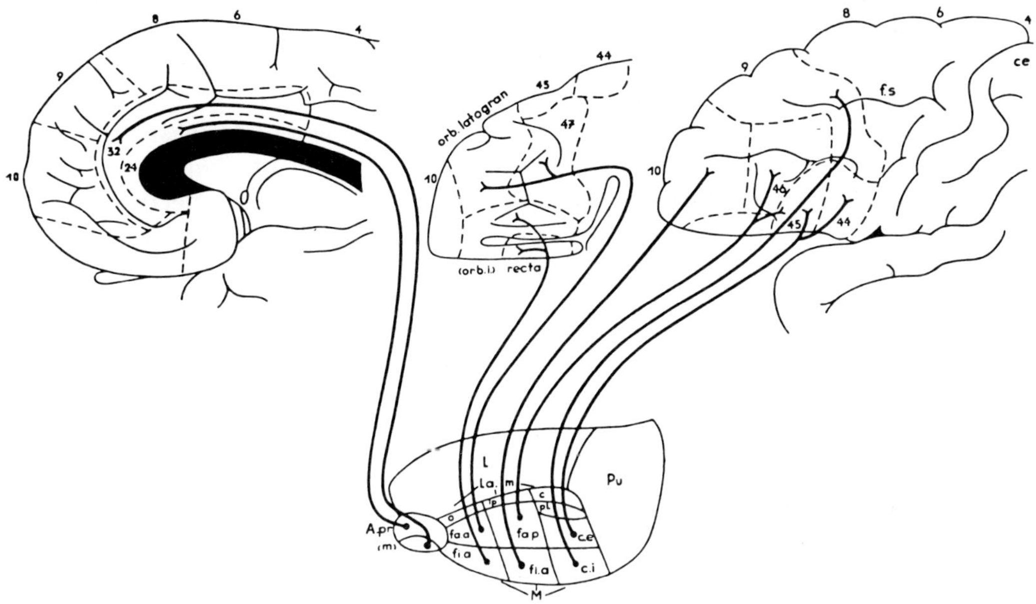

Fig. 16/5. Scheme of the thalamus — frontal lobe — connections. Below schematic drawing of longitudinal section of thalamus, with subdivisions of the medial nuclear region and the nc. anterior principalis (A.pr.). The single thalamic nuclei are drawn with one representative fiber to their cortical projection area. Areas of frontal lobe according to Brodmann. Upper left medial plane, center orbital plane, upper right convexity of frontal lobe. From Hassler [1948].

capsule. They reasoned that lesions of the dorsomedian nucleus also destroy pathways connecting the amygdala and the hippocampus with the anteromesial portion of the dorsomedian nucleus and hence the posterior hypothalamus. They thought therefore that anterior limb section would produce less side effects. They report in 26 cases of intractable pain, not further specified, 65% excellent and 10% satisfactory relief. They did not mention whether the lesions were unilateral or bilateral.

Thalamotomy of Anterior Nuclei

The thalamic relay nuclei for the limbic system in man are the nuclei of the anterior group with the chief afferent fibers in the Vicq d'Azyr bundle, and the principal efferent fiber projections to the anterior parts of the gyrus cinguli (fig. 16/5).

Evidence of involvement of the limbic system in some psychiatric conditions and the basis for cingulotomy have been extensively documented for psychosurgical interventions. More germane to our topic here has been its use in cases of intractable pain, with the intention of eliminating the emotional aspect of pain and suffering (chapter 19). Anterior nuclei thalamotomy seems to have been performed rarely. Andy [1973] has reported one case of a patient with hysterical pain who one year after a unilateral anterior thalamotomy was still pain-free.

Conclusions

Tasker's [1982a] conclusion, reasonable in our view, was that the risks of failure and of complications are significantly greater for these procedures than for more peripheral operations so that these should usually be reserved for patients 'with cancer pain in the head and neck and certain other selected cases'. As does mesencephalotomy, thalamotomy competes with deep brain stimulation and drugs by intraventricular and other routes in the management of these difficult problems.

The foregoing observations and lucubrations thereon have been sharply challenged in the thoughtful critique of Jones [1985, p. 818]. He points out that although nociceptive receptors at the periphery have their impulses conveyed via spino- and quintothalamic tracts and portions of the ventral-posterior nucleus of the thalamus, these cells lack the substance P, enkephalin and opiate receptor constituents characterizing the substantia gelatinosa of the cord and nucleus caudalis. He points out that the other major region of the thalamus to which cells with high-threshold mechanoreceptors project is the rostral group of intralaminar nuclei and not the centrum medianum and parafascicular nuclei which have been the main neurosurgical targets. He also points out that although these cells are well supplied with opiate receptors, their striatal projection is much heavier than their light, diffuse projection to the cerebral cortex. We may have been barking up the wrong tree in our inferoposteromedial thalamic efforts. The knowledge of cerebral neurotransmitters and their function at their various sites is still fragmentary. We have a long way to go.

Chapter 17. Hypothalamotomy

In 1976, Fairman published his results of stereotactic hypothalamotomy for the alleviation of pain in malignant tumors. His working hypothesis was that 'the archithalamus, which includes the thalamic intralaminar nuclei, is closely related to the hypothalamic periventricular system, and that this periventricular system is the most important efferent path of the hypothalamus projecting to the thalamus'; hence, it might be 'possible to interrupt at the hypothalamic level with a small lesion the ascending pain pathways to the thalamic intralaminar nuclei'. He made electrolytic lesions in the hypothalamic periventricular nucleus in 54 cancer patients, describing relief of pain to the point of no narcotic requirement in 76%, which was maintained until death at 2–15 months. There was no operative mortality and complications occurring in 10% were reversible. No sensory disturbance was seen in any of the patients with pain relief; nor was a change in tactile, thermal or pain sensitivity found on examination. The absence of any further accounts points to the likelihood of subsequent disappointment.

Sano, having demonstrated the feasibility of posteromedial hypothalamotomy in 1962, started to perform this operation for intractable pain in 1971 [Sano, 1977]. His rationale was his finding that this is the part of the hypothalamus to which A-delta fibers project, and that since painful stimuli typically cause signs of sympathetic discharges, there must be connections between the sympathetic or ergotropic area of the hypothalamus and pain pathways. This concept has recently been confirmed by the discovery of a spinohypothalamic tract which gives nociceptive information to the lateral hypothalamus and probably thence direct access to limbic circuits [Burstein et al., 1987]. Pituitary and autonomic functions may thereby be influenced.

The 'posteromedial hypothalamus' is defined by Sano in man as the triangle whose sides are the lines connecting the midcommissural point, the

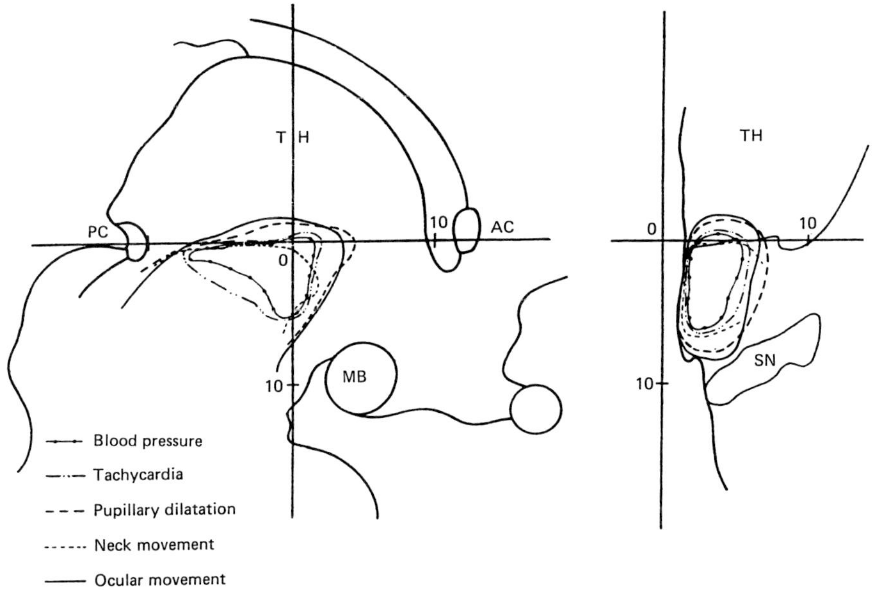

Fig. 17/1. In the lateral view at the left, a small triangle in the posterior hypothalamus outlined by the midcommissural point (0) the mammillary body (MB) and the posterior commissure (PC) delineates an area from which stimulation evokes autonomic and motor responses. In the antero-posterior view at the right this area is situated 2–5 mm lateral from the third ventricle wall. From Mayanagi et al. [1978].

mammillary body and the posterior commissure, lying 2–5 mm from the third ventricular wall (fig. 17/1).

Stimulation in this region produces signs of sympathetic discharge (such as rise in blood pressure, tachycardia, pupillary dilatation) and in addition neck tilting to the side of stimulation, ocular movements, EEG desynchronization or high-voltage slow waves and unpleasant feelings, such as fear and horror, but no pain. He calls this area the ergotropic triangle. Stimulation here also elevates temporarily the plasma level of growth hormone [Mayanagi et al., 1978]. Lesions here in 20 patients gave complete or almost complete relief of pain in 66% of them. These good results were concentrated in the 13 patients with cancer; the 7 with central or other neurogenic pain did poorly. According to Tasker's [1982a] review, two thirds of 66 patients with pain caused by cancer were helped by hypothalamotomy with a 10% incidence of complications. The procedure was ineffective in 5 patients with 'deafferentation pain'. No sensory deficit is noted after the lesion and no clinical manifestations of serious endocrine disturbances have been found. Several cases have shown a relatively low value of urinary 11-OHCS and 17-KS, but no substitutional therapy has been necessary [Mayanagi et al., 1978].

Conclusions

Such important functions are concentrated in the hypothalamus that this has little appeal to most neurosurgeons as a stereotactic target despite the low complication rate described to date.

Section VII. Pituitary Destruction

Chapter 18. Pituitary Destruction

Historical Note

On the basis of the then-known correlation between hormones and cancer, Luft and Olivecrona in 1953 performed hypophysectomy in patients with advanced carcinoma of the breast and the prostate. They not only confirmed that not all patients responded to hypophysectomy as far as tumor regression is concerned, but also observed that relief of pain was the most constant effect, the more surprising in that it could appear within hours after the completion of the procedure. There was no direct correlation between the amount of tumor regression and pain relief; in fact, '40–60% of the patients whose pain is relieved ultimately show no obvious tumor regression' [Ramirez and Levin, 1984]. These observations suggested that pain relief by hypophysectomy may not be limited to patients with endocrine-sensitive tumors, such as those from the breast and prostate gland, but might occur in patients with other neoplasms, caused by hormone-independent tumors, a hope soon borne out by experience.

Pituitary destruction has been performed by different techniques, such as transcranial and transphenoidal approaches classically used for access to the pituitary in neurosurgery, transcranial pituitary stalk section [Ehni and Eckles, 1959], destruction by RF [Zervas, 1969], cold [Rand, 1964; Bleasel and Lazarus, 1965] and interstitial irradiation [Talairach et al., 1956; Benabid et al., 1978]. The technique of injecting alcohol in the pituitary gland, often referred to as neuroadenolysis, was first described by Greco et al. [1957]. By 1965 he and his colleagues were able to report, in a series of 7 articles in a single issue of one medical journal, on 180 cancer patients treated for their tumors and associated pain in this fashion [Greco, 1965]. These long antedate any other on this procedure. Because of its simplicity, low cost, low risk and repeatability, it has been widely used.

Technique of Chemical Pituitary Destruction

Several reports of minor technical variations for chemical pituitary destruction have been published [Greco et al., 1957; Katz and Levin, 1977; Lipton et al., 1978; Lipton, 1983; Gianasi, 1984; Miles, 1984]. The procedure is performed either with local anesthesia, or the patients are lightly anesthesized in such a way that the pupils still react to light, and they can easily be awakened. With the aid of X-ray control, a sturdy cannula (gauge ranging from 15 to 20) is placed through one of the nasal passages, through the sphenoidal sinus and tapped through the anterior wall or floor of the pituitary fossa at the midline. If the tip of the cannula is in the subarachnoid space, this is shown by filling with radio-contrast of the periglandular position of that space in the sella turcica, with eventually an overflow into the general subarachnoidal space. The desired position within the gland shows up as a gradually extending bolus therein. As demonstrated initially by Lipton et al. [1979] the alcohol may soon spread up the pituitary stalk into the region of the hypothalamus and even third ventricle. When the cannula is situated in the hypophysis, pure alcohol is injected, usually in increments of about 0.1 ml and usually not to exceed 2 ml, although 5–6 ml has been used by Katz and Levin [1977]. Of course injections can be made in different parts of the pituitary, and it seems logical to inject different regions of the gland to obtain maximal destruction. It should also be remembered that the cannula has a certain volume which should be accounted for when calculating the amount of alcohol delivered to the pituitary. During stepwise injection, pupillary diameter is monitored between each 0.1-ml increment. In case of increasing pupillary diameter without return to normal within 3 min., the injection is stopped completely and prednisone 25 mg is promptly injected into the spinal subarachnoid space. This is done preferably by a lateral approach at the C1–C2 level [Miles, 1984]. More recently Lipton has been using injections in the uppermost cervical spinal fluid of hydrocortisone prophylactically. In 35 patients this injection immediately following the intrapituitary placement of the alcohol has eliminated significant ocular problems in all of them. When the patient will tolerate the procedure under local anesthesia, ocular movements and visual acuity are also constantly checked. Some authors introduce only one needle; others, in order to induce a more widespread necrosis, introduce two or more needles in different areas of the pituitary. If the pain relief is insufficient a second or even a third injection can be made with an interval of a few days between the different injections.

Results of Pituitary Destruction

Pain relief after hypophysectomy has been reviewed in detail by Ramircz and Levin [1984]. They collected six studies describing the results of cryohypophysectomy [West et al., 1979]; transcranial hypophysectomy [Thompson et al., 1974]; or open microsurgical hypophysectomy [Gros et al., 1975; Tindall et al., 1976, 1979; Silverberg, 1977]; all performed specifically for the relief of pain. They noted also four studies in which pain relief after hypophysectomy, although not the primary goal, was discussed [Scott and Schirmer, 1962; Kapur and Dalton, 1969; Zervas, 1969; Maddy et al., 1971]. From the 334 patients so collected, 43% presented with metastatic mammary carcinoma and 57% with metastatic prostatic carcinoma. Significant pain relief was obtained in 70% of these cancer patients; in half of them pain relief occurred without apparent tumor regression.

This same review discussed the results of 3 series of chemical transphenoidal adenolysis [Madrid, 1979; Miles, 1979; Levin et al., 1980], comprising 533 patients of which 24% had cancer other than from breast or prostate. Pain relief to the point of discontinuance of narcotics was secured in 71% of 106 patients of Miles [1984] and in 84% of 82 patients of Levin et al. [Ramirez and Levin, 1984]. Complete relief occurred in 67% of Madrid's [1979] 329 cases. Lipton [1983] has further data on the amount of pain relief. In his series of 192 patients 30% of them had partial relief and 30% no relief at all. The remaining 40% had complete relief for some period of time, but only half of these had complete relief which lasted for 4 months or more.

Surgical and chemical hypophysectomy similarly relieved pain in a comparable percentage of cases and there is clearly evidence that this pain relief is not directly related to the expected fall in levels of known pituitary hormones [Ramirez and Levin, 1984]. There is a lone report of relief of thalamic pain (unrelated to cancer) in 3 patients following the operation [Levin et al., 1983].

Complications of Chemical Pituitary Destruction

Pituitary hormonal deficiencies leading to diabetes insipidus, hypoadrenalism, hypothyroidism, etc., are of course a necessary consequence of pituitary destruction and should not be considered as complications. Such sequelae have included rhinorrhea, meningitis, puncture of an aberrant carotid artery, hypothalamic injury, visual field loss and third nerve palsy.

Mortality has been low. Lipton [1983], in a series of 192 patients, reported 10 cases (5%) in whom death was 'from causes associated with the pituitary injection' of 1–2 ml of alcohol. Levin et al. [1980], who usually inject 5–6 ml at a session, have secured four postmortem studies, all of which showed damage to the median eminence and considerable cell loss in the supraoptic and paraventricular nuclei. These findings suggest that the more cautious use of less alcohol per session may be preferable.

Mode of Action

When removal of normal pituitary gland was performed to reduce tumor growth on the basis of the influence of endocrine activity on this tumor growth, it was inferred that pain relief was due to this reduction of tumor bulk. However, evidence was accumulated that pituitary destruction can have a pain-suppressive effect without tumor reduction [Schwarz et al., 1981]. The mechanism by which pain can be relieved without invoking tumor regression is far from clear, but three main explanations are offered.

(1) The first relates to the influence of certain hormones on pain. There is some experimental evidence [Kawakami and Terasawa, 1967; Endroczi et al., 1968] that certain hormones, such as estrogen and progesterone, can influence activity in the somatosensory system. However, there are cases in which complete pain relief is observed after pituitary destruction even when no hormonal abnormality can be found, while in other cases no pain relief occurs after endocrinologically complete pituitary ablation [Williams et al., 1980]. Most of the endocrinological work on pituitary destruction and cancer has addressed the issue of tumor regression, but even when the issue of pain is specifically considered no clear picture emerges [LaRossa et al., 1978; Takeda et al., 1978; Lipton et al., 1979; Tindall et al., 1979; Williams et al., 1980; Deshpande et al., 1981]. Some authors [Takeda et al., 1978] conclude that it is necessary to aim for a major anterior pituitary dysfunction in order to get pain relief, while for others this is unnecessary [Williams et al., 1980].

(2) After the discovery of the endogenous opiates and the presence of endorphins in the anterior lobe and pars intermedia, but not in the neurohypophysis [Bloom et al., 1977], several authors have hypothesized that pain relief is due to the release of endogenous opiates. Tindall et al. [1979] speculate that the loss of short-loop feedback control due to pituitary ablation is followed by release of beta-endorphin, while Williams et al. [1980] invoke the possibility that autolysis by alcohol could release opioid frag-

ments which travel to appropriate receptor areas in the CNS. However, the relationship between pituitary function and the endogenous beta-endorphin system remains speculative [Goldstein, 1976]. Thus, some workers find no increase in CSF endorphins in a few cases after pituitary adenolysis [Lipton et al., 1978]; but plasma titers of beta-endorphin after this procedure show a significant increase over pre-adenolysis levels in one study [Deshpande et al., 1981]. Naloxone reversal of analgesia did not occur in 5 patients with pain relief tested by Levin et al. [1980].

(3) A third explanation of the effect of pituitary adenolysis on pain calls on a neural mechanism. Although the majority of patients after adenolysis experience pain relief gradually over a period of a few days, a minority noted complete pain relief within minutes of the injection, suggesting a neural mechanism. Miles and Lipton [1976] found, when using a contrast medium to localize the point of the needle, that in 20% of patients radio-contrast could be seen to ascend in the pituitary stalk into the hypothalamic region and in many cases eventually breaking through into the third ventricle. This raises the possibility that pain relief might be due to hypothalamic injury (chapter 17). They extended these observations to autopsy studies in which they injected in the pituitary of 13 cadavers a mixture of India ink and contrast material [Miles and Lipton, 1976; Miles, 1984]. They observed histologically that the contrast was present in the stalk, mainly in the portal vessels and in all 13 cases in the hypothalamus as well. They suggested that injury to the hypothalamus by direct fixation with alcohol or indirectly by thrombosis and infarction could result in interference with pain perception and suffering, possibly by interrupting hypothalamo-thalamic connections. These observations have been confirmed by some authors [Madrid, 1979] while others deny them [Katz and Levin, 1977; Takeda et al., 1978].

Competing with alcohol injection in terms of low cost, risk and complexity and associated with immediate destruction of the gland is the RF method developed by Zervas [1969]. Pain relief, usually immediate and protected, occurred in 31% of his 66 patients with cancer. Whether this lower percentage than with alcohol is statistically significant and possibly related to no hypothalamic injury is not known.

Conclusions

The percentage of pain relief and low complication rate following the relatively low stress procedure of intrasellar alcohol injection in reputable centers suggest that it is underutilized in the treatment of severe cancer pain. This is another example of the complexities attendant upon the suppression of chronic pain of which we have become aware only following critical observations in man.

Section VIII. Lesions in the Telencephalon

Chapter 19. Frontal Lobe Lesions

Historical Note

Moniz [1936], stimulated by Fulton's 'cure' of disabling neuroses in 2 trained chimpanzees by frontal lobectomy, in 1935 began [Fulton and Jacobsen, 1935] to treat incapacitated psychotics by cutting spherical cones in their mid-frontal lobes. Freeman and Watts [1942] modified this to transections in the coronal plane of the mid-frontal lobe white matter which they called prefrontal lobotomies. They noted that some of their several psychotics, who were also complaining bitterly of pain before operation, no longer did so after the lobotomy. This was a sufficiently striking observation so that in the second edition [Freeman and Watts, 1950] of their monograph, Psychosurgery, they added the further title 'in the treatment of mental disorders and intractable pain'. They state, 'Probably the most important discovery (since their first, 1942, edition) is that unbearable pain can be favorably influenced by lobotomy and that comfort of the body can be added to peace of mind for those dying from malignant disease and other distressing conditions.' By 1943 they began to do the operation for unbearable pain due to organic diseases of many types — a tactic rapidly taken up by many others. It soon became apparent that extensive bilateral divisions of frontal lobe white matter produced unacceptable deficits and systematic attempts were made to maintain the benefits while reducing the damaging sequelae by more limited ablations — both for psychosis and for pain. The adverse effects have been more conspicuous in the pain patients so that their reduction has been especially needed for this group. By 1954, LeBeau and collaborators published in excellent detail 86 operations on 68 pain patients including a wide variety of neurogenic and somatic painful disorders treated by 8 different types of destructive procedures on various parts of the frontal lobes. Among their successes were cases of atypical facial pain and facial anesthesia dolorosa which have represented especially difficult problems. They described 13 such cases followed for from one to 6 years; 8 of them complained of pain only when asked; 4 were nearly free of pain; one was not helped. The history and evaluation of the various loci for lesions to treat both psychosis and pain have been summarized elsewhere [Sweet, 1973; Bouckoms, 1984]. We shall point out here both problems and surprising discoveries, concentrating on the current state of knowledge regarding the management of pain.

Clinical Data

The behavior of the patient with a major leukotomy freed of his chronic severe pain has tended to go through stages. In the first period after operation he might forget he had had any pain and deny it on direct questioning; later he could remember having had it, but would state it was now gone; still later he would not complain of pain or ask for relief, but respond affirmatively to inquiries about its presence. In many patients this degree of relief would gradually give way to more complaints and need for treatment.

The relief of pain from more extensive lesions seemed to be correlated with the memory loss and other disturbed cognitive functions. Although these deficits recovered toward normal one was concerned that the pain relief lasted only as long as the psychological sequelae persisted [White and Sweet, 1969; Walsh, 1977]. Moreover, the pain seemed better relieved in those in whom agitation, depression or anxiety was also present than when such affective symptoms were absent [Elithorn et al., 1958]. 'A fixed state of tortured self-concern', Arnot's [1949] description of the best candidate for leukotomy for psychosis, seemed also to describe the frame of mind of those in pain most likely to benefit. Both the pain and the affective symptoms represented 'stereotypy of an excessive futile response'. However, more precise selection and reduction in the amount of frontal lobe white matter destroyed have enhanced the benefit:risk ratio.

Correlated with and perhaps a component of this calmer mental state has been the reduction or elimination of the general psychological suffering and distress so often accompanying the other nonpainful symptoms which are another disturbing feature of the downhill course of malignant neoplastic disease. This is a major special advantage of leukotomy not enjoyed by the normal neurosurgical procedures which are directed only toward the symptom of pain.

Two other anomalous features of the responses are: (1) the lowered threshold to motor behavior such as wincing and withdrawal in response to new injurious individual stimuli. For example, venepuncture or removal of skin stitches would lead to excessive protests. Chapman et al. [1948] did the first semiquantitative study of the phenomenon using the Hardy-Wolff-Goodell apparatus to apply a measured amount of heat to a 2.5 cm^2 area at the midline of the forehead blackened with india ink. The level of heat at which the individual winced or pulled away dropped after operation to a half to three quarters the preoperative value in nearly all of 23 patients. The behavior was especially striking in a patient whose reactive depression was accompanied by steady right maxillary pain unrelieved by trigeminal posterior rhizotomy. Massage of the right cheek had caused unbearable burning. After the lobotomy she stopped complaining of pain and this massage caused little or no discomfort, but her level of heat tolerated on the forehead before she withdrew dropped to two thirds the preoperative level! This exaggerated response persisted at 10 months as did likewise her relief from both depression and facial pain. In general, these patients complain unduly of new externally or internally generated stimuli yet tend to ignore the previous steady internally arising pain. Hardy et al. [1952] using their own technique to measure subjective pain thresholds found that these averaged about the same before and after operation.

The second anomalous feature is that after the leukotomy new internally generated pain, whatever its cause, accidental or surgical trauma or advancing disease, is likely to be painful. Thus, the cancer patient of LeBeau [1954, p. 2351], while maintaining relief of his original pain, 3 months later began to develop pain in another area newly involved by cancer.

Rationale for Selection of Brain Target

The early recognition that the affective psychoses involving anxiety, depression and agitation are much more favorably treated by lesions of the frontal white matter than the schizophrenics, led to the surmise that those areas related to emotional expression might be the most fruitful to destroy. Just what parts of the brain are most involved in emotions is debatable. Suffice it to say that a medial group of cerebral cortical structures, the cingulate, medial orbital, anterior temporal and hippocampal gyri and their connections to the deeper hippocampus, fornix, amygdala, mammillary bodies and anterior thalamic nuclei have been so implicated, beginning with Pàpez [1937] and MacLean [1949]. Figure 19/1 illustrates some of these areas, some of their relevant connections and the most favored current sites for lesions.

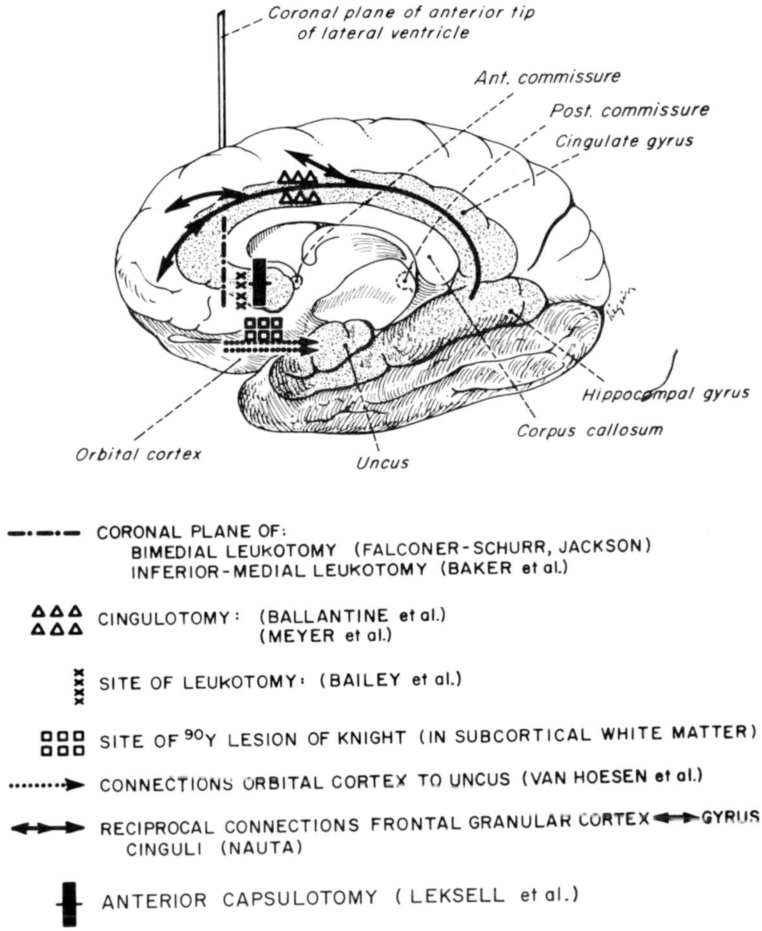

Fig. 19/1. Sites of frontal lobe lesions for psychoses and pain. Indications of some relevant cortico-cortical projections. From Sweet [1973].

Lesion of Supracallosal Gyrus Cinguli or White Matter Cingulum

Based on the foregoing meager rationale lesions were first confined to removal of the anterior 4 cm in the cingulate gyri on each side by Cairns [Lewin, 1961] and by LeBeau et al. [1948]. Lewin [1961], after Cairn's death, gave a late follow-up on the 52 patients the two of them had thus treated, drawing attention to 'the mild but definite personality and other changes as well as the benefits'. To reduce the undesirable effects and the operative risks,

Foltz and White [1962] began in 1955 to make stereotactically electrical lesions in the white matter of the anterior cingulum in patients with a primary complaint of severe pain but with superimposed major anxiety, depression or emotional lability. By 1966 they could report in 26 patients 22 excellent and good results — i.e. no or only occasional mention of pain.

Attempts to select areas for making the lesion in the cingulum on the basis of responses to electrical stimulation have yielded a wealth of responses most often of affective or autonomic nature but in some, complex motor or sensory and other verbal responses occur. Speech arrest or arrest of contralateral body movement have been noted. One patient said repeatedly on stimulation of a specific point, 'Forgive them, Father, for they know not what they do.' Presumably one would be well advised not to destroy this area. Of Meyer's [1973] 7 pain patients, who all had a prominent affective component of anxiety or depression, 4 had 'worthwhile improvement'. Atkinson [1973] selected an etiologically widely varied group of 24 patients, all on narcotics, for his stereotactically placed RF lesions in the cingulum. Some type of useful work for others was achieved by 8 patients and 12 helped more with their own care, but typically made little advance in the level of function despite going off narcotics. Atkinson joins many others in emphasizing the necessity for formal systematic rehabilitation, carried on both by the family and outside agencies, to break the preoperative habit pattern of fruitless inactivity. Other shorter series of cingulotomies for pain include the stereotactic lesions of Gutierrez-Lara [1973] in 14 cases of 'causalgia' with complete relief in 10; and the 23 cancer patients of Wilson and Chang [1974] whose open 8-cm-long bilateral anterior cingulectomies yielded 'such disappointing results' that they 'cannot recommend this operation for the relief of pain'. Voris and Whisler [1975] on the other hand describe relief until death in all 5 of their cingulotomized cancer patients. The relief after this operation lasted over 12 months, however, in only 2 of their 11 patients without cancer. Hurt and Ballantine [1974] cite many of the other series.

Ballantine began in 1962 to use stereotactic methods to make similar lesions. This he has developed during the last quarter century to one of the largest series in the world of 485 patients treated by limited frontal white matter lesions for affective psychoses and/or pain. He took a major step to deal with the bias of the general public against 'lobotomy'. Since both psychiatrists and neurosurgeons were accused of self-serving motives in selecting patients and describing their results, he enlisted the interest of the world famous psychologists at the MIT under the leadership of H.L. Teuber [1977]. They studied the patients in an MIT Clinical Research Center which was geographically, administratively and financially independent of the psychiatrists, neurologists and neurosurgeons who were clinically responsible for the patients. Hence the MIT group had nothing to gain or lose no matter how things turned out. They studied patients intensively before and after operation, each patient serving as his own control. In addition a psychiatrist and a neurologist not involved in the patient's care assessed the patient's status and the adequacy of the previous therapies as one of the prerequisites to the cingulotomy. Patients, relatives and close friends were interviewed and a full day was devoted to psychological and other testing in the week before operation. The follow-up assessments were even more extensive, involving a 3- or 4-day admission to the MIT center. A substantial series of reports describes the results of 85 exhaustively studied cingulotomy patients — 26 of them for pain. In an initial group of 16 patients the late result was of marked improvement in 9 and moderate in 3. The most striking result is that for some years not a single one of the extensive battery of performance tests and other studies revealed any postoperative 'visible impairment of the patient's capacity to perform a wide variety of tasks in the laboratory or in real life' [Teuber et al., 1977]. Recently two esoteric tests have revealed small postoperative deficits only in those over 30 years of age. Corkin [1980] has provided a summary of this massive documentation.

In the 23 years ending September 1987, Ballantine et al. [1987] carried out their bilateral cingulotomy in 139 patients for the treatment of chronic pain. Their RF lesions in the anterior supracallosal white matter as assessed by postoperative CT scans are in the coronal plane 0–4 mm behind the anterior ends of the lateral ventricles. Each lesion is a cylinder about 2 cm high and 1 cm in diameter, made by a temperature of 80–85 °C for 100 s (fig. 19/2).

'Severe persistent, disabling pain refractory to all commonly accepted treatments' was the primary indication for the operation, with the presence of clinical depression as a factor also favoring its choice. There were no 'postoperative deaths and the only serious complication was a severe Landry-Guillain-Barré syndrome (idiopathic polyneuritis)'. With respect to pain relief results were classified as shown in table 19/I [Ballantine, unpublished data]. Of the 35 patients with terminal cancer 25 lived 3 months or less; 57% of them had moderate to complete relief. Only 2 of the 10 who survived more than 3 months had such relief. Of the 95 patients with nonmalignant pain followed for 1–21 years and an average of 7 years after operation, the pain in 61 was related to the 'failed low back syndrome'. Complete or marked pain relief was sustained in 26%, and moderate relief continued in another 36% of

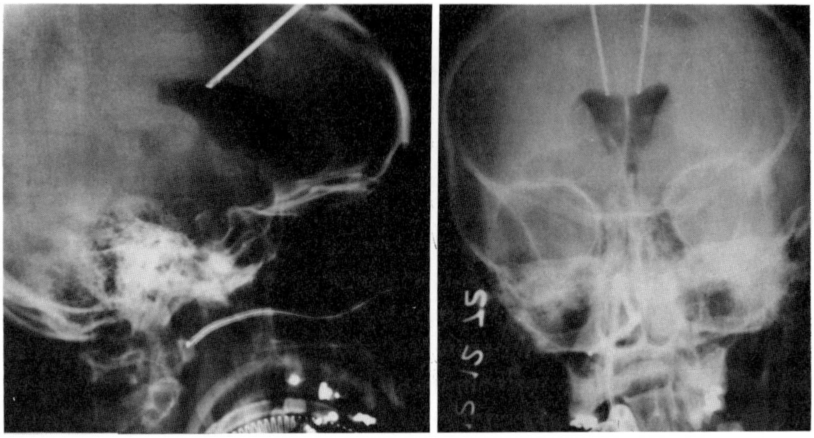

Fig. 19/2. Locus of lesions for Ballantine's supracallosal cingulotomy. Lowest 1 cm of 17-gauge needle serves as bared electrode. From Hurt and Ballantine [1974].

Table 19/I. Outcome rating of cingulate surgery for pain

Status	Pain relief	Normal function, %	Medications
V	complete	90–100	none
IV	marked	70–90	minor psychotropics
III	moderate	40–60	nonnarcotic analgesics psychotropics
II	slight	10–30	analgesics (all types) psychotropics
I	none	0–10	same as preop.
0	worse	−10–0	more than preop.
S	suicide		

this difficult group. In this same group 4 other patients later committed suicide; 3 of them had carried the diagnosis of clinical depression. In 6 patients with persistent abdominal and flank pain after abdominal surgery moderate or better relief was maintained in 5. Of 5 patients with pain in a phantom limb there was one each in the complete, marked and moderate relief category, whereas in the 6 post-herpetics there was only one with even moderate relief. In 17 others in 6 miscellaneous categories only 3 had moderate or marked relief.

Conclusions

The principal conclusion of practical importance from this long-term critical study is that cingulotomy for low back pain secondary to multiple operative interventions and/or arachnoiditis is a valuable addition to the armamentarium. Despite the uneasiness in the USA about malpractice actions following such surgery these operations continue at the Massachusetts General Hospital under the rigorous conditions of patient selection and care described, because they have a proven place in the treatment repertoire. The unequivocal absence of anything approaching significant deficit of basic function and the low complication rate of the stereotactic procedure are particularly attractive. We would precede any performance of cingulotomy in such cases by a full range of nondestructive operations.

Subcaudate Tractotomy, Inferior Fronto-Medial Leukotomy

Again on the assumption that some cerebral component of the limbic system is an appropriate target for these problems, lesions have been made in the white matter of the postero-medial orbital cortex just below the head of the caudate nucleus. These lesions destroying connections between deeper structures and orbital as well as medial cortex might be expected to produce evidence of more deficits and so it has proved — although not much more. The lesions in the largest series, that of Knight [1965] begun in 1960, were made by inserting two rows of three or four ^{90}Y seeds in this area on each side. The flat horizontal lesion in the posterior orbital white matter is about 2 cm from front to back, 1 cm wide and 0.5 cm high. Ström-Olsen and Carlisle [1971] reported their late follow-up on 210 of these psychiatric patients, 150 of whom were interviewed along with their relatives. Follow-up was at 2–6 years in 100 of them. There were only 4 of the 150 who developed 'troublesome, lasting behavioral change'. A still later follow-up of this group by Goktepe et al. [1975] revealed that none of the side effects was sufficient to cause incapacity. Nor did this occur when supplemental ^{90}Y lesions were made later [Bartlett and Bridges, 1977].

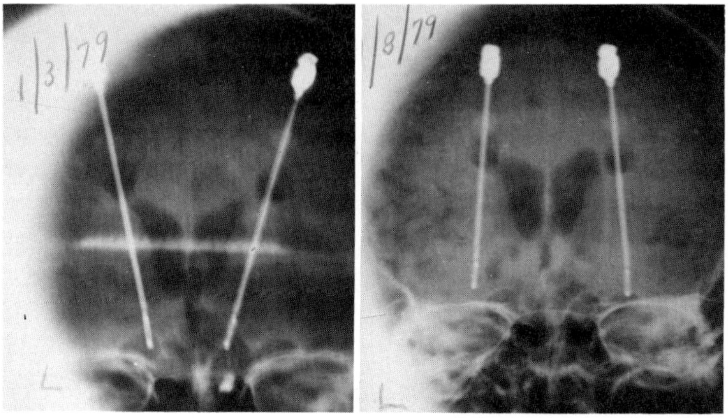

Fig. 19/3. Locus of lesions for subcaudate tractotomy. *a* Site of initial pair of lesions — electrode 1 cm long. *b* Site of second pair of lateral lesions — if needed. From Sweet et al. [1982].

Sweet et al. [1982] have made RF lesions in the subcaudate region because of their immediate effect in contrast to the slower acting ^{90}Y. The hope was that this lesion site would yield more lasting relief than cingulotomy in the 35 cancer patients so treated. Initially 2 pairs of lesions are made at the subcaudate sites of figure 19/3a adjoining medial orbital cortex. If these did not suffice a unilateral or bilateral lesion was made more laterally as shown in figure 19/3b. A second open operation is not necessary, the electrodes being introduced in the radiographic suite through the closed scalp incisions. The sicker the patient the fewer lesions needed for relief. The procedure was not accepted by many patients and their families until the patient was desperate for relief of pain and near death. In general these patients were all too ill and deteriorating too rapidly for it to be fruitful or feasible for the Teuber-Corkin group to study them. When clinical relief occurred, not only was focal pain of organic origin but psychological distress as well was allayed. Flattening of affect, lethargy and mental changes beyond a minor degree did not occur except in 2 of the 3 patients in whom we made a third pair of lesions. Thus, two intelligent, critical sisters of one patient noted, as evidence of personality change in him after operation, that he was no longer diffident about speaking to them without his dentures or using a urinal beneath the bed clothes in their presence as he would have been before his tractotomy. However, they warmly agreed that this was a small price to pay for his relief from pain. Another favorable feature is the abruptness with which the massive doses of narcotics can be stopped with no withdrawal symptoms. In the 4 patients who were so ill that death occurred in less than 2 weeks appraisal of pain was uncertain, but in the other 31 whose status could be assessed 22 (71%) had good to excellent relief after the last operation. This persisted until death or terminal stupor in 17 of the 22. By good relief we mean that the patients took little or no analgesics even though they might describe pain on direct question. The patient who lived the longest had excellent relief for the first year, but used percodan for her terminal 3.5 months.

We are presently using intrathecal or intraventricular morphine for this group of patients but Gybels has employed RF subcaudate tractotomy for intractable atypical facial neuralgia. He makes a more complete destruction of the medial orbital white matter by inserting the electrode through the low forehead parallel to these fibers similar to the ^{90}Y lesions.

Conclusions

Earlier conclusions were: 'that the patients leukotomized for pain seem to suffer much more deficit than those leukotomized for psychosis' [White and Sweet, 1969, p. 835]. This turns out to be wrong for appropriately placed and circumscribed lesions, which may be gratifyingly beneficial.

Chapter 20. Pre- and Postcentral Gyrectomy

Two distinguished groups of investigators, Head and Holmes [1911] and Penfield and Jasper [1954], concluded that the cerebral hemispheres were relatively unimportant in the mediation of pain. Massive documentation has been assembled from many lines of evidence proving that the reverse is true; much of this was cited by Sweet [1982a]. In fact, not only both somatic sensory areas I and II have been shown to be involved in pain perception, but the plasticity of the brain is such that nearby areas in primary and secondary motor and supplementary sensory cortex have all been shown on stimulation of normal cerebral cortex in persons afflicted with disabling chronic pain to give rise to pain in the affected parts (fig. 20/1) [Woolsey et al., 1979]. This is probably the reason for the high percentage of failures of postcentral gyrectomy of somatic sensory area I to give relief. Of 30 early successes in 38

Fig. 20/1. Diagram of responses from cerebral cortex evoked at operation. Pain in phantom leg amputated above knee. Heavy broken line to right marks anterior limit of exposure; heavy continuous curving line to left of this is central sulcus; thin curving line to left of this is postcentral sulcus; heavy continuous horizontal line is superomedial border of hemisphere; thin curving line above this is sulcus cinguli. Monopolar stimulation of the 3 points related to the foot all caused sensations in the phantom like her clinical phantom pain. From the more caudal point on the medial wall was evoked pain in the medial side of the sole. From the point just rostral to this, she had less severe pain on the lateral side of the foot. From the point at the junction of medial and superolateral cerebral surfaces, she had pain 'just like somebody took a knife and slit the center of the sole'. It is noteworthy that all five of the responsive points in the top left of the diagram lay behind the expected extent of Brodmann's areas 3, 1, and 2. From a fourth point, the most anterior in the diagram on the medial surface of the cortex, there occurred flexion of the stump at the hip, a sense of flexion at the phantom knee and of plantar flexion of the phantom foot plus a 'pain, mildly like the usual pain' in the phantom foot. Inset on smaller scale: o shows sites of monopolar stimulation. From Woolsey et al. [1979]

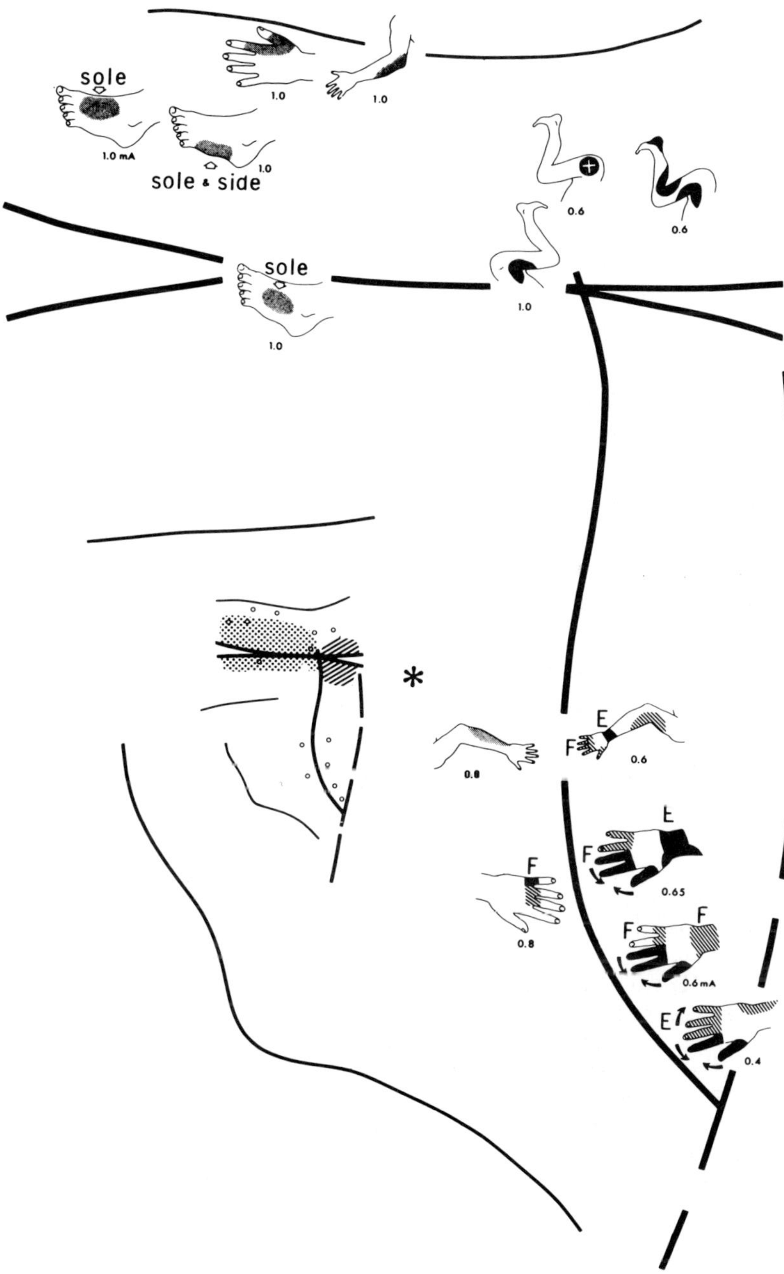
sole
1.0
1.0
1.0 mA
1.0
sole & side
0.6
0.6
sole
1.0
1.0
*
E
F
0.6
0.8
E
F
0.65
F
0.8
F
F
0.6 mA
E
0.4

cases from 23 centers only 7 persisted with relief of pain at 10 or more months [White and Sweet, 1969, pp.835–842]. Only in the rare cases of a painful cerebral scar involving sensory cortex is a resection likely to give sustained benefits. Lewin and Phillip's [1952] case 1 is an example of pain relief maintained at 4 years.

There is, however, a better chance of relief if all or both motor and sensory areas I and II can be removed. This is possible without disfiguring motor deficit in the face and has been reported by Lende et al. [1971] in 2 cases. In one, burning facial pain following a brain stem stroke was not relieved by total trigeminal rhizotomy, but remained relieved after the corticectomy for the 20 months until death from a heart attack. In the second case anesthesia dolorosa following trigeminal rhizotomy for trigeminal neuralgia was not helped by frontal lobotomy but the corticectomy stopped the pain at once for the 20 months of follow-up. In both cases the cortical removal extended up to the border of the motor and sensory representation of the hand area and down to the Sylvian fissure with excision of the operculi of the pre- and postcentral gyri so that the insular gyri were exposed. The pain in both patients was left-sided so that the postoperative dysarthria in both was transient.

We have found only one other report of a patient thus treated [Sano, 1977]. His left facial pain due to cancer was poorly relieved by trigeminal rhizotomy and for only 6 months by 'bilateral stereotaxic destruction of the CM-Pf complex'. A corticectomy similar to that of Lende included some of the hand area and yielded 'a marked decrease in the pain' with no new sensory or motor deficit. The patient died 5 months later.

Conclusions

Three cases of pre- and postcentral gyrectomy with pain relief are encouraging but too few upon which to base a recommendation, especially when the successful surgeons have themselves described no more.

Section IX. Lesions in the Autonomic Nervous System

Chapter 21. Sympathectomy for Pain

Introduction

At present sympathetic denervation for pain is carried out at three main sites: the limbs, the heart, and the abdominal viscera. An at least tentative determination of the probability of pain relief by such denervation is achievable by the accessibility in all of these areas to the tactic of repeated transitory anesthetic blocks in conjunction with placebo blocks. These may not only establish the essential role of the sympathetic pathway in genesis of the pain but upon repetition of effective blocks one may actually stop the pain and obviate the need for destructive surgery. The increasing knowledge of sympathetic blocking pharmaceuticals and new methods of applying them are decreasing the need for operative sympathectomy.

Sympathectomy of Limbs

Painful disorders in the limbs are the commonest of those for which sympathectomy is indicated. These include causalgia, (reflex) sympathetic dystrophy or Sudeck's atrophy, and painful ischemic states of vascular occlusive disorders.

Causalgia

This word may be translated as 'burning pain' and was introduced by Mitchell [1872] as his term for the sharply limited dramatic syndrome of intense pain coming on after a small minority of the injuries to peripheral nerves. His patients were wounded soldiers in the United States Civil War. In general, it is missile injuries to major peripheral nerves in the limbs which have been the principal causes of 'major causalgia'.

Leriche [1939] is the first to conceive that the pain has its origin in the sympathetic nervous system. He considered vasomotor abnormalities to be the main cause of the pain and advocated through the years high periarterial sympathectomy. He cites at least 18 other surgeons who joined him in reporting many cures of causalgia by such an operation in soldiers wounded in World War I. However, removal of the appropriate portion of the sympathetic chain has since then become the most definitive treatment because of its more complete sympathetic denervation and correspondingly higher success rate. The first three case reports all came independently from Flothow [1930], Pieri [1930], and Spurling [1930].

Clinical Features. Although commonly the pain is described as burning, this has little diagnostic value because of the frequency with which pains with a wide variety of causes are so described. Moreover, in causalgia such adjectives as 'throbbing', 'aching', 'pressure', 'knife-like stabbing' and 'twisting, crushing' were used in from 10 to 48% of the 52 patients of Kirklin et al. [1947]. The word 'burning', however, was used in 89% of their patients to describe the pain. This appears in the overwhelming majority of the patients within 24 h of the injury. The worst pain is likely to be in the hand or foot although the cause of the wound is usually more proximal. The pain, spontaneous and persistent, may attain extreme severity and cause such amazing behavior that the physician is likely to regard it as unreasonably exaggerated. For instance, the entire affected limb will be insistently held immobile and any examination of the part may be resisted. Frequently, the patient applies cold wet cloths or less often warm cloths to the painful area of the hand or foot. In a few patients either warmth or cold worsens the pain. Any sensory stimulus in the extreme case may exacerbate the pain so that the afflicted person becomes a recluse, avoiding any light touch, vibration, even a loud sound or bright light. Emotional or other psychic stimuli may join minimal physical stimuli in becoming intolerable. Not only stressful or neutral stimuli but even those which are normally pleasurable such as enjoyment of a television program or a book may worsen the pain. Spread of the pain up into the forearm or leg and well beyond the territory of the injured nerve or nerves may occur as the disorder worsens. In those in whom the clinical picture is of much less devastating intensity, the expression minor causalgia has been used.

If the wound initially provokes numbness, the pain may not appear until the numbness goes away hours or days later. The pain came on in the first 3 days in 83% of Barnes' [1954] 48 patients. The onset was instantaneous in about half of Mayfield's (1951) 105 patients. Although Barnes described a slow spontaneous improvement of the pain in some patients, he, Leriche [1939], Livingston [1943], and many others point out that the the pain may continue for many years. Sunderland [1976] is alone in stating that the pain usually 'subsides and vanishes' within 6 months, rarely persisting for more than a year. When the pain is severe and worsening, nearly all authors recommend early aggressive treatment.

The vascular changes in the limb which led Leriche to implicate the sympathetic nervous system may be of either vasodilator or vasoconstrictor character. Thus, the limb may be either warm and pink or cold and mottled blue. The initial state may be of vasodilatation for days or weeks, succeeded then by a vasoconstricted appearance. Trophic changes in the untreated patient include dry scaly skin, stiffening of the joints, thin tapering fingers, uncut nails and increased hairiness or loss of hair over involved parts. Sweating may likewise vary from anhidrosis to extreme hyperhidrosis. Although there is no correlation between skin temperature and degree of sweating, on the one hand, with a sense of burning, on the other hand, the severity of the vasomotor and trophic changes tends to parallel that of the pain.

Although hypersensitivity may preclude a sensory and motor examination, once effective treatment has been instituted one finds that the syndrome developed in the great majority only after partial nerve injuries. Thus, Carayon and Bourrel [1963] found only 17% total nerve sections in their 150 cases and Barnes had none in his 48 cases. Since injury of more than one nerve appears to predispose to the syndrome, the causative wounds are more likely to involve the proximal neurovascular bundle in the arm or the thigh.

The features of the pain of spontaneity, severity and remarkable aggravation by physical and especially psychological stimuli do not suffice to make the diagnosis. This requires the crucial diagnostic criterion of relief by proven blockade of the appropriate sympathetic pathways. As in all other forms of diagnostic block, one is well advised to repeat this and accompany it by at least one placebo block. The latter is likely to give less complete relief for a shorter period. The simplest objective test for completeness of the block is the measurement of the skin potential response (psychogalvanic or sympathogalvanic reflex). Chemical tests (starch, iodine or quinazarin) for anhidrosis throughout the limb provide more complete information but are more cumbersome. If a successful sympathetic block does not stop or greatly reduce the pain, many of us do not use the diagnostic term causalgia; some other pathogenesis, such as direct irritation of somatic afferent fibers related to the lesion, seems more likely. This has been developed in great detail by Campbell et al. [1988] in a thoughtful study concerned with the painful sequelae of nerve injury. Ochoa et al. [1987] have described a 'specific neuropathic pain entity' in a limb with vasomotor features in which warming aggravates both spontaneous and induced pain and a sympathetic block by warming the limb actually worsens the pain. The mechanism of the pain appears related to antidromic release of a neurotransmitter (perhaps substance P) leading to sensitization of nociceptors. We classify the pain on the basis of the principal sympathetic pathogenesis because this determines the treatment and as well because some patients will have in addition to the primary sympathetic abnormality, some other additional cause and require some other form of treatment.

Causalgia occurs in only 2–5% of the peripheral nerve injuries in wartime.

Psychological Factors. A predisposition to autonomic disturbances or an unstable personality are found only infrequently in a study of the pre-injury personalities of these military personnel. This is correlated with a relatively prompt return to duty as soon as the pain has been relieved. A temperamental predisposition to this syndrome seems to be more likely after civilian injuries and illness as noted under sympathetic dystrophy. The syndrome can rarely be simulated by predominantly psychogenic mechanisms, as was graphically demonstrated in a detailed case report of Lidz and Payne [1945]. Distress of a young soldier over a judgment that he had deliberately shot himself through the palm of his right hand led to the development of a remarkable, full-blown picture of causalgia of the limb. An astute psychiatrist discovered the patient's anxiety that he had unintentionally disgraced himself and psychological and physiotherapeutic support resulted in prompt subsidence of the pain and the florid objective signs.

Local Procedures. Perineural infusions of lidocaine with epinephrine into trigger or irritated areas at the site of the injury have relieved the pain when such injections are continued every few hours for several weeks if necessary. The most encouraging reports of this maneuver have been those of Omer and Thomas [1971] who said that 14 of their 17 patients thus treated had had satisfying results. The remainder of their 70 patients, however, have not had areas of irritation at the site of injury and have been treated by other methods. In general, the results of local neurolysis, repair of the damaged nerve segments, resection of occluded arteries or radiotherapy have been grossly inferior to those of sympathectomy.

Sympathetic Blocks in Diagnosis and Treatment. One of the simplest ways to achieve general sympathetic blockade is to give phenoxybenzamine. This drug is about 100 times as potent a blocker of adrenergic receptors in the postsynaptic (alpha-1) category as it is of the presynaptic (alpha-2) type. It has long been known that this produces 'an irreversible and insurmountable type of blockade' when given frequently by mouth [Gilman et al., 1980]. Only recently has this agent been given a clinical trial — in 40 consecutive cases of causalgia from war wounds in Lebanon [Ghostine et al., 1984]. Enough detail is given to support the diagnosis of typical causalgia; in this group the pain came on within 2 days in all but 4 cases. The median nerve alone or with other nerves in the upper limb was involved in 14 cases, the sciatic nerve in 12, the brachial plexus in 7, the cauda equina in 5 and the greater occipital nerve in 2 cases. The doses began at 10 mg 3 times per day gradually increasing to a maximum of 120 mg/day if needed — a level required by only 4 patients. 'Total resolution of causalgic pain was achieved in all cases within 18 days', whether they were treated early or weeks after the injury. Full doses needed to be continued for only 6 weeks; the dose was then slowly tapered with recurrence of pain in only 4 of the cases. Resumption of the effective dose restored the relief. At follow-up of 6 months to 6 years relief has been maintained in all 40 cases. The complication of orthostatic hypotension in 17 cases required the wearing of leg stockinettes in 8 or an abdominal girdle only during the treatment in another 8 patients.

Sympathetic Trunk. Diagnostic blocks at the stellate ganglion or the lumbar sympathetic trunk may become effective treatment in many of the patients with less severe pain. Bonica [1979] found satisfactory lasting relief of pain from a succession of sympathetic blocks reported in 10 of 17 publications in 18–25% of the cases. The remaining seven articles report that permanent relief from such blocks was only rarely occurring. Rasmussen and Freedman [1946] have probably disclosed the basis for this discrepancy inasmuch as their patients in moderate pain — 48 in number — achieved satisfactory relief in all but 10 of the patients by one or several sympathetic blocks. However, in their 43 patients with severe pain only 2 had sustained relief long outlasting that at the height of the block.

Intravenous Regional Sympathetic Block. A major contribution in the form of a more lasting and localized type of sympathetic block was introduced by Hannington-Kiff in 1974. He demonstrated its clinical utility in a series of articles [1974, 1977, 1979, 1982, 1984]. Despite this contribution winning for him [1980] the Jacksonian Prize of the Royal College of Surgeons of England, the procedure has not yet been approved for general use by the Federal Drug Administration of the USA. His contribution was to point out that a regional sympathetic block to a limb could be an effective lasting one when such an agent as guanethidine was used. Confinement of the drug to the limb was achieved by placing a cannula into a distal vein thereof and then inflating a proximal blood pressure cuff on the limb to 50–100 mm Hg above the systolic pressure. Guanethidine sulfate, 10–30 mg, was then injected into the venous cannula and a period of 20–25 min of circulatory blockade with a tourniquet was maintained. The guanethidine displaces norepinephrine (NE), the transmitter of the sympathetic nerves from their endings. It then occupies the storage sites for the NE in the nerve terminals precluding the reuptake of this neurotransmitter from the synaptic cleft and the normal storage of NE. It binds so strongly that its complete elimination requires a number of days as shown by the persistence of an elevated skin temperature in some treated limbs for days or a few weeks. The guanethidine is fixed in the sympathetic nerve endings in less than half an hour and hence maintains a 'chemical sympathectomy'. He describes the relevant details of the method in two comprehensive chapters [1984, 1988].

Each of his first 10 patients with causalgia received two guanethidine blocks at 3-week intervals with an average of about 80% relief being maintained at 15 weeks in the 5 who had had causalgic pain for 5 weeks or less. In the 5 whose pain had persisted an average of 15 weeks before the treatment he achieved less than 50% relief after the treatment began. The more lasting modes of treatment will be discussed near the end of the chapter.

Sympathetic Dystrophy (Sudeck's Atrophy)

Clinical Features. An enormous number of terms has been used in the literature to indicate the syndrome we are describing under the above heading. Ascherl and Blümel [1981] collected a list of 26 German, 28 English and 9 French terms which are apparently synonymous. These disorders include the same variety of clinical features already described under causalgia but with additional manifestations. In those patients with a predominance of muscular or joint symptoms designations such as pseudorheumatism and pseudoarthritis have been used. Osteoporosis of the affected part may develop surprisingly early leading to the term acute bone atrophy. Sudeck emphasized the osteoporosis among other aspects of the picture in a comprehensive series of papers beginning in 1900 and extending over 42 years [Sudeck 1900, 1942]. The common denominator in most of these clinical pictures is as in classical causalgia, relief by effective sympathetic blockade. By 1943, Livingston had concluded that 'the post-traumatic pain syndrome seemed to be identical in type with the minor causalgias'. We agree with Bonica that effective treatment by sympathetic denervation warrants classification of the entire group under one heading.

Unlike major causalgia these patients exhibit a varied clinical presentation often with no suggestion of sympathetic hyperactivity. A period of protracted futile therapy often ensues with nearly irreversible trophic changes developing before the diagnosis is made. A burning or dull pain worse on motion or other modest stimuli often appears in the early stages of the disorder in some portion of a limb although not necessarily distally. The skin may be red, warm, sweating and edematous with an increased growth of the nails and hair and decreased muscle tone. Radiographs as soon as one or 2 months may show some rarefaction in the subchondral spongiosa as compared with its normal side. Within a few months there may be subsidence of the spontaneous pain, although motion or weight-bearing may cause enough pain to readily provoke the immobilization of the limb. The skin may alter to become reddish gray or pale as well as shiny dry and cool. Brittle nails, loss of hair, edema becoming sclerotic, and atonic atrophic muscles may develop. The radiographs are likely to show many bony rarefactions with coarse residual lines of bone in the shafts and the epiphyses. Extraordinarily wide-ranging factors seem to predispose to such a picture. Almost any type of trauma to joints, bones, nerves or other soft tissues may seem to be the minor factors leading to this astonishing train of events. Predisposing factors may include phlebothromboses or phlebitis, angina pectoris, myocardial infarction (shoulder-hand syndrome), pulmonary embolism, skin disorders, such as scleroderma, and various drug toxicities. It often seems that the more minor the injury the greater is the abnormality. White and Sweet [1969] had a patient who developed the syndrome successively in three limbs after trivial injuries to each. She had a long history of cool cyanotic sweaty hands and feet, a picture confirming Leriche's [1939] conclusion that the disorder is 'a disease which must be regarded as a function of the temperament of the individual'. The exciting event frequently sets off the adverse train of events only days or weeks later and there is a more gradual buildup of symptoms and signs than with causalgia. Some of the cases develop as complications of injection therapy into or near nerves, tight-fitting casts or other minor procedures. Clearly the number of patients in these categories vastly exceeds the number with major causalgia. However, the definitive diagnosis requires a careful analysis of each case.

Psychological Factors. Psychogenic manifestations are frequent. Mounting jury or Workmen's Compensation awards after injury make an appraisal of the role of the focal organic factors the more difficult. Shaw [1964] has presented a warning account of 'pathological malingering' simulating the painful disabled extremity. Likewise Arieff et al. [1964] reported 7 cases in whom determination to secure financial compensation was maintaining atrophic disturbances and disability. The magnitude of this aspect of the problem is only too familiar to all of us working in the field of chronic pain in our two centers as well as in many others. A stunning success of psychotherapy was described by Brihaye and Violon [1978] in a patient after 2.5 years of useless focal treatment for pain of a finger wound. We do have the valuable tool of sympathetic blockade which will prove the presence of a sympathalgia rather than a psychalgia if the results are consistent.

Sympathetic Blocks in Diagnosis and Treatment. The sympathetic dystrophies are more likely to be cured by single or often-repeated blocks than the major causalgias if this therapy is initiated soon enough. Thus, Bonica [1979] estimates as much as an 80% cure rate as gleaned from 7 publications when such blocks are supplemented by vigorous physical therapy. Of Hannington-Kiff's 17 patients treated by his regional intravenous guanethidine method, 7 maintained improvement after one session and 5 more did so after the second session. Schwartzman and McLellan's [1987] recent review collects the evidence for this treatment both with and without an indwelling catheter. They reemphasize the need for early diagnosis and treatment since those with long standing disease have a lower recovery rate. Relief following blocks should ensue before sympathectomy is advised. Indeed, many more temporary sympathetic blocks are advisable for diagnosis and advice for sympathectomy than are required in major causalgias. Even full relief of pain after several technically successful sympathetic blocks is not necessarily an adequate basis to recommend the operation. We have made the mistake ourselves of moving too soon to surgery and have seen many other patients in whom surgical sympathetic denervation has failed despite temporary relief after 1 or 2 blocks.

Results of Surgical Sympathectomy

When a minor injury gives rise to severe pain in a limb one should not conclude at once that sympathectomy is in order. Nor should vasomotor disturbances lead to the diagnosis of causalgia. Thus, in one patient in whom digital puncture with a rose thorn produced a hot, dry, painful hand the syndrome was unrelieved by sympathectomy from T2–8. However, if temporary sympathetic blocks are consistently beneficial and repetitions thereof do not give adequate protracted relief, the same firm recommendation for sympathectomy that applies in major causalgia is appropriate here. Thus, a summary of five reports in this type of patient by Wirth and Rutherford [1980] revealed that 95 of 108 patients were either significantly improved or totally relieved. In Thompson's [1979] series of 120 patients sympathetic blocks had sufficed as definitive treatment in 49%; 5% needed only medical measures and 46% required surgical sympathectomy of the T2–3 ganglia for the upper limb and of L2–3 for the lower limb. The frank diagnosis of causalgia in 27 required surgical treatment in all, of whom 89% had excellent relief of their pain. Other residual symptoms related to limitation of motion, stiffness of joints and other trophic changes were present, however, in one third of the causalgia patients and in 30% of the whole group. The greater the delay between trauma and diagnosis (which averaged 5 months), the greater was the number of residua, although in some, good results ensued whenever the proper treatment was begun. Excellent pain relief was the final outcome in 87% of the cases in the entire group. Varying criteria for the diagnosis of causalgia and sympathetic dystrophy make it difficult to compare the efficacy of sympathetic denervation in different groups of cases. Some authors include many categories of burning or other pain and others include patients whose pain is accompanied by vasomotor manifestations without regard to relief from temporary sympathetic denervation. For example, a report of 11 'causalgia' cases describes sympathetic blocks in only 4 — all without relief [Horowitz, 1984]. 'Burning post-traumatic pain with or without trophic skin changes' sufficed for the diagnosis of causalgia by Manart et al. [1985]. Their upper dorsal sympathectomy achieved even an early good result in only 59% of 22 procedures. They do not mention preoperative sympathetic blocks.

Pathogenesis of Causalgia and Sympathetic Dystrophy

The pain of causalgia cannot be attributed to a slowly evolving process such as fibrosis or neuroma formation because it sets in so soon after injury.

Likewise, ischemic lesions in the tissues as hypothesized by many have not been shown to be etiologic. For example, the associated artery was damaged in only 23% of Barnes' cases of causalgia [1954], in 31% of those of Omer and Thomas [1971] and 25% reported by Carayon and Bourrel [1963]. However, causalgia developed in two thirds of the patients with combined vasculo-neural lesions in the series of the latter authors. Just how the arterial injury affects the nerve has not yet been elucidated. Infection is one of the factors predisposing to sympathetic dystrophy.

A famous experiment of Granit et al. [1944] demonstrated 'the artificial synapse' of injury. Moderate crush of a mixed motor sensory nerve permitted efferent impulses descending the nerve to initiate at the site of injury an afferent discharge recordable from the sensory root when the motor root was stimulated. This artificial synapse of injury was suggested as the site at which tonic efferent sympathetic impulses in a nerve jumped to the adjoining poorly myelinated sensory fibers including those mediating pain [Doupe et al., 1944]. Such activity would be consonant with the increase in tonic efferent sympathetic discharge accompanying physical or emotional stress and would explain the characteristic increase in pain with such stress. The possibility that the pain arises from impulses in afferent fibers from the limbs traversing sympathetic neural pathways seems dubious since two groups [Walker and Nulsen, 1948; White and Sweet, 1969] have only been able on rare instances to elicit pain in an upper limb in patients without causalgia by stimulation of the upper thoracic sympathetic trunk or ganglia. However, Walker and Nulsen demonstrated in 3 patients with causalgia that stimulation of the decentralized upper thoracic sympathetic ganglia did cause a tingling burning which developed slowly over 4–20 s in parallel with the pilomotor response. Barnes has added the idea that antidromic conduction may also occur in the sympathetic fibers at the artificial synapse, causing release of a vasodilator substance at the periphery. He suggests that these might reduce the threshold of sensory stimulation or even set up centripetal impulses to account for the extreme sensitivity of the skin. This theory does not explain the following facts:

(1) Excision of the entire zone of a nerve injury carried out on a few of the patients with a complete lesion has not always relieved the pain. In the series of Kirklin et al. [1947] this operation completely relieved only 2 of 5 patients.

(2) The pain may spread well beyond the domain of the nerves impaired in some instances to include the whole forequarter of a body from the lesion of a single nerve [Leriche, 1939; Loh and Nathan, 1978].

(3) A crucial observation is that a regional guanethidine block has relieved the pain even when the sphygmomanometer cuff has been applied distal to the lesion on the peripheral nerve [Loh and Nathan, 1978]. Artificial synapses at the site of injury would then be unaffected by the distally injected drug and the pain should continue if these were responsible for it.

A more likely explanation may prove to be that NE acts abnormally at peripheral sympathetic terminals producing hyperpathia and hyperesthesia. Regenerating fibers after transection of a rat sciatic nerve may fire constantly and this response is increased by NE as demonstrated by Wall and Gutnick [1974a]. A spreading hypersensitivity to peripherally secreted NE is suggested by the fact that the guanethidine replacing the NE at these terminals distal to the constricting cuff stops all abnormal sensitivity below the cuff — not merely that in the domain of the injured nerves. The slow buildup of pain over 4–20 s in the 3 causalgic patients of Walker and Nulsen upon stimulation of the upper thoracic sympathetic ganglia is better explained by a slow buildup of NE at the nerve terminals than by an instantaneous electrical excitation at the artificial synapse which would have initiated prompt conduction back into the posterior root. Hannington-Kiff points out that not only patients with causalgia, but those with the less focal injuries of Sudeck's atrophy and sympathetic dystrophy, are often successfully treated by regional blocks with guanethidine. Hence an abnormal mechanism for nerve terminals appears to be operative in both types of patients and a new mechanism need not be hypothesized to account for this result in the sympathetic dystrophies. There is also an unusual case of Gordon [1961] in whom the successful surgical treatment was all distal to the wound and which consequently also suggests abnormal response to NE.

An even more general tendency to abnormal responses to NE as the cause of some painful states in the limbs is suggested by the observations of Loh and Nathan [1978]. In two thirds of 31 patients with a variety of hyperpathic states the pain and hyperpathia were both relieved by sympathetic block. Peripheral nerves, posterior root ganglia, nerve roots or the spinal cord were involved in these various patients. Such relief occurred in only 2 of 15 similar patients in whom the pain was not accompanied by hyperpathia.

The next task of identifying the structure responding abnormally to NE was attacked by Torebjörk and Hallin [1979]. In a patient with causalgia they found her thresholds for pain upon changes in temperature, both up and down, were greatly reduced in the painful hand as compared with the normal one. These low thresholds were still further reduced by an intracutaneous injection of only 1 μg of NE. In fact this provoked a severe attack of pain in the entire limb for hours despite large i.m. doses of morphine. No such reaction was provoked from the normal hand or in normal people. After anesthesia of superficial cutaneous nerve endings was induced in her by topical application of ketocaine, an intracutaneous injection of NE no longer caused an attack of pain or a reduction in the thresholds for temperature change causing pain. The cutaneous nerve endings were thus established as one major site of action of the NE. Further direct records from peripheral nerves of this patient showed that populations of A and C fibers were abnormally reactive to NE at their endings. In 4 more causalgia patients whose pain had been relieved by sympathectomy, intracutaneous injections of NE into the previously painful areas of skin still strikingly reduced the pain thresholds both to mechanical and cold cutaneous stimuli. This hyperalgesia was abolished after perceptions of touch and cold had disappeared upon compression of the limb nerves by an inflated blood pressure cuff. Both warmth and delayed pain were still perceived. These results point to myelinated A fibers as signaling pain from the NE-sensitized skin. This is contrary to the observations of Meyer and Fields [1972] in 8 patients with causalgia, 6 of whom obtained significant relief by electrical stimulation selective for the large fibers in the injured peripheral nerve proximal to the lesion. Hence the identification of the afferent fibers responsible for the pain and hyperpathia related to the peripherally secreted NE remains uncertain.

The pathways for the impulses causing the pain may shift after regeneration which follows sympathectomy in some patients. Thus, our patient Lillian T. whose causalgic ulnar pain was temporarily completely relieved after each of a series of five upper thoracic sympathectomies and a cervicothoracic ganglionectomy finally secured lasting relief from our posterior rhizotomy at the C8–T1 levels. This relief persists at a recent follow-up 35 years later.

The neural impulses for pain in this disorder may travel over the central pathways for somatic pain as indicated by the patient of Birkenfeld and Fisher [1963]. When an incomplete sympathectomy did not relieve pain in the upper limb, they carried out a bulbar spinothalamic tractotomy producing contralateral analgesia up to the C1 level with relief of pain.

Livingston [1943], Sunderland [1976] and Loh and Nathan [1978] among many others have hypothesized that abnormal central excitatory states in the spinal cord worsen and sustain the problem. Although objective studies to support these hypotheses remain to be carried out, one must concede that the ease with which a huge variety of physical and psychic stimuli trigger worsening of the pain in major causalgia do point to a role of the CNS in these patients. Happily, the prompt success that follows upon peripheral sympathetic denervation in many instances makes it clear that this hyperexcitability may be subject to a decisive, easily achieved peripheral control.

Vascular Occlusive Disorders

When angiography fails to demonstrate proximal focal lesions susceptible to direct surgical attack but reveals instead distal arterial occlusion, the painful structural occlusion or vasospastic lesions of these small distal vessels of the limbs may benefit from temporary blocks of the sympathetic trunk. If more lasting types of chemical sympathectomy fail, then surgical destruction of the sympathetic pathway may be advisable.

Primary and Secondary Raynaud's Disease

A discouraging late follow-up after 104 dorsal sympathectomies for primary Raynaud's disease has been provided by Baddeley in 1965. This agrees with the much later comprehensive report by Mattassi et al. [1981] that the operation should be restricted to those with severely painful progressive lesions in whom trophic changes threaten the viability of a digit. These two reports, as well as that of Touati et al. [1982], all describe poor results when Raynaud's phenomenon was secondary to scleroderma. The two Italian groups did have better results in the traumatically caused syndrome related to workers with vibrating tools. Their best results and those of Arnulf [1979] have occurred in those with distal arterial occlusive disease. The latter author ascribes a particular efficacy to the operation when frostbite injuries with ulceration are the problem.

Other Structural Occlusive Disease

The Upper Limbs

The cases classified as secondary Raynaud's phenomenon overlap with those in this group. The outcome of sympathetic blocks correlates poorly with the results of sympathectomy both in a positive and a negative direction. For example, in one series 2 of 9 patients whose symptoms did not improve after stellate block were relieved after sympathectomy [Berguer and

Smit, 1981]. They had 3 of 4 good results from a T2,3,4 ganglionectomy in patients with arterial occlusion in the wrist, hand or fingers. In every one of 12 similar patients Dale and Lewis [1970] achieved success upon excising the sympathetic trunk from the caudal part of T1 through T3 ganglia. The lone significant complication was one patient with intercostal pain for several months. In a somewhat similar group of patients, a group of 16 patients with Raynaud's phenomenon secondary to arteriosclerotic arterial occlusions, Mattassi et al. [1981] report good results after a T2–3 thoracic sympathectomy upon a 2- to 11-year follow-up; recurrence had taken place in only one. In a different 16 of their patients in whom the disorder was secondary to scleroderma, their results were exactly reversed — all but one experienced a recurrence.

The Lower Limbs

Sympathectomies for the legs, now often carried out by way of an anterior extraperitoneal approach, have been reevaluated extensively in the last 10 years. Many centers have combined to publish two major groups of articles [Goldstein et al., 1977; Simeone, 1979]: (1) the first 8 pages of Acta chirg. belg. (vol. 76, 1977), and (2) '50 Years of Lumbar Sympathectomy' (vol. 20, 1979). Firmer conclusions with respect to the lower limbs are now tenable because of the greater volume of data.

A recent terse but comprehensive review of Cotton and Cross [1985] includes their own randomized prospective report on lumbar sympathectomy for ischemic rest pain. They cite the mounting evidence that intermittent claudication and its pain are not helped by lumbar sympathectomy. Evidence presented by the prospective controlled study of Fyfe and Quin [1975] demonstrating this failure in 27 patients is especially convincing. The fundamental reason appears to be that an increase in muscle blood flow does not take place [Duff, 1951] nor does vascular resistance in muscle diminish after sympathectomy [Dornhorst et al., 1951]. Moreover, sympathectomy may not even increase capillary blood flow in the skin inasmuch as it dilates the dermal arteriovenous anastomoses, thereby shunting more blood directly into the veins [Dornhorst, 1963]. Similarly, Uhrenholdt et al. [1971] have collected and added to the evidence that a paradoxical reduction in blood flow is caused by lumbar sympathetic blockade in patients with severe arterial obstruction. This is probably due to the 'steal' proximally in the limb.

Capillary blood flow appears to be improved significantly by exercise which closes the dermal arteriovenous anastomoses as a consequence of released metabolic products. Many preoperative tests to aid in patient selection for the operation have proved disappointing. An exception appears to be the result of comparing ankle with brachial systolic pressure. If this ratio is less than 0.35 [Yao and Bergan, 1973] or less than 0.3 [Walker and Johnston, 1980; Persson et al., 1985], sympathectomy is unlikely to succeed. Persson et al. report complete relief of rest pain in 27 of the 33 limbs meeting this criterion — relief maintained until death or the last follow-up.

Evidence that the ischemic rest pain is relieved consequent upon destruction of nociceptive afferents in the sympathetic trunk and not by virtue of improving the circulation has been adduced by Cross and Cotton. We summarize this in the section on percutaneous lumbar sympathectomy with phenol. The striking conclusion which emerges is that sympathectomy's principal value in vascular occlusive disease is to stop the pain with minor fruitful results from any vasodilatation.

Post-Amputation Pain

After digital amputations sympathetic block and sympathectomy may stop persisting pain. The late J.C. White had 7 such cases with good results in 2 of them and excellent results in 5 [White and Sweet, 1969]. One was followed for 20 years. Neither of us has found sympathetic denervation helpful for pain in amputations at or above the wrist and ankle. In the most comprehensive report, that of Kallio [1950], sympathectomy in 68 patients for phantom or stump pain resulted in a recurrence usually within 6 months, in all but 6 patients. Even when there is vascular insufficiency in the stump the results are poor according to Jensen and Rasmussen [1984].

Open Sympathectomy of Limbs

Extent of Ganglionectomy

Appropriate preoperative studies have usually permitted determination of the required extent of denervation both for the upper and the lower limb. As will be discussed further under causalgia, the upper level of removal of the sympathetic chain to relieve pain in the lower limb is particularly likely to require special study. Perhaps the most accurate of the tactics for determining this level is that proposed by Erdemir et al. [1982]. They injected slowly 1% lidocaine into the mid-lumbar posterior epidural space, ascertaining the upper level of the somatosensory block required to give complete relief of pain. They cite 2 patients in whom the unusually high sensory level to T10 was required for temporary pain relief. Both then maintained relief of their post-traumatic sympathetic dystrophic pain for many years after thoraco-lumbar sympathectomies carried up to the T10 level.

Pre-Ganglionic versus Post-Ganglionic Denervation

In two series the value of each of these two types of procedure has been compared in the treatment of causalgia. The pre-ganglionic sympathectomy of the upper limb involved cutting the rami communicantes to the second and third thoracic sympathetic ganglia and dividing trunk below the third ganglion; this was compared with the post-ganglionic operation which includes the stellate ganglion (fig. 21/1). Barnes [1954] compared 8 pre-ganglionic with 9 post-ganglionic procedures noting a slight edge in favor of the pre-ganglionic procedures in terms of pain relief. In these 17 patients complete denervation was achieved in about equal numbers in the two groups to a total of 14; 3 of these had persistent hyperalgesia in relationship to the operative site. In the larger series of Rasmussen and Freedman [1946] all of the 14 pre-ganglionic operations yielded complete relief of pain whereas only 10 of 21 in the post-ganglionic group had complete relief. The post-ganglionic operation then has the disadvantage of a lower success rate and includes the minor annoyance of Horner's syndrome. The more extensive removal via a transthoracic approach recommended by Buker et al. [1972] involves removal from the lower half of the stellate ganglion through the fourth or fifth thoracic ganglia. This, probably pre-ganglionic, procedure relieved all of his 9 patients, none of whom had Horner's syndrome. The customary procedure in the lower limb of removing no ganglia below L3 is a pre-ganglionic operation.

Completeness of Denervation

Failure to accomplish complete sympathetic denervation caused the only 3 failures in Barnes' [1954] 30 cases and 3 of Whitcomb's [Mayfield, 1951]. Completion of the denervation by a second operation in 4 of 5 of these patients did then give relief in all 4. Likewise, Mayfield [1951], by completing the denervation in 9 of his incompletely sympathectomized patients, then gave all of them relief. Denervation is especially likely to be a problem in the lower limb; the standard removal of the second and third or the second, third and fourth lumbar ganglia may still permit sweating in the foot as an indication of the incompleteness of the operation. Mayfield [1951] completed the denervation in 3 of these patients by removal of the L1 ganglion,

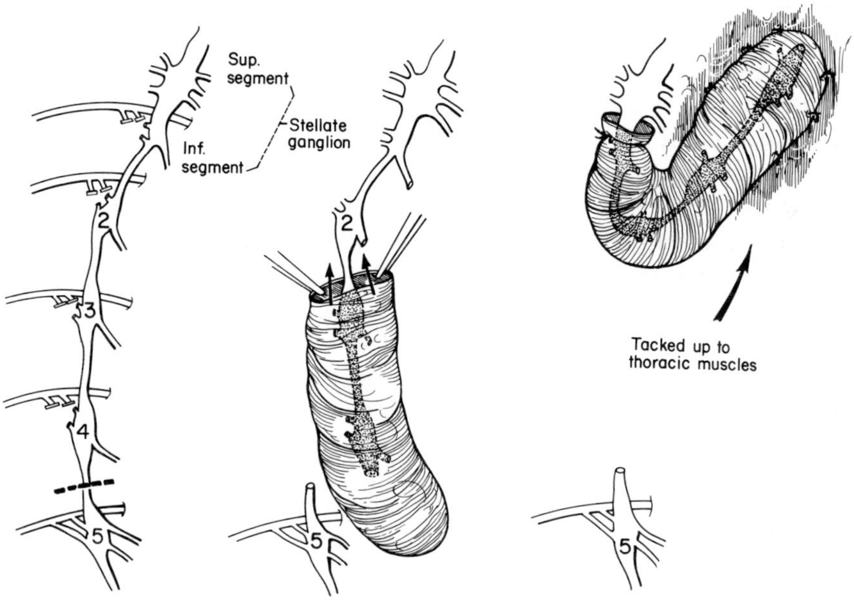

Fig. 21/1. Stages in pre-ganglionic upper thoracic sympathectomy. On the left the rami communicantes from thoracic sympathetic ganglia 1 through 4 have been cut and their ends joining the somatic trunks clipped to discourage regeneration. The middle illustration shows the sympathetic trunk divided below the T4 ganglion and the freed trunk and ganglia inserted into a cylindrical plastic sac. On the right the sac's opening has been tied below the superior aspect of the stellate ganglion and the blind end carried out and tied into the muscles of the back to preclude regeneration in the chest.

but in the other 4 he had also to remove D11 and D12 ganglia before the limb was finally denervated — with complete relief. Bonica [1979] cites similar examples. However, Carayon and Bourrel [1963] did not turn the tide to success in 2 patients — one after a T2–3 ganglionectomy was supplemented by stellate ganglion removal and in another after the reverse sequence of operations. Complete sympathetic denervation was accomplished by Ray and Console [1949] in some cases only by adding anterior rhizotomy of T12, L1 and L2 to lumbar ganglionectomy.

Regeneration

A stubborn tendency of the sympathetic nerves to regrow can be remarkably complete. A patient of Mattassi et al. [1981] had recurrent pain after the first histologically proven sympathectomy and at reoperation, what proved histologically to be another essentially normal sympathetic chain, was again removed from the lower T1 through T3 ganglia. Consequently, encasement of the disconnected ganglia in a nylon or other plastic sleeve, the closed end of which is sutured well into the muscles of the back, seeks to guide regenerating fibers into areas remote from their normal habitat. One should routinely check the completeness of the sympathectomy in a month or so after operation by sweating tests, sympathogalvanic potentials or skin resistance measurements [Van der Stricht, 1972; Benassy, 1977]. If the pain recurs the possibility of regeneration should be checked in the same fashion. We have had one patient with causalgia whose persistent sympathetic regeneration finally required posterior rhizotomy to give the patient relief. Inasmuch as recurrences in the lower limbs are less of a problem special measures at operation are usually not carried out in order to preclude them, although Simeone prefers to remove L2 through L4 ganglia in order to make regeneration 'much less likely'.

Complications

The supraclavicular, transaxillary or posterior costotransversectomy approaches for the open upper thoracic operations all have a low rate of complications. For example, only 3 of Adar's [1979] 456 such sympathectomies by the supraclavicular approach had severe brachial plexus injuries. Even these 3 recovered after 4–6 months. The transaxillary approach [Atkins, 1954] gives the best view of the entire length of the upper thoracic trunk but is accompanied by more minor complications such as pneumothorax, pain or dysesthesias in the chest or medial arm.

The complications following lumbar sympathectomies likewise are almost always transient. This was the case, for example, in the 1,344 such operations by Goldstein et al. [1977] whose mortality of 0.6% was principally in elderly advanced arteriosclerotics. In that group 3 patients had a prolonged paralytic ileus lasting 5, 6 and 12 days, respectively. A paradoxical but temporary partial ischemia of a sympathectomized lower limb rarely occurs and is usually effectively treated medically.

'Postsympathectomy neuralgia' is the most frequent complication of the operation and appears to be correlated with no particular operative technique. The pain is referred to the proximal part of the limb only, i.e. shoulder and upper arm after the upper thoracic and groin and anterior thigh after the lumbar procedures. This deep aching or burning comes on abruptly but typically only during the second week after operation — usually after the patient has left the hospital. Increased sympathetic activity in the area of the pain in the anterior thigh was demonstrated by the lowered skin resistance of increased sudomotor activity in the study of Tracy and Cockett [1957]. In those patients who did not develop this puzzling pain the increased sweating over the anterior thigh did not occur. Litwin [1962] and Longoni et al. [1981] summarizing about 20 publications note that the pain appears in about 20% of the patients with about equal frequency in the upper and lower limbs. This neuralgia subsides in nearly all cases in from 12 days to 6 months — unlike many pain syndromes associated with some form of deafferentation.

It is important to warn males that major sexual dysfunction may occur after bilateral removal of the first or second lumbar ganglia or of the presacral plexus. Our most informative data on this score come from the comprehensive report of Whitelaw and Smithwick [1951] after their study of a massive series of sympathectomies for hypertension which were bilateral and included upper lumbar ganglia. Only 3 of the 8 patients with the most extensive bilateral removals, which included the lower thoracic chain, the splanchnic nerves and the first two lumbar ganglia had a significant disturbance of erection or a permanent loss of ejaculation. When this operation did not include the second lumbar ganglia such loss of sexual function occurred in only 20% of 66 patients. When the bilateral removals included only L2 with various combinations of L1 and L3 ganglia there was disturbed erection in 63% and permanent elimination of ejaculation in 54% of 11 cases. When the removals were only unilateral the disturbances of erection were confined to 2 of 12 cases.

Simplified Sympathectomies of Limbs

Thermal RF Lesions of Upper Thoracic Sympathetic Trunk

Wilkinson [1984] has pioneered the percutaneous introduction of electrodes against the bodies of the upper thoracic vertebrae at the site of the sympathetic chain. Using only local anesthesia external to the ribs plus neurolept analgesia, he places the electrodes under radiographic control and in accordance with responses to electrical stimulation and gentle RF heating in order to ensure that the electrode is not near enough to an intercostal nerve to provoke pain and far enough from the stellate ganglion so that Horner's syndrome does not occur. Destruction of two or three ganglia on one or both sides can be carried out at the same session. The patient is usually discharged from the hospital on the day of the procedure. The minor complications of one small pneumothorax and pain in chest or medial arm occurred in 4 patients lasting 2–3 months. Initial failure in 8 of 65 procedures (111 limbs) has been improved to failure in but one of 65 limbs more recently [Wilkinson, 1989] by alterations in the technique. None of 20 patients with recurrences or failure came back for a repeat percutaneous operation. Circulatory problems in an upper limb, such as Raynaud's phenomenon, have been followed by sustained sympathectomy in all 7 of these patients but satisfactory limb perfusion was maintained in only 4. Causalgia or sympathetic dystrophy in 7 other patients was followed by persistent sympathetic denervation in only 5, one of whom was operated on a second time. Unfortunately, pain relief has been maintained in only 2 of them (the great majority — 37 patients — were treated by the procedure for hyperhidrosis).

Upper Thoracic Endoscopic Sympathectomy

This procedure begins with collapse of the lung via introduction of air into a pneumothorax needle in the mid-axillary line. Then, a 1.5-cm incision caudal to the angle of the scapula is used to introduce a special endoscope. This permits dissection of the sympathetic ganglia from T2 down through T6 if needed. Reinflation of the lung is usually followed by discharge of the patient within 48 h. This operation had been performed by Kux of Vienna 166 times by 1977. Twenty-three patients with Raynaud's syndrome followed by Rösner and Goldberg [1979] for a minimum of 6 years after this operation had no significant complications but there were no lasting cures in contrast to 35% cures after open sympathectomy. Use of the endoscope to destroy the sympathetic trunk by electrocoagulation under direct vision has been the tactic of Weale [1980], 10 cases, and Malone et al. [1982], 30 cases.

Percutaneous Lumbar Sympathectomy with Phenol

Treatment of occlusive arterial disease of the lower limbs by this method was introduced by Haxton [1949] and by Boyd et al. [1949]. They used it primarily for the treatment of ischemic rest pain but had useful results as well in decreasing tissue necrosis and intermittent claudication. The operation has been used mainly in older patients with advanced disease thought to be unsuitable for vascular reconstruction. By 1970, Reid et al. were able to report on 5,000 such procedures at various levels of the sympathetic chain. Ischemic rest pain was relieved initially in 77% of one series of 189 male patients. Sixty percent of these remained relieved until they died or were last followed.

Method. Modern image intensifiers have improved the accuracy of the procedure and were used by Scott and Littlewood [1982] in 350 lumbar operations from 1980 to 1982. Assurance that the 6–10% phenol is to be injected correctly closely applied to the anterolateral surface of the second to fourth lumbar vertebral bodies is provided by preliminary injection of a contrast medium into the lumbar needle. This also precludes injection into a vein although it may not prevent the phenol from moving into a periureteric position. CT to guide needle placement and injection also increases the precision of the maneuver [Schild et al., 1984; Redman et al., 1986]. Spotting of the position of the ureters in the CT scan by a previous i.v. injection of 50 ml of contrast medium is the contribution of Dondelinger and Kurdziel [1984]. Löfström et al. [1980] have provided excellent illustrations of misplacements and current methods.

Complications. Pain referred to groin or thigh is the most frequent difficulty. The locus and the usual duration of about 6–8 weeks are similar to the postsympathectomy neuralgia seen after the open operations. The pain has also been ascribed to spread of phenol to the genito-femoral or other nerve if the injection is too close to the side of a vertebral body [Cousins and Bridenbaugh, 1980]. This complication was reported in 9% of 1,666 lumbar injections of phenol by Reid et al. [1970] and was seen in 'many' of the 53 patients of Dondelinger and Kurdziel [1984]. Walsh et al. [1984] treated the 6 of their 31 patients who developed pain in groin or thigh by transcutaneous nerve stimulation, usually with resolution in 3 weeks. The low incidence of only 6% described by Hatangdi and Boas [1985] was associated with no incidence of lateral or dorsal spread of the contrast upon reassessment of the radiographs. Hence they concluded the somatic nerve supply could not have been involved but they did not assess the completeness of the sympathectomy. At least 3 cases of protracted severe pain have been described [Löfström et al., 1980; Hughes-Davies and Redman, 1976]. Renal or ureteric injuries are more serious complications. Fraser et al. [1984] had 3 such nonfatal lesions in patients with a clinically demonstrable sympathectomy. In the series of Reid et al. [1970] there were 5 renal or ureteric lesions and 6 intrapleural injections. In the one report of ejaculatory failure after chemical sympathectomy the symptom persisted for only 2 weeks [Baxter and O'Kafo, 1984]. On the whole complication rates are low.

Results. Although Dondelinger and Kurdziel [1984] describe substantial pain relief in 60% of their patients initially, after a mean follow-up of 8 months only 33% showed improvement. They cite four other similar reports.

Better results were documented in a randomized prospective controlled study of Cross and Cotton [1985]. In 41 limbs of 37 patients unsuitable for open arterial surgery a lumbar sympathetic block with bupivacaine was given to 20 in a control group. Only 24% of these had relief of pain at one week whereas this occurred in 84% of the phenol group. A spontaneous remission rate of roughly 24% in a group of nonprogressing patients at one week is intimated by these results. In the phenol group 67% continued with significant relief of their rest pain at 6 months. By that time many of the bupivacaine control group had required other treatment so were no longer available as controls. The sympathogalvanic or psychogalvanic reflex in the foot was not lost in 7 of the 24 limbs in the phenol group — evidence of failure of sympathetic denervation therein. Consequently, these were not included in the assessment of the results in that group. Unfortunately, an appraisal as to the effectiveness of the chemical denervation is not a feature of most of the reports. The Cross and Cotton [1985] study also involved appraisal of three hemodynamic factors: (1) the ankle — brachial systolic pressure index and strain gauge plethysmographic measurements of (2) resting blood flow and of (3) reactive hyperemic peak blood flow in the foot. None of these three parameters became better in either group, leading the authors to conclude that the absence of improvement in peripheral blood flow means that the relief of pain had to be related to destruction of nociceptive pathways in the sympathetic trunk. Two other studies have found that the relief of rest pain corresponded to the duration of the lumbar sympathetic blockade by drug [Cousins et al., 1979b; Omer and Thomas, 1971].

Improvement of the results of chemical sympathectomy would probably follow the same kind of detailed analysis of failures to which open operations have been subjected.

Cardiac Sympathectomy

In the middle third of this century upper thoracic sympathectomy proved to be an effective treatment for medically intractable angina pectoris. Better drugs and the operation of coronary artery graft to bypass occluded segments of the arteries have replaced this operation. The form of cardiac ischemia associated with coronary arterial spasm, 'Prinzmetal's angina', has not responded as well to the bypass grafts as has classic angina. Consequently, a number of cardiac denervation procedures have been tried — with variable results. Two other dangerous cardiac disorders associated with syncope and sudden death, also treated by sympathectomy, are refractory ventricular tachycardias and the 'long QT syndrome'. Trunk denervation from the stellate through the T7 ganglia on both sides appears tentatively to be desirable, and to be more beneficial than direct cardiac plexectomies which have the undesirable feature of including vagal denervation. The sympathetic fibers appear to be less able to reinnervate the heart after denervation than is the case with other structures. Indeed, there are at least three reports of many patients who have undergone cardiac transplantation who failed to show evidence of cardiac reinnervation up to 9 years after operation. The percutaneous RF procedure of Wilkinson should be brought to the attention of cardiologists since it carries a far lower risk than open sympathectomy in these high-risk patients. The neurosurgeon and his cardiologic colleagues can be brought up to date in this highly specialized area by the review of Kadowaki and Levett [1986].

Sympathectomy of Abdominal Viscera

Open Excisions

Unlike the limbs, the upper abdominal viscera send enormous numbers of nociceptive afferents into the spinal cord by way of the greater, lesser and least splanchnic nerves. Consequently, the pain from nonresectable cancers of such upper abdominal viscera as the pancreas, stomach, liver and gall bladder can be treated effectively by sympathectomy of these nerves. Painful chronic relapsing pancreatitis, often with calculi obstructing the ducts, has also been so treated. Bilateral removal of all three splanchnic nerves and the lower four thoracic sympathetic ganglia is a simple extrapleural 1-hour procedure devised by Max Peet for the treatment of essential hypertension. The results of eight groups with a total of 26 cases were summarized by White and Sweet [1969] and again by Vosschulte and Wagner [1970]. The latter authors found that in 25 publications reporting 141 cases 67% had initial satisfactory results, and in the 84 cases followed from one to several years 64% were still satisfactory. In the smaller group of 39 cases followed 5 or more years 69% were still in this gratifying category. Although a group of French surgeons [Michotey et al., 1983] secured relief in all 12 of their patients with chronic pancreatitis subjected to bilateral splanchnicectomy,

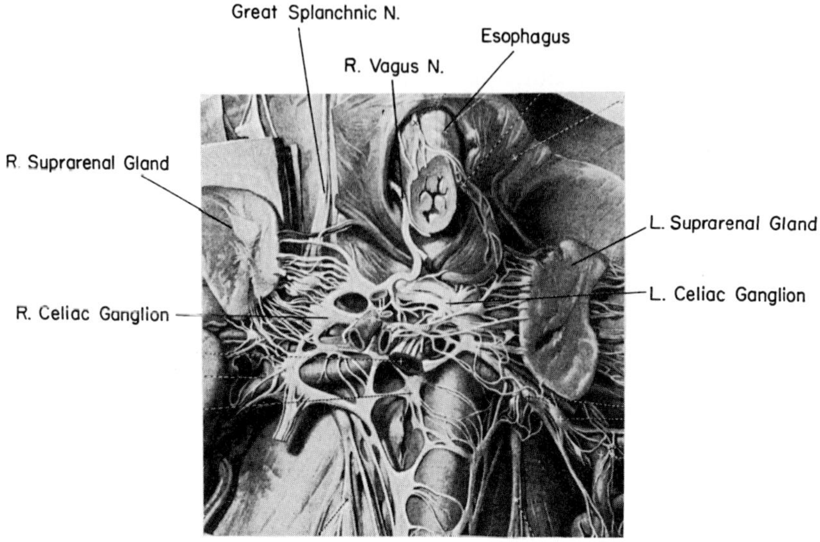

Fig. 21/2. Upper abdominal sympathetic ganglia and plexuses. Note the many unlabeled and often unnamed small ganglia and their gross preponderance to the right of the midline in this person. The lower four ganglia in the field to the right of the aorta are all mesenteric ganglia. From Spalteholz [1940].

the experience of surgeons in the USA has been much less gratifying. We find no articles on this subject from North America in the last 15 years.

However, the Peet type of bilateral extensive sympathectomy carried out in the low thoracic extrapleural space has been used since 1950 by Sadar and Hardy [1978] in the management of 56 patients with pancreatic carcinoma. Their operation begins with a laparotomy at which any feasible palliative procedure is done and the patient is then turned to the prone position for the sympathectomy. Although the operative mortality in this high-risk group was 7%, 70% had an initial good or complete relief, the pain recurred to some extent in 23% of that 70%. The French group [Michotey et al., 1983] also had 100% early pain relief in their 11 cancer cases although they do not indicate their later results.

Chemical Sympathectomy of Celiac Plexus and Splanchnic Nerves

Injection of phenol or 50% alcohol into the general region of the junction of splanchnic nerves and celiac ganglia may be performed either at the time of exploratory laparotomy or percutaneously with radiographic guidance. The 41 cancer patients of Flanigan and Kraft [1978] experienced a 15% operative mortality, and the initial relief in 88% of the survivors lasted only an average of 4.3 months. The 37 cancer patients of Gardner and Solomou [1984] had a 70% relief of pain until death with an accompanying 5% operative mortality.

We have summarized elsewhere [Sweet, 1988b] the troublesome features experienced by others using this general method. There are no precise radiographic landmarks and the diffuse dispersal into many tissue planes of the enormous plexuses of the celiac ganglion and the scattering into many small clusters of what is described as a single celiac ganglion seem to us to constitute a poorly localizable and too diffuse target to have a reasonable hope of a useful result by a blind injection into it (fig. 21/2).

Conclusions

The indications for open sympathectomy have decreased steadily consequent upon the increasingly valuable sympatholytic drugs which may be given either by mouth or by intravenous regional injections into limbs. Radiographic procedures have greatly increased the precision of percutaneous RF and chemical procedures as well. The ease of execution of percutaneous approaches has led to a somewhat cavalier assessment of the completeness of denervation they achieve. The success rates of the newer methods still require critical appraisal.

Part II. Electrical Stimulation of 'Pain-Suppressive' Systems

Introduction

Although the production of analgesia by electrical energy has a long history [for review, see Kane and Taub, 1975], neurosurgeons became really interested in neurostimulation for the treatment of 'intractable pain' in the late 1960s. The immediate reason for this was the formulation of the gate control theory [Melzack and Wall, 1965] followed by Reynolds' discovery [1969] that electrical stimulation of midbrain structures could provoke profound analgesia. The possibility of activating more or less selectively pain inhibitory pathways without destruction of nervous tissue had indeed tremendous appeal and this mainly for three reasons. Unwanted side effects, which are a burden with destructive procedures, can be avoided; the effects of electrical stimulation are reversible, and before implanting a stimulating device a temporary test stimulation is worthwhile.

Before neural stimulation by means of an implanted electrode system can legitimately be applied clinically, a number of requirements have to be met. Problems related to neural damage caused by the local electrochemical reactions at the electrode-tissue interface and the use of electric currents have been largely solved [Rowland et al., 1960; Lilly, 1961; Miller et al., 1961; Weinman, 1965; Mortimer et al., 1970; Pudenz et al., 1975; Brummer and Turner, 1977a–c; Swiontek et al., 1980; Sances et al., 1981; Yuen et al., 1981] and with proper selection of electrodes, parameters of stimulation and careful implantation technique, neural injury is not a real problem in the clinical situation [for review, see Sheer, 1961; Hambrecht and Reswick, 1977; Myklebust et al., 1985]. Kindling, a phenomenon in which convulsions develop in response to repeated low-level electrical stimulation of the brain and which has been extensively observed in animals [Goddard, 1967], might theoretically pose a threat for the safety of electrical stimulation of the human brain [Cain, 1979] but has in practice not been a complication. Materials and instrumentation have been gradually developed to activate the electrodes safely — leading to totally implantable and programmable stimulating devices — and different electrode configurations are available. Although neurostimulation is still plagued with technical difficulties, such as electrode migration, fibrosis around electrodes in the epidural space or around peripheral nerves with, as a consequence, increased stimulation thresholds and power consumption, lead breakage, faulty devices, rejection reaction, infection etc., the real difficulties are not technical, but lie, as we shall see in the next chapters, in the physiological and pathophysiological domain.

Indeed, multiple endogenous opiate and nonopiate analgesia systems seem to exist [Mayer and Watkins, 1984] and their physiology is very complex and far from unraveled. More disturbing, activation of these systems, which in experimental animals have a strong analgesic effect on tests for acute pain, does not necessarily lead to suppression of pathological pain. The divorce between 'douleur laboratoire' and 'douleur maladie' to use Leriche's terminology, is here also part of the problem.

Chapter 22. Peripheral Nerve Stimulation

Historical Note

Wall and Sweet [1967], in order to test in man the predictions of the gate control theory [Melzack and Wall, 1965], stimulated the infraorbital nerve on themselves producing brief hypalgesia. They then observed that stimulation either of peripheral nerves (5 cases) or spinal roots (3 cases) caused temporary abolition of clinical chronic pain outlasting briefly the duration of the stimulation. In 1968, Sweet and Wepsic reported relief of pain in patients with pathological pain with peripheral nerve stimulation (PNS), performed with the use of permanently implanted peripheral nerve electrodes. It became gradually clear that the best results for pain relief were obtained in those conditions in which the pain was due to an injury to a peripheral nerve and the goal was to induce paresthesias in the distribution area of the injured nerve while avoiding motor responses. This led to technical advances permitting electrode contacts to be positioned in such a way that maximum stimulation is available to the injured afferents [Nashold et al., 1979, 1980]. Compared to transcutaneous nerve stimulation, dorsal column stimulation and deep brain stimulation, peripheral nerve stimulation by means of implanted electrodes seems to be less frequently performed.

Mechanism for Pain Relief by Peripheral Nerve Stimulation

The mechanism of effective pain relief is uncertain and many possibilities can be proposed. At the peripheral level, it has been shown that electrical stimulation can induce a peripheral blockade of nociceptive afferents [Campbell and Taub, 1973; Torebjörk and Hallin, 1974; Ignelzi and Nyquist, 1976, 1979; Van Hees, 1979; Myklebust et al., 1984]. In pathological situations such a blockade might become particularly significant: among the physiological properties of experimentally produced neuromas [Wall and Gutnick,

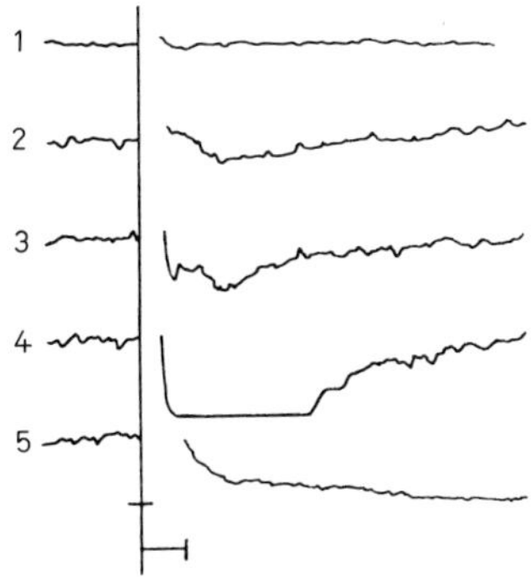

Fig. 22/1. Rate of ongoing activity in dorsal root filaments. *1* From normal intact nerve; *2–5* from neuromas. Combined rate of 4–6 single units. At the vertical line, the rootlet from which recordings were taken was stimulated for 6 s with a maximal stimulus square wave of 0.1 ms duration at 100 Hz. Time mark, 12 s; rate mark, 30 impulses per second. From Wall and Gutnick [1974a].

1974a, b; Scadding, 1981; Korenman and Devor, 1981; Blumberg and Jänig, 1982, 1984; Devor, 1983], spontaneous ongoing activity in both A and C fiber afferents is a common feature, although it may well be that due to the action of potassium channel-blocking agents, such as gallamine as anesthetics, the amount of spontaneous electrical activity in experimental neuromas has been overestimated [Burchiel and Russell, 1987]. It has been shown that a short period of repetitive electrical stimulation of the nerve in which a neuroma has been produced, at a strength above threshold for the single fiber under study, may completely stop the ongoing discharge for several minutes [Wall and Gutnick, 1974a, b] (fig. 22/1).

The reason for this turnoff following antidromic invasion is not known, but it has been hypothesized that the tetanic stimulation hyperpolarizes the terminals and raises the threshold, thereby decreasing their tendency to generate impulses spontaneously. It has been shown in man by microneurography techniques that sensitized C fibers can be responsible for hyperalgesia [Cline et al., 1987] but it is not known how those sensitized nociceptors are influenced by peripheral nerve stimulation. The results of tetanic stimulation on the ongoing activity in the experimental neuroma model, and their interpretation as a prolonged turnoff of the abnormal pulse generator, cannot only explain the prolonged effect but also the localization of the therapeutic effect. However, there are problems with this explanation. In the clinical situation it is a common experience that the intensity of the stimulating current for pain relief is below the threshold for activation of small fibers, and the post-stimulation effects may be very long lasting, of the order of days and on a few occasions of weeks.

The pain-suppressive effects of peripheral nerve stimulation have also been explained by a central mechanism. Most attention has been paid to inhibitory mechanisms in the dorsal horn and it is on the basis of the concept of the gate control theory [Nathan and Rudge, 1974] that the modern era of peripheral nerve stimulation for pain relief was initiated. There is experimental evidence in the intact animal that prolonged inhibition of spinothalamic tract neurons can be obtained by peripheral nerve stimulation (fig. 22/2).

This inhibition was also observed in spinalized animals, indicating that it must depend in part on spinal cord neural circuitry. This inhibition was only slightly affected by naloxone, and not affected by blockers of GABA, serotonine, catecholamine, and substance P [Chung et al., 1984a]. Moreover, the A-delta fiber group was most important for producing this inhibition, although significant additional effects were also produced by activation of the A-alpha-beta and C fiber group [Chung et al., 1984b]. Both from an experimental and clinical point of view there is clear evidence that peripheral nerve lesions induce profound changes centrally, which may be instrumental in producing pain, but there are almost no data available on how those central changes are modulated by peripheral nerve stimulation. However, in recent years it has become increasingly clear that different pathophysiological mechanisms form the basis of painful sequelae of nerve injury [Campbell et al., 1988], and therefore one cannot expect that peripheral nerve stimulation will influence these painful sequelae in a uniform way.

Surgical Technique

The details of the surgical technique for placing electrodes around peripheral nerves and implanting a stimulating device have been described in several publications [Long, 1973, 1983; Picaza et al., 1975; Nashold and Goldner, 1975; Nashold et al., 1980].

Before implantation, it is necessary to determine whether an implanted nerve stimulator will be able to suppress the pain by trial stimulation, either by stimulating the nerve by means of electrodes applied on the skin over the nerve or when the nerve cannot be activated transcutaneously because of its deep location, by inserting through the skin electrodes close to the nerve with the use of guiding needles. When the trial stimuation performed for several

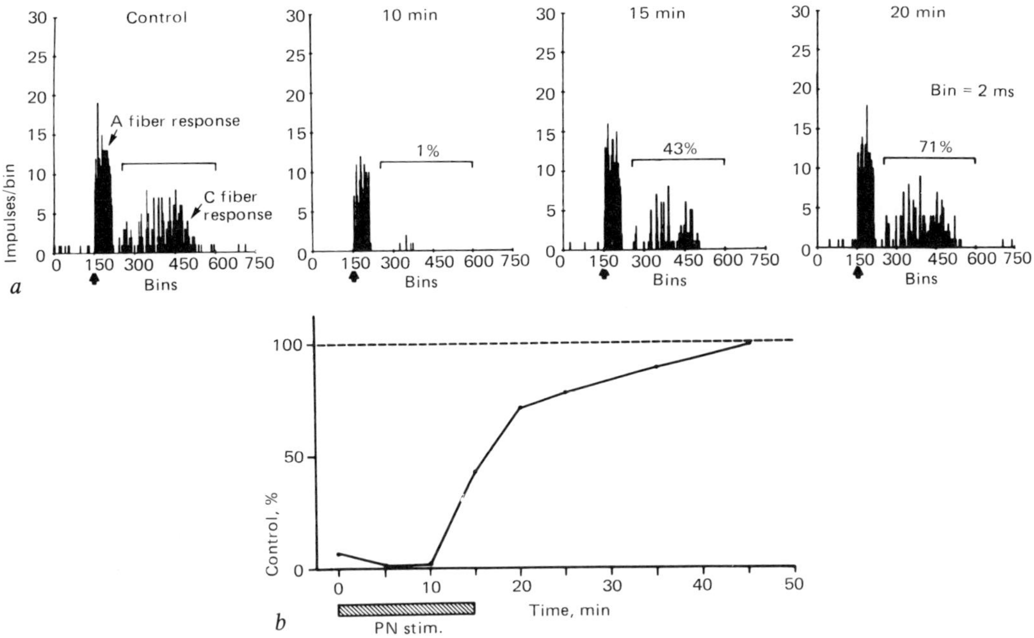

Fig. 22/2. An example of the inhibition of a spinothalamic tract cell produced by peripheral nerve stimulation. *a* Post-stimulus time histograms showing A and C fiber responses following stimulation (arrow at bottom) of the sural nerve. Histograms were formed from 10 consecutive stimuli. The C fiber response, was inhibited to 1, 43 and 71% of control value during, immediately after, and 5 min after 15 min of conditioning stimulation, respectively. *b* The C fiber evoked response was plotted to show the full time course of recovery. PN stim = Peripheral nerve stimulation. From Chung et al. [1984b].

days gives a favorable result, a definitive implant is made. Several types of electrodes and stimulating devices are commercially available. Usually silastic cuffs with platinum contact points are used, and several sizes of cuffs can be chosen, depending on the diameter of a given nerve. Some authors prefer to suture small single electrodes to the nerve in order to avoid constriction of the nerve. Significant constriction by the electrode cuff should by all means be avoided, since it may lead to fibrosis of the nerve with impairment of its function and failure of the therapeutic effect of the stimulation. Performing the surgery under local anesthesia will allow one to manipulate the electrode so as to obtain the paresthesias in the most appropriate area. Once appropriate paresthesias can be elicited, the electrode is connected to a stimulating device as described in chapter 23.

Results

The results of peripheral nerve stimulation obtained with a permanent implant are summarized in table 22/I. (The numbers cited in this table, as well as in table 23/I and 24/I are only approximately correct, due to incomplete information by the different authors.) The study of the literature cited in table 22/I leads to the following comments. The best results are reported with implants in the upper extremities and in cases of peripheral nerve injury; the worst results in cases of low back pain with sciatica and in pain due to metastatic disease. The success rate varies widely between different authors but this seems partly to be due to the fact that certain authors have implanted a large proportion of patients with low back pain and sciatic neuralgia. Nerve block does not seem to have a prognostic value while transcutaneous nerve stimulation has. Necessary conditions to obtain a satisfactory result include the provisos that the paresthesias evoked by the stimulation cover the painful area and that the electrodes be placed proximal to the nerve lesion. It is often noted that in the favorable cases, as time passes, the patients have to stimulate less and less to obtain the same pain suppressor effect.

Complications

There are few complications. Besides the usual complications proper to implanted neurostimulation devices specific complications are: (1) constriction of the nerve by too tight an electrode cuff which may lead to impairment of nerve function and failure of stimulation; (2) rotation of the electrode cuff with failure of adequate stimulation, and (3) tenderness in the area where the electrode is fixed to the nerve.

Stimulation of the Ganglion of Gasser

Meyerson and Håkanson reported in 1980 a method to stimulate the ganglion of Gasser by means of a bipolar electrode sutured to the dura over the ganglion exposed through a subtemporal approach. They applied this technique in a condition which they refer to as painful trigeminal neuropathy, in which facial pain results from injury to the peripheral part of the trigeminal nerve and which is also often labeled as atypical trigeminal neuralgia. For our different use of this term please see chapter 1.A., p. 41. The

Table 22/I. Results of peripheral nerve stimulation: N_t=total number of patients tested; N_i=total number of implantations

Author	Year	N_t/N_i	Follow-up	Pain syndrome: terms used by the authors	Results success (≥50% pain relief) (%)
Meyer and Fields	1972	?/10	?	pain after nerve injury	75
Long	1973	?/10	3–13 months	pain after nerve injury	80
Kirsch et al.	1975	?/32	>1 year	?	initially 90 after 1 year 53
Nashold and Goldner	1975	20/22	6–48 months	pain after nerve injury	60
Picaza et al.	1975	?/23	6–20 months	neurogenic/deafferentation	87
Campbell and Long	1976	?/33	3–17 months	multiple (esp. low back)	25
Sweet	1976c	?/69	1–5 years	esp. traumatic neuropathy	initially 43 after 1–5 years 25
Picaza et al.	1977–78	?/37	12–46 months	esp. postop. disc surgery	49
Law et al.	1980	?/22	9–88 months	esp. post-traumatic neuropathy	62
Long et al.	1981	?/34	9 years	neurogenic	initially 41 after 9 years 32
Nashold et al.	1982	?/35	4–9 years	neurogenic	
				upper extremity	52
				lower extremity	31
Gybels and Kupers	1987	7/7	1–7 years	pain after nerve injury	89

pain is confined to the territory of the trigeminal nerve, and the presence of dysesthesia, hyperalgesia and sometimes allodynia are characteristic features. In these cases there is often a history of interventions on the sinuses, facial fractures, dental surgery, alcohol blocks of branches of the trigeminal nerve and thermal trigeminal rhizotomy. Usually this type of pain responds well to transcutaneous stimulation of the branches of the trigeminal nerve, but since this method is bothersome to apply in the face, direct stimulation of the ganglion of Gasser was developed as an alternative to TENS (Transcutaneous Electrical Nerve Stimulation) and a possible way of improving the efficiency of the stimulation. It is interesting to note that as early as 1966 Shelden described 3 patients with trigeminal neuralgia who had temporary but not useful relief with such stimulation. A percutaneous technique for implantation of a chronic electrode in the Gasserian ganglion has also been developed, in which the lead has a helically curved section designed to prevent traction on the tip with the movement of the jaw [Meglio, 1984; Steude, 1984]. As with other forms of nerve stimulation the paresthesias evoked by stimulation must cover the painful area and therefore the extent of retroganglionic fiber degeneration is of importance for the possibility of obtaining pain relief by trigeminal ganglion and root stimulation. Judging from the few data available, the results of this technique for treating painful trigeminal neuropathy have been very rewarding. In 1986, Meyerson and Håkanson reported long-term results (mean follow-up of 4 years) in 14 cases; 11 patients had retained the pain-suppressive effect of the stimulation. This is all the more remarkable since this type of pain is notoriously difficult to manage. Gorecki et al. [1987] have used ganglion of Gasser stimulation both in central neurogenic and in peripheral neurogenic pain. In their 15 patients of which 11 had permanent stimulators inserted, there was no clear distinction in success rate between central neurogenic and peripheral neurogenic pain. Six of these 11 patients were using their stimulators successfully after 1–60 months of follow-up.

Conclusions

In view of the rather favorable long-term results of peripheral nerve stimulation and the simple low-risk technique it is surprising that peripheral nerve implantation is rarely performed (we found only 335 reported cases).

Chapter 23. Spinal Cord Stimulation

Historical Note

Spinal cord stimulation (SCS) for control of pain was introduced by Shealy et al. in 1967. They reasoned that the greatest concentration of A-beta fibers lay in the dorsal columns and that stimulation there would, according to the gate control theory, provoke inhibition of C fibers better than stimulation from any other area.

A prerequisite for successful pain relief by SCS has usually been a coinciding or blanketing of the painful area by the generalized paresthesias. The assumption that the crucial area affected is the posterior white columns gave rise to the name 'dorsal column stimulation' (DCS). However, pain reduction without paresthesias, for instance by placement of the electrodes over the anterior cord surface, has been reported as well [Larson et al., 1974; Campbell, 1981], and therefore has challenged the mediation of the dorsal column or even of the lemniscal pathways, generally speaking, in spinal stimulation for pain.

The remaining uncertainty about the real target of the current applied, for pain alleviation within the cord, led to the use of 'spinal cord stimulation' as a general designation of the technique instead of the earlier term 'dorsal column stimulation', although both terms are indiscriminately used.

SCS was adopted with enthusiasm by many neurosurgeons and the more recent percutaneously implantable forms also by nonneurosurgical pain clinics. It was estimated in 1985 [Maiman et al., 1985] that since the initial report of Shealy et al. [1967] more than 10,000 patients have had electrodes implanted in the spinal canal for pain management. There were more than 2,000 spinal stimulators implanted each year in the USA and 3,400 in the rest of the world. From 1975 to 1985 the number of implants performed each year has grown at an annual rate of 20%. As SCS came into use in Europe a few years after the method was introduced in the USA, European clinicians, on the basis of reports from several North American centers of a high percentage of late failures, have applied SCS a bit more discriminately than their North American colleagues, and SCS is recognized as a valuable but not ideal therapeutic method. The target group has included patients suffering from chronic low back pain after so-called failed back surgery, phantom pain, post-herpetic neuralgia, cramping pain in multiple sclerosis, pain due to peripheral vasculopathic ischemia, and to a lesser degree pain due to cancer.

Mechanisms of Pain Relief by Spinal Cord Stimulation

It is not possible, with the evidence available, to point out what might be the physiological mechanisms underlying the chronic pain-suppressor effects of SCS, but different hypotheses can be formulated.

The initial theory postulated an antidromic activation of A-beta afferents and SCS was seen as a clinical application of the gate control theory [Shealy et al., 1967]. This explanation was, however, controversial because some details of the gate control theory were challenged [Franz and Iggo, 1968; Gregor and Zimmermann, 1973; Whitehorn and Burgess, 1973]. An important frequent clinical characteristic of SCS, a long-lasting after effect of pain relief for hours after a period of stimulation [Nashold and Friedman, 1972; Sweet and Wepsic, 1974a; Nielson et al., 1975a] did not find a counterpart in animal experiments in which dorsal column stimulation usually induced only a brief inhibition of dorsal horn nociceptive neurons [Hillman and Wall, 1969; Handwerker et al., 1975; Feldman, 1975; Foreman et al., 1976].

It has been argued that SCS blocks transmission in the spinothalamic tract [Larson et al., 1974] because with electrodes placed on the anterior part of the spinal cord pain was reduced even though no paresthesias were experienced, but this again cannot account for the extended post-stimulation pain relief seen in many patients. The same objection applies to a proposed masking effect [Larson et al., 1974]. It is tempting to speculate that SCS activates fibers in the dorsolateral funiculus which contains an important descending naloxone-reversible pathway for inhibiting nociceptive input [Basbaum and Fields, 1979], but naloxone does not reverse SCS-induced pain relief, and spinal cord stimulation does not increase spinal fluid endorphine [Meyerson, 1983].

Rather than, or in addition to, an inhibition at the level of the dorsal horn, some authors have postulated an inhibition at supraspinal levels

[Nashold et al., 1972; Nyquist and Greenhoot, 1973; Bantli et al., 1975; Modesti and Waszak, 1975; Gildenberg and Murthy, 1980; Atweh et al., 1985; Saadé et al., 1985, 1986], particularly on the basis that when the dorsal columns are destroyed distal to the stimulating electrodes there is still evidence of activation of pain-suppressing mechanisms.

It has also been suggested that SCS might activate central inhibitory mechanisms influencing sympathetic efferent neurons [Meyerson, 1983] and there is much clinical evidence that spinal cord stimulation can favorably influence the ischemia as well as the pain of vascular diseases of the extremities [Cook et al., 1976; Tallis et al., 1983; Augustinsson et al., 1985]. It is not known, though, whether the pain-reducing effect and the autonomic effects share a common neural mechanism. Finally, neurohumoral mechanisms are often invoked in the pain-suppressive effect of spinal cord stimulation, because a large number of known and putative neurotransmitters and neuromodulators are implicated in nociception and antinociception, and the pain-suppressor effects of SCS may outlast the stimulation period for several hours and occasionally several days. Not many data are available in patients regarding biochemical correlates with pain suppression after spinal cord stimulation. An increase has been shown of epinephrine [Levin and Hubschmann, 1980] and substance-P-like immunoreactivity in CSF [Meyerson et al., 1985] with SCS, while somatostatin, cholecystokinin, vasoactive intestinal polypeptide, neurotensin and monamine metabolites showed no change related to stimulation and the ensuing pain relief [Meyerson et al., 1985]. The limited number of data and the technical difficulties inherent to this type of approach do not allow one to draw any conclusions with respect to the involvement of neurochemical mechanisms in the pain-suppressor effects of SCS.

Surgical Technique

The technique for SCS has been described by several authors. In the early years, a laminectomy was needed in order to place electrodes extra-, endo- and intradurally over the midline of the spinal cord [Shealy et al. 1967, 1970; Nashold and Friedman, 1972; Burton, 1973, 1975; Sweet and Wepsic, 1974a; Krainick et al., 1975; Pineda, 1975; Shelden et al., 1975].

Connections were made with a device implanted subcutaneously, usually in the subcostal or subclavicular region. The first and most widely used RF-linked arrangement allowed the electric power supply to be transmitted to the electrodes from an external source, by placing the doughnut-shaped antenna of a transmitter device over the skin that covers the implanted receiver. The external miniaturized battery-powered transmitter generates rectangular electric pulses and permits their different parameters to be varied within certain ranges. The electrodes are uncoupled from the power supply and its control, both because of the high power requirements of SCS, about two orders of magnitude greater than those for cardiac pacing, and the demand for maximal adjustability of stimulation parameters.

In spite of the higher energy requirements as compared with cardiac pacemakers, totally implantable and programmable systems for neurostimulation have been produced, employing lithium batteries that provide several years of service. The stimulator and electrode system can be interrogated for impedance and parameters in use. The patient's compliance for the totally implantable system was reported to be much better than for the RF-linked systems (with external parts), the inconvenience of the former being the dependence on an attending doctor for reprogramming [Davis and Gray, 1981]. Cathodal stimulation proved to be the more effective and energy-saving type [Ranck, 1975; Sherwood, 1981; Davis and Gray, 1981; Law, 1983]. So the option of reversible polarity could be omitted. The remaining degrees of freedom were voltage, frequency and pulse width, respectively, ranging in the order of 1–10 V, 20–200 cps and 100–500 μs.

Since 1972 the less invasive percutaneous installation of wire leads into the epidural space by means of a puncture needle (type 'Tuohy-Huber' and 'Hustead') achieved widespread usage, first as a preliminary selection procedure and then as a definitive implant [Hosobuchi et al., 1972; Long and Hagfors, 1975; Long et al., 1981; North et al., 1977, 1977/78; Doerr et al., 1978; Young, 1978a; Richardson et al., 1979]. To do this the patient is placed prone on an X-ray permeable operating table, with a pillow under his thorax or abdomen, in accordance with the intended site of puncture. An X-ray image amplifier system visualizes the tip of the puncture needle and enables one to follow the electrode as it is passed upward within the spinal canal. Local anesthesia is applied to the skin and the soft parts overlying the interspinous space to be punctured. A small incision is made, and then an epidural 15- or 16-gauge needle with upward angulation and provided with a stylet is introduced between two chosen spinous processes, through the fascia and interspinous ligament. Although the needle meets more resistance if it is advanced all the way through the interspinous ligament in the midline, this course yields an optimal position of the needle tip at the dorsal midline notch of the spinal canal. When the needle tip enters the epidural space by perforating the yellow ligament, a sudden decrease in resistance is felt.

Intermittent X-ray control with sagittal beam direction is helpful in maintaining the epidural needle in the midsagittal plane. The negative pressure within the epidural space is a final criterion of correct needle position. The audible aspiration of air or that of a drop of sterile saline placed into the open hub of the needle, or otherwise the unresisting injectability of a small amount of saline without aspiration of blood or CSF, indicate an epidural placement. The very flexible coil-wire lead is straightened by inserting a less flexible wire stylet, the front tip of which can be gently bent. This makes the lead steerable by axial rotation, once it is advanced through the needle and maneuvered in a cephalad direction through the epidural space. Sideward rotations of the needle tip may also contribute to overcome initial obstructions the lead may encounter on its way up. The electrode is positioned over the dorsal aspect of the cord in such a way that cathodal test stimulation (e.g. 0.5–5 V, 100 Hz and 200 μs pulse width) generates a tingling or other painless sensation within the painful body parts. The anodal electrode is then applied to an indifferent skin area. After successful lead placement, the wire stylet and then the epidural needle are prudently retracted, leaving only the coil-wire lead at its target. These procedures are monitored by fluoroscopic control and by continuous test stimulation. By means of sutures and a silicone cuff or a plastic button, the lead is anchored at the fascia. Subsequently, it is plugged on a percutaneous extension. The percutaneously implanted wire electrode is not attached to any intraspinal structure and is only subsequently held in place by adhesions due to minor local tissue reactions. This technique is therefore burdened with a higher incidence of electrode displacements than the open surgical implantation, which for this reason remains a useful option.

For the sake of gradual fixation of the — in principle mobile — electrode at its correct target, it may be helpful to impose confinement of the patient to bed with limited spinal motion for a few days after the intervention. The percutaneous stimulation test usually lasts 7–10 days. If adequate pain relief is produced over this period of time, the system is internalized. For permanent implantation or secondary internalization, the lead is connected with a receiver or a totally implantable power-supply and control device. The latter is placed in a bluntly dissected subcutaneous pocket in the subclavicular or subcostal region, under local or general anesthesia (fig. 23/1).

The subcutaneous tunneling from the pocket to the mid-back incision, harboring the connection leads, can indeed cause severe discomfort to the patient, in spite of ample local infiltration and the use of an appropriate tunneling instrument, so that for this intervention general anesthesia should be considered as an alternative, depending on the patient's individual

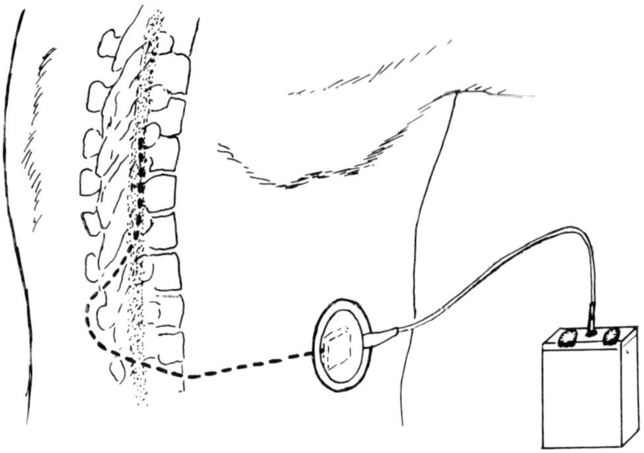

Fig. 23/I. Scheme of an SCS device.

compliance and tolerance. A Teflon bag may be wrapped around the connection plugs, in order to avoid adhesions to the subcutaneous tissue, and rendering easier possible later operative revisions.

Wire electrodes for percutaneous insertion have been used in various forms: one single-lead electrode acting as a cathode in a monopolar arrangement, the device case serving as the anode; two single-lead electrodes in a bipolar arrangement, and one multiple-lead electrode in a bipolar arrangement with many possible combinations. The latter assembly allows multi-level trials over a chosen part of the spinal cord. The early unit was composed of four disc electrodes in linear array, spaced 1 cm apart, molded in Dacron mesh and silicone rubber, connected to a plug housing, requiring a partial laminectomy and percutaneous testing prior to permanent receiver implantation. A newer four-electrode catheter assembly can be installed through an epidural needle and connected with a computerized receiver which allows the lead combinations to be monitored on a continual basis through an external transmitter [Waltz, 1982; Waltz and Davis, 1983]. Minor variations from the above technique, such as operating in the sitting position, are certainly possible without affecting the essential principles [Ray, 1981; Siegfried and Hood, 1983].

Results

Table 23/I summarizes the results of SCS with a permanent implant; the literature cited here can be summarized as follows: There is a decrease with time of the efficacy of the pain-suppressor effect of SCS. Of a total of 1,219 patients at short-term the success rate was 66%, at long-term 52%. Moreover, when a distinction is made between studies in which a thorough patient selection has taken place, and these are the more recent studies, versus studies in which this was not the case, it appears that in studies without thorough patient screening the success rate at short-term is 50%, at long-term 36%, while in studies with a 'good' patient screening, the success rate at short-term is 83%, at long-term 65%. A thorough case selection includes the evaluation of psychological factors and trial stimulation during a variable period. These results show that although a 'good' screening yields a much higher success rate than a 'bad' screening, it cannot prevent the fall in initial success rate over time. The reasons given for this decline of efficacy are: stimulation system dysfunction due to technical factors; insufficient stimulation because of increased electrode resistance due to scarring, and migration of the electrode tip, which precludes production of paresthesias in the painful area, usually a necessary condition to obtain pain suppression. It may well be that besides these technical factors, more fundamental physiopathological factors are responsible for the late failures, but these factors are not known. Pain associated with spinal cord injury and confined to a completely denervated area is unlikely to be attenuated, since no fibers are available for stimulation in such a condition. The same may apply in plexus avulsion, where the lesion is proximal to the ganglion, and therefore dorsal column fibers will degenerate. It is not easy to correlate a particular pain condition with an expected success rate, but SCS is more effective for pain of neurogenic origin and particularly effective in those cases where vascular disorders are present [Cook et al., 1976; Meglio et al., 1981; Tallis et al., 1983; Augustinsson et al., 1985; Broseta et al., 1986]. As can be seen in table 23/I, SCS has been applied in a large number of patients with 'low back pain'. In most of these cases there were multiple lumbar operations, with a diagnosis of epidural fibrosis or arachnoiditis, and different pain loci, including lumbar pain and radicular pain. The major studies, with a follow-up from 1 to 5 years, report that more than 50% of the patients experienced pain relief that was classified as excellent, good, or more than 50% relief, a result that in these difficult cases has to be judged as useful.

Table 23/I. Results of dorsal column stimulation. N_t = Total number of patients tested; N_i = Total number of implantations

Author	Year	N_t/N_i	Follow-up	Pain syndrome: terms used by authors	Results success (≥50% pain relief)	%
Nashold and Friedman	1972	?/30	9–18 months	neurogenic	initially	40
					after 3 years	28
Krainick et al.	1975	?/73	?	neurogenic (esp. post-amputation		38
Long and Erickson	1975	?/69	7 years	multiple	initially	81
					after 1 year	49
					after 7 years	33
Nielson et al.	1975b	221/130	5 years	multiple (esp. low back	initially	67
					after 5 years	49
Hunt et al.	1975	?/13	2–6 years	neurogenic		31
Pineda	1975	?/79	?	multiple (esp. failed disc surg.)		44
Shelden et al.	1975	?/27	3 years	somatic (17)		47
				neurogenic (10)		80
Urban and Nashold	1978	?/20	2 years	multiple (esp. low back)	initially	35
					after 2 years	21
Young	1978a	?/51	12–67 months	multiple (esp. lumbar disc)	immediately	78
					after 3 years	47
Krainick et al.	1980	?/84	2.5–5.5 years	postamputation	initially	39
					after 2.5–5.5 years	18
Richardson et al.	1980	?/19	1 year	paraplegic pain	initially	50
					after 1 year	30

Table 23/I. (cont.)

Author	Year	N_t/N_i	Follow-up	Pain syndrome: terms used by authors	Results success (≥50% pain relief)	%
Long et al.	1981	?/30	7 years	multiple	after 6 months	77
					after 7 years	73
Winkelmüller	1981	89/81	4 months–7 years	neurogenic (esp. low back)	immediately	88
					after 4 months–7 years	68
Le Roy	1981	?/49	5 years	low back		59
Blume et al.	1982	?/28	?	low back		70
Siegfried and Lazorthes	1982	191/89	3 months–8 years	low back (esp. lumbar disc)	after 3 months	91
					after 2 years	66
					after 4–8 years	60
Ray et al.	1982	?/50	5 years	low back		54
De la Porte and Siegfried	1983	94/38	3–96 months	spinal arachnoiditis	immediately	95
					after 1 year	68
					after 2 years	57
Siegfried	1983b	291/146	1–4 years	deafferentation (84)	initially	81
					after 1–4 years	71
				somatic (62)	initially	74
					after 1–4 years	71
Hood and Siegfried	1984	16/8	56 months	brachial plexus avulsion		6
Augustinsson et al.	1985	?/34	16 months	severe limb ischemia		61
Waisbrod and Gerbershagen	1985	?/16	6–30 months	battered root syndrome		75
Vogel et al.	1986	50/44	>3 years	multiple (esp. sciatica)		9

Complications

In the early days, several cases were reported of complete or partial transverse spinal syndromes, which have usually been reversible after removal of the electrode system. With electrodes placed subdurally, spinal fluid leak along the lead wire is rather common. With the percutaneous technique, electrode displacement can be expected in 10% or more of the cases, although the use of the newer multipolar leads may partly compensate for electrode migration [Leclercq, 1984; Law, 1986]. Lead breakage, eventually with current leakage, will also occur in some 10% of the cases. Epidural fibrosis may have as a consequence, insufficient current intensity to stimulate the spinal cord and changes in current strength to the spinal cord related to changes in posture and root stimulation may be bothersome.

Conclusions

Spinal cord stimulation for pain is frequently not a single and simple but a time-consuming and rather expensive technique. It is as yet not possible to correlate a particular pain condition with an expected success rate, but spinal cord stimulation is probably more effective for pain of neurogenic than somatic origin and particularly effective in those cases in which a vascular disorder is present. It has probably been overused but its reversible character has largely avoided unwanted side effects.

Chapter 24. Deep Brain Stimulation

Historical Note

Prompted by the observations of Olds and Milner [1954], who described a rewarding effect of deep cerebral stimulation in animals, a few surgeons attempted to treat pain by the use of temporary implanted electrodes, particularly in the septal area [Heath and Mickle, 1960; Gol, 1967]. Apart from these early attempts, two lines of development can be distinguished in the history of deep brain stimulation (DBS). One is a direct consequence of physiological work, starting from the discovery of Reynolds [1969] demonstrating that stimulation of the lateral margin of the periaqueductal gray (PAG) prevented nociceptive responses of rats during abdominal surgery without concomitant drug administration, and progressively unfolding the story of an endogenous pain control system. This has led to a characterization of the neural structures capable of what is termed stimulation-produced analgesia (SPA), and in which much emphasis was initially placed on the role played by certain neurotransmitters, such as serotonin and NE, and the endogenous opioids. It is now clear that the 'analgesia systems' are much more complex than was initially thought [for recent review, Hammond, 1986]. The first observation in man that stimulation of the periventricular gray (PVG) could suppress pain was made in 1973 by Richardson and Akil [1977c] and during the late 1970s PAG-PVG stimulation was systematically developed for clinical use [Hosobuchi et al., 1977].

A second line of development of DBS can be traced to the formulation of the gate control theory [Melzack and Wall, 1965]. This formulation offered a conceptual framework to attempt pain control in humans by means of electrical stimulation of the skin, peripheral nerves and dorsal columns. This paved the way to stimulation of the VPM-VPL nuclei in the thalamus [Hosobuchi et al., 1973] and the sensory part of the internal capsule [Adams et al., 1974] in those cases in which, because of lesions, fibers in the peripheral nerves and dorsal columns were no longer available, and supraspinal stimulation offered an alternative to activate the lemniscal system. However, several years before the formulation of the gate control theory Mazars et al. [1973] had introduced VPL-VPM stimulation on the basis of the classical theory of Head and Holmes [1911], who had postulated that pain results from a release of the protopathic system from the epicritic system. Stimulation of the thalamic sensory relay nuclei would presumably increase the epicritic component of the sensation.

Central Nervous System Mechanisms for Pain Modulation

The PVG-PAG Area

Figure 24/1 represents a model proposed by Basbaum and Fields [1978] of the descending pathways believed to modulate pain transmission which is still reasonably valid.

Neurons in the PAG and nucleus raphe magnus (NRM) form a pathway from the midbrain to the dorsal horn that is instrumental in inhibiting nociceptive neurons. In this descending inhibitory control system are also included the locus coeruleus (LC), the subcoeruleus-parabrachial complex (Sc-PB) and the magnocellular part of the n. reticularis gigantocellularis (Rmc). There is moreover evidence suggesting that centrifugal control of nociceptive information is not restricted to the dorsal horn but is also operating at supraspinal levels, such as the thalamus. From the anatomical point of view, projections from the n. raphe magnus to the intralaminar nuclei and the n. submedius have been demonstrated [Peschanski and Besson, 1984]; from the physiological point of view, stimulation of the dorsal raphe nucleus inhibits the responses to noxious stimuli of neurons in the n. parafascicularis [Anderson and Dafny, 1983]; from a pharmacological point of view, micro-injection of morphine in PAG is followed by a naloxone-reversible reduction in the responses of neurons in the ventrobasal complex, even with doses which do not depress the responses of dorsal horn nociceptive neurons [Benoist et al., 1983].

The VPM-VPL Area

There is much evidence for the existence of nonopioid analgesic systems [Cannon et al., 1982; Watkins and Mayer, 1982; Mayer and Watkins, 1984; Terman et al., 1984]. In particular, stimulation of the ventral

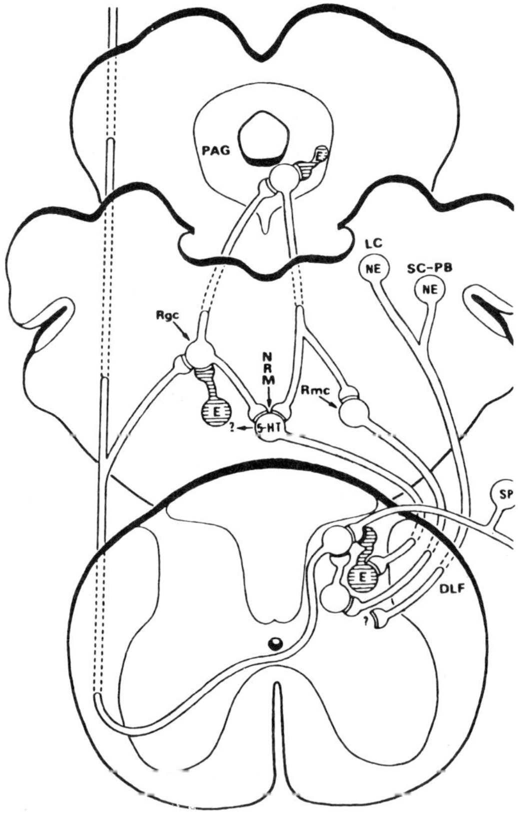

Fig. 24/1. Neural circuits thought to be involved in the endogenous analgesia system. NRM = N. raphe magnus; LC = locus coeruleus; SC-PB = subcoeruleus-parabrachial complex; Rgc = n. reticularis gigantocellularis; Rmc = magnocellular part of Rgc; NE = norepinephrine; E = enkephalin; DLF = dorsolateral funiculus; cross-hatched neurons contain endogenous opioid substances. From Basbaum and Fields [1978].

posterior medial and lateral nuclei of the thalamus can, as is the case with PAG stimulation, also inhibit the evoked responses of wide dynamic range and high threshold spinothalamic tract neurons [Gerhart et al., 1981; Dickenson, 1983], and although stimulation of these primary somatosensory relay nuclei does not preferentially inhibit the responses to nonnoxious or noxious natural stimuli, the response to C fiber volleys is reduced to a greater extent than the response to A fiber volleys [Gerhart et al.,

1983]. Possibly antidromic activation of collaterals of the spinothalamic fibers to the medullary reticular formation and PAG could fire neurons in those structures which participate in the previously described centrifugal control of nociceptive transmission in the spinal cord [Tsubokawa et al., 1982]. However, the inhibition of dorsal horn neurons by stimulation of VPM-VPL is not influenced by the administration of naloxone [Tsubokawa et al., 1985]. Moreover, the inhibition of nociceptive responses of neurons in the Pf nucleus by VPL stimulation is also not affected by naloxone [Benabid et al., 1983]. Thus, the pathways that mediate the inhibitory effects of VPM-VPL stimulation on nociceptive input remain to a large extent to be elucidated.

As was argued by Willis [1984], even if it can be asserted that a given neuron transmits nociceptive information from the spinal cord to the brain, the exact role of a given neuron in the evocation of conscious sensation is not known. Nevertheless, from the few data available in man there is evidence that VPL stimulation can suppress an experimentally induced acute pain sensation [Gybels et al., 1976] (fig. 24/2).

Surgical Technique

Useful information regarding technique can be found in several publications [Adams and Hosobuchi, 1977; Sedan and Lazorthes, 1978; Hosobuchi, 1982a; Dieckmann et al., 1982; Siegfried et al., 1983; Meyerson, 1985].

Stimulation Site PVG-PAG

Usually, multipolar electrodes are used which, during a period of trial stimulation, allow one, via wires passed through the skin of the scalp, to explore the region along the electrode and to choose that combination of stimulation sites which offers a maximal pain-suppressive effect (fig. 24/3a, b).

The crucial point in the technique is to reach the correct target, since there are many indications that the region in the medial diencephalic-mesencephalic junction zone, from which stimulation-produced pain relief can be obtained, is small [Meyerson et al., 1979; Gybels et al., 1980; Boivie and Meyerson, 1982; Baskin et al., 1986]. Commonly used target points for PVG are those defined by Richardson and Akil [1977c]: X = 10 mm posterior to the midpoint of the AC-PC line; Y = the AC-PC line,

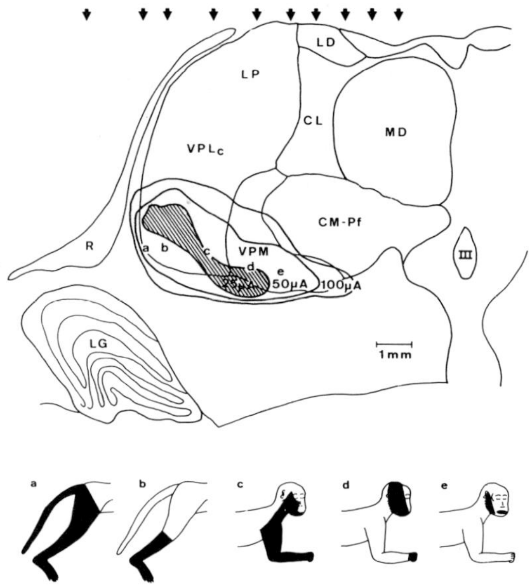

Structure	Number of cases	Number of stim. (100 cs, 1 ms, 10 s; 0.5–2 mA	$S_2 < S_1$	$S_2 = S_1$	$S_2 > S_1$
Frontal cortex (area 9 ?)	9	160	24	102	34
Parietal cortex (area 19 ? – 39 ?)	12	119	39	50	30
Nucleus caudatus and fundus striati	4	31	1	28	2
VPL and V.c.p.c.	17] 2] 19	290] 16] 306	141] 12] 153	112] 2] 114	37] 2] 39
CM–Pf	3	23	2	19	2
VL	10	79	20	52	7

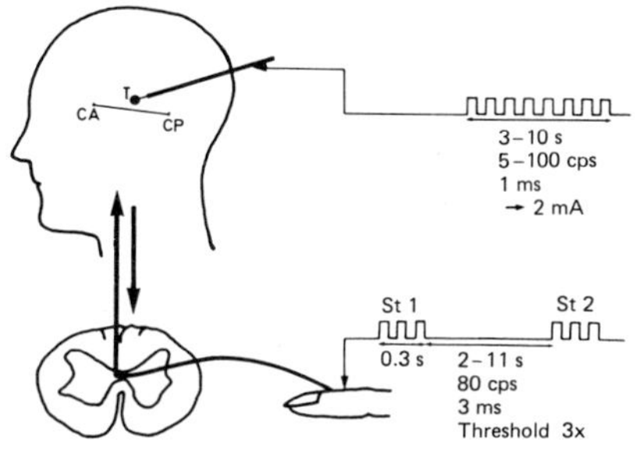

Fig. 24/2. Left side: Monkey; results of an ipsilateral thalamic mapping experiment. The ipsilateral thalamic stimulating electrode was moved to each of the medial-lateral locations indicated by the vertical arrows and then advanced through the thalamus in 1-mm steps. At each point on the tracking grid, long trains (several seconds duration, 100-µs pulses, 333 Hz, 200 µA) were delivered through the electrode to test the effect of such stimulation on the activity of a wide dynamic range STT (spinothalamic tract) neuron. When stimuli of 200 µA were found to inhibit STT cell responses, lower strengths were tested. The circled areas in and ventral to the VPLc and VPM nuclei show regions in which pulses at 100 µA or less caused inhibition of STT cell activity, with the cross-hatched (innermost) region being effective at 25 µA or less. Figurines at the bottom show the cutaneous receptive fields that were mapped at each of the corresponding points (a–e) in the VPLc and VPM nuclei. Fields were mapped by recording multi-unit activity through the thalamic electrode. From Gerhart et al. [1983]. Right side: Results from 26 patients who underwent stereotactic surgery for a variety of diseases, mostly parkinsonism. The subject has to make comparisons of the subjective intensity of two equally noxious electrical skin stimuli St1 and St2. A brain structure is stimulated during the second noxious stimuli. Three categories of judgment are permitted: the sensation (S2) provoked by the second stimulus is equal to (S2 = S1), greater (S2>S1) or smaller (S2<S1) than the sensation (S1) provoked by the first stimulus. From Gybels et al. [1976]. The figure shows that VPL-VPM stimulation inhibits spinothalamic tract neurons in monkey and acute pain sensation in man.

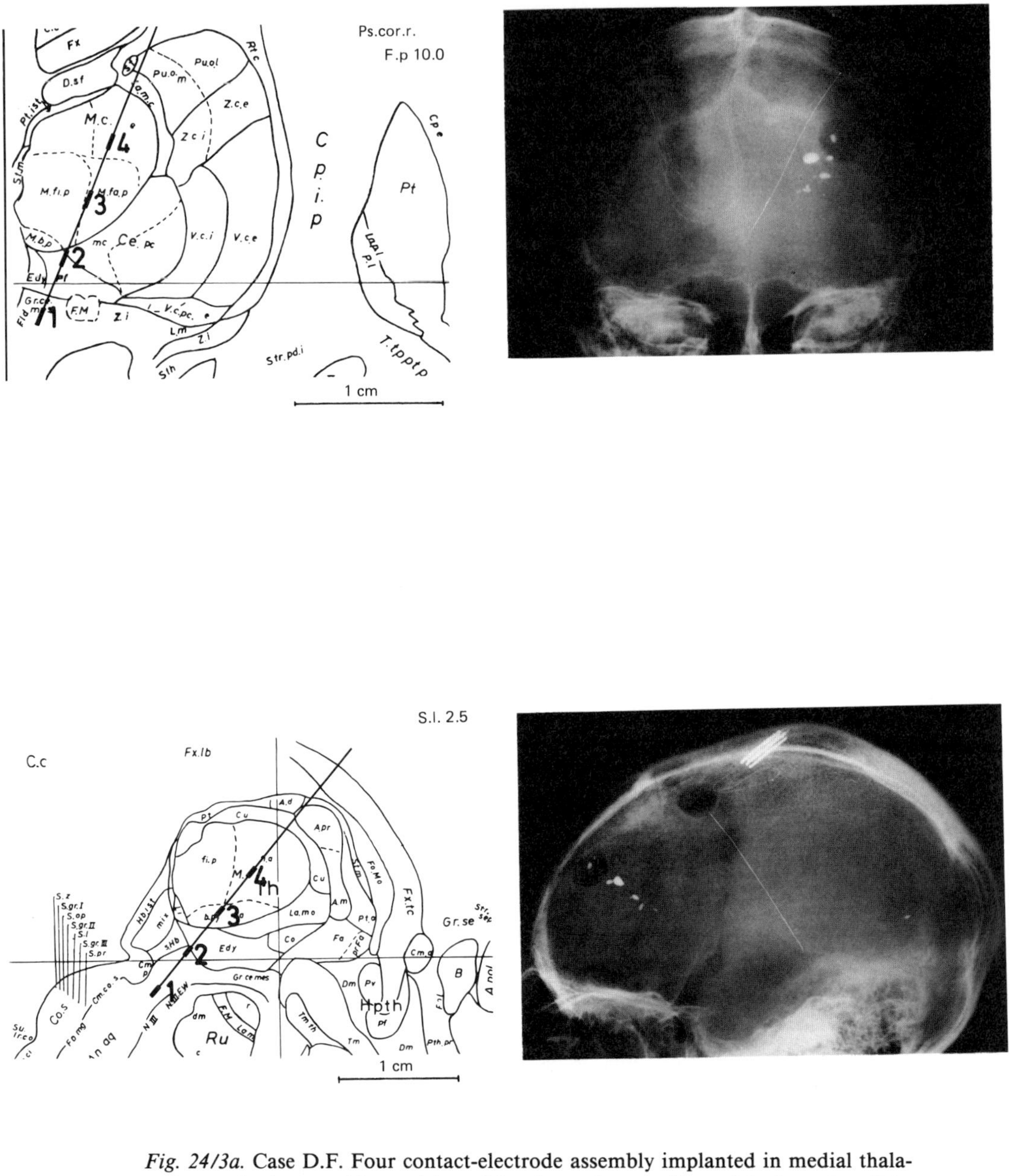

Fig. 24/3a. Case D.F. Four contact-electrode assembly implanted in medial thalamus and upper brain stem. The position of the electrode assembly and the bare tips of the 4 electrodes are projected, respectively, on frontal plane 10 and sagittal plane 2.5 of Schaltenbrand and Bailey's [1959] atlas. From Gybels and Cosyns [1976].

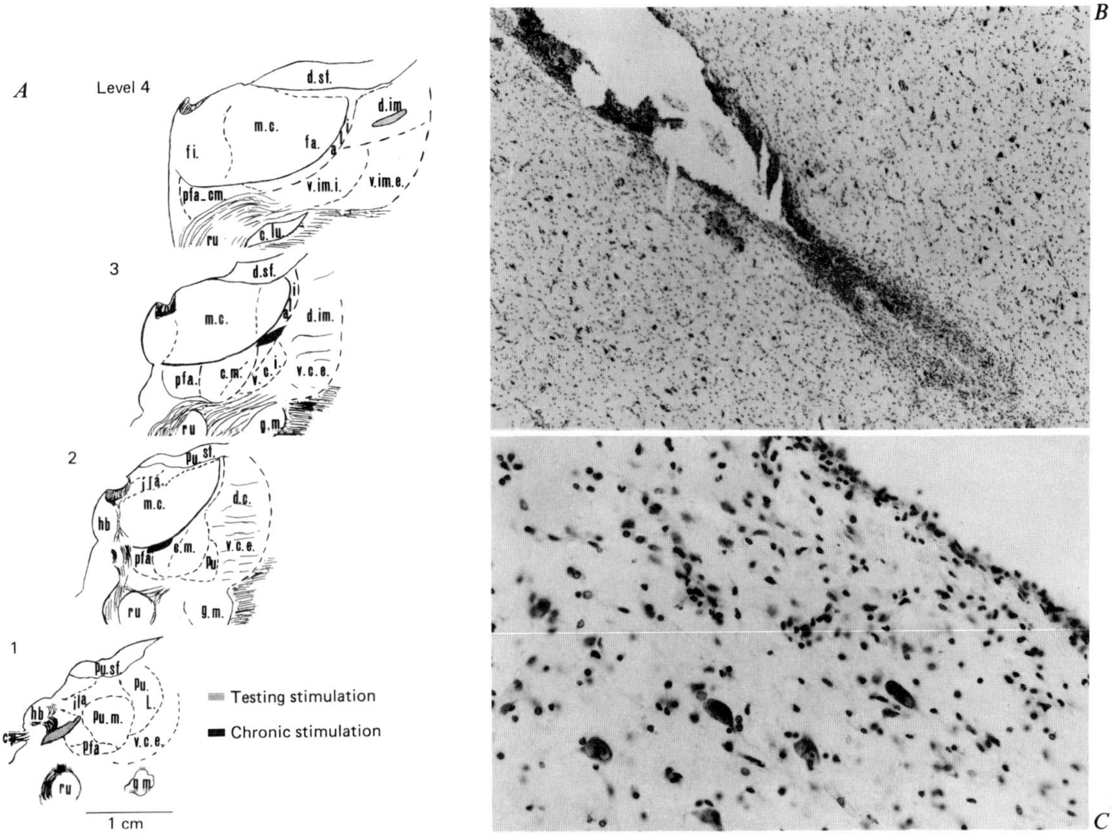

Fig. 24/3b. Casae D.F. Autopsy material. *A* Four vertico-frontal sections, level 1 most caudal, level 4 most rostral. From Gybels et al. [1980]. The small electrode sites moving from superio-laterally to infero-medially are just visible. Microscopic examination in *B* and *C*. *B* The most distal part of the electrode trajectory is seen in the upper left-hand corner. There is a slight chronic inflammatory reaction with lympho-histiocytic proliferation and some glial reaction in the immediate vicinity. At the tip end of the electrode, a mild tissue reaction can be observed: some lymphocytes and histiocytes and a slight gliosis with disappearaance of neurons. The normal architecture of the surrounding thalamic intralaminar nuclei should be noticed. HE. × 125. *C* In the upper right-hand corner, the wall of the electrode trajectory in its middle portion is shown. There is only minimal tissue reaction: some histiocytes, occasional lymphocytes and some spongioblastic astrglial reaction. The nervous tissue in close proximity to the electrode has a normal appearance. HE. × 400. *B* and *C* are unpublished data.

and Z = 2–3 mm lateral to the midline, depending on the width of the posterior part of the third ventricle. Commonly used target points for PAG are those defined by Hosobuchi et al. [1977]: X and Y = the iter of the aqueduct, and Z = 2.5–3.5 mm lateral to the midline of the iter of the aqueduct. Both these targets seem to be equally effective as far as the pain-suppressive effect is concerned, but patients seem to prefer the PVG locus, stimulation of which often provides a diffuse sensation of warmth and well-being, while PAG stimulation tends to elicit a feeling of apprehension, impending doom and oscillopsia [Young et al., 1984].

Stimulation parameters and regimens differ among different authors but usual values might be 25–50 cs, 0.1–1 ms, intensity 0.5–2 mA (below the behavioral threshold), 15–20 min, to be repeated 3–4 times a day. If during trial stimulation of a few weeks good relief of pain is obtained for a given pair of electrodes, the extracranial end of the electrode lead is internalized and the appropriate connections established with a stimulating device subcutaneously implanted (usually in the subclavicular area). This device may be an RF receiver which can be activated by induction through an external stimulator or a totally implanted stimulator which can be programmed by a radiolink operated by the physician expert or the patient after tutelage.

Stimulation Site VPM-VPL

Often a monopolar electrode is used for this target, since during operation, correct electrode positioning is signaled by the evoked paresthesias. The technical advantage of the monopolar electrode is that it is commercially available with a central stylet. This assembly is less traumatizing for the brain than an electrode which has to be introduced with a laterally placed insertion tool and in which an injury can be caused by the angle between the electrode and the insertion tool. A monopolar stimulation arrangement seems to be as efficient for stimulation as a bipolar design [Comte, 1982] although it has been claimed that the design of the electrode is important for inducing 'adequate' nervous tissue activation [Mazars, 1976].

Some authors, instead of aiming for the primary sensory thalamic relay nuclei, place the electrode in the afferent or efferent pathways of these nuclei, either because they are of the opinion that lemniscal stimulation is more effective [Mundinger and Salomao, 1980] or that due to tissue destruction, such as in a thalamic syndrome, there is in these nuclei an insufficient number of neurons available to serve as substratum for the stimulation [Hosobuchi et al., 1973].

Results

Table 24/I gives a survey of what we considered the most relevant series of DBS either because of the number of patients, details on patients, or discussion in depth.

According to this survey, 57% had a pain relief which was estimated 50% or more in the total of 1,539 patients. (This number is greater than the number of implanted patients, since several patients have been reported more than once). Looking at the individual series, it is striking that the results vary considerably among different authors. As a rule, somatic pain responds better to PV–PAG stimulation, while neurogenic pain responds better to VPM-VPL stimulation. A combined stimulation of PV–PAG and VPM-VPL may be useful in those cases in which there is a mixture of somatic and neurogenic pain. For this reason, some authors implant an electrode in the same patient both in PVG-PAG and VP targets [Hosobuchi, 1986]. In table 24/I cases of somatic pain include pain associated with malignant disease and low back pain. It is in this last condition that with long-term follow-up the higher success rates have been reported. In one such study with a follow-up of 2–14 years 80% of 49 patients were classified as successful. In 20 patients the target was PVG-PAG, in 19 both PVG-PAG and VP were stimulated [Hosobuchi, 1986]. Cases of neurogenic pain include anesthesia dolorosa, post-herpetic facial pain, post-injury peripheral nerve pain, phantom limb pain, brachial plexus lesions, pain due to spinal cord injury and thalamic pain. Exceptionally favorable results have been reported by Mazars et al. [1979] with VPL stimulation in phantom limb pain, which they think are due to the particular design of the electrode they use and in which the stimulating pole has a surface of 4 mm^2 and the interpolar distance is 4 mm [Mazars, 1976]. To help determine which patients may benefit from PV–PAG stimulation, some authors advise the use of a morphine test [Hosobuchi, 1982a]. Opiate analgesics are withheld 2 h before the test. A baseline pain assessment is then made. Thereafter, morphine is injected in divided doses over a period of 35–45 min (up to 30 mg i.v.). A dose-response curve is established. When the pain relief due to the morphine administration is reversed by naloxone, the patient is considered a good candidate for PVG-PAG stimulation. If the patient experiences only partial relief with 30 mg of i.v. morphine, withholding surgery is advised until tolerance is reversed by the administration of *L*-tryptophan. As we shall see in the next paragraphs, the value of this test has been challenged [Young and Chambi, 1987; Arnér et al., 1986].

Table 24/I. Results of DBS: N_t = total number of patients tested; N_i = total number of implantations

Author	Year	N_t/N_i	Follow-up	Target	Pain syndrome: terms used by authors	Results: success (≥50% pain relief) %
Richardson and Akil	1977a	30/27	1–46 months	PVG	multiple	70
Gybels	1979	?/7	6–27 months	PAG/PVG	multiple (esp. cancer)	16
Lazorthes	1979	226/130	1 year	PVG	deafferentation (76)	25
					neurogenic (31)	77
					cancer (36)	47
				VPM-IC	mainly deafferentation (83)	28
Mazars et al.	1979	?/205	?/17 years	VPL/VPM	deafferentation (99)	84
					nociception (22)	0
				PVG	nociception (17)	0
				PAG	cancer (67)	22
Hosobuchi	1980a	62/43	6 months to 9.5 years	IC,VPL,VPM,LM	deafferentation (21)	71
				PAG	peripheral (22)	73
Mundinger and Salomao	1980	?/32	47 months	LM	deafferentation	53
Schvarcz	1980	6/4	?–42 months	PAG/PVG	deafferentation	100
Turnbull et al.	1980	18/14	?–5 years	VPL,VPM	neuropathic	57
Dieckmann and Witzman	1982	52/46	6 months to 4.5 years	PVG or VPL, VPM	mainly deafferentation	28
Boivie and Meyerson	1982	?/5	3–17 months	PVG	cancer	80
Groth et al.	1982	339/252	1–108 months	multiple	multiple	76
Plotkin	1982	?/60	?–4.5 years	VPL,VPM,PAG	deafferentation (12)	33
					multiple (48) (esp. failed low back syndrome)	79
Shulman et al.	1982	?/24	2 years	VPL,VPM	neuropathic	67
Lazorthes et al.	1983	?/8	<1–12 months	PVG	cancer	87
Meyerson	1983	?/41	?	VPL,VPM	neurogenic (13)	17
				PVG	deafferentation (11)	0
					cancer (18)	50
Siegfried	1983b	61/44	5 months to 2.5 years	VPL,VPM	deafferentation (41)	78
				PAG	somatic (3)	100

Table 24/I. (cont.)

Author	Year	N_t/N_i	Follow-up	Target	Pain syndrome: terms used by authors	Results: success (⩾50% pain relief) %
Hood and Siegfried	1984	?/8	21 months	VPL,VPM	brachial plexus avulsion	50
Levy et al.	1984	?/145	?–12 years	VPL,VPM and/ or PVG,PAG	neurogenic (84) nociception (57)	41
Tsubokawa et al.	1984	?/14	2 months	VPL,IC	multiple	64
Young et al.	1984	29/31	2–54 months	PAG,PVG and/ or VPL,VPM	multiple	45
Kumar and Wyant	1985	18/21	8 months to 4 years	PVG (20) VPL,VPM (3)	esp. failed back	78
Schvarcz	1985b	?/10	1–42 months	septal area	neurogenic	60
Young et al.	1985	48/71	2–60 months	PVG,PAG IC and VPL/VPM	multiple	73
Baskin et al.	1986	?/9	2–7 months	PVG,PAG	esp. cancer	89
Hosobuchi	1986	122/141	2–14 years	PAG,PVG	peripheral (65)	82 (initially) 77 (more than 2 years)
				VPL,VPM	deafferentation (76)	68 (initially) 58 (more than 2 years)
Young and Brechner	1986	?/17	1–21 months	PAG/PVG and VPL,VPM (6) PVG/PAG (11)	cancer pain ass. with neural deficit cancer pain not ass. with neural deficit	94 (initially) 59 (at long term)
Young and Chambi	1987	52/47	12–86 months	PAG/PVG	?	100 (initially) 64 (after 1 year)
		?/27	?	VPL/VPM	?	44

IC = Internal capsule.

Mechanism of DBS According to Clinical Data

The PVG-PAG Target

The discovery of endogenous substances with opiate properties in the nervous system of animals, and the demonstration that both morphine analgesia and analgesia by PVG-PAG stimulation depended on the integrity of cerebral monoamine systems, provided a powerful tool for understanding how this stimulation might have a pain-suppressing action in man [for the evidence, see Mayer and Price, 1976]. Indeed, in the early years of DBS in man, a number of observations made in patients fit well with this hypothesis: PVG-PAG stimulation increases the endorphin content in ventricular fluid [Akil et al., 1978; Hosobuchi et al., 1979]; there is a cross-tolerance between stimulation-produced analgesia and narcotic-induced analgesia [Hosobuchi, 1978]; PVG-PAG stimulation-induced suppression of chronic pain is reversed by naloxone [Hosobuchi et al., 1977]. The tolerance to analgesia induced by central gray stimulation in humans is inhibited by disulfiram [Hosobuchi and Wemmer, 1977] and is reversed by a daily 3-gram dietary supplement of *L*-tryptophan [Hosobuchi, 1978]. These data are in favor of an opioid-mediated pain-suppressive mechanism, but they have been challenged. In a study comprising 45 patients who were followed for at least one year after placement of the electrode in the central gray, the development of tolerance to stimulation, the possibility of cross-tolerance to morphine and the reversibility of stimulation-induced pain relief by naloxone were critically assessed; no evidence was found for an opioid mechanism [Young and Chambi, 1987]. Moreover, the early data in favor of an opioid mechanism should be interpreted with caution. The observation that the morphine antagonist, naloxone, may reverse the effect of periventricular stimulation is considered as an argument for postulating common mechanism for SPA and morphine analgesia. In a pathological pain situation, however, both in man [Levine et al., 1979] and in arthritic rats [Kayser and Guilbaud, 1981], naloxone will act in a different way than in the absence of pathology. In the pathological condition, low doses of naloxone produce hypoalgesia, high doses hyperalgesia. It has also been reported that PVG-PAG stimulation in man can produce an increased release of beta-endorphin without pain suppression [Amano et al., 1980, 1982] and conversely that no consistent elevation is found in ventricular fluid with PVG-PAG stimulation in spite of satisfactory pain relief [Young et al., 1984]. Moreover, the contrast medium used for ventriculography, which in most cases is required for correct electrode placement, by itself may cause a release of beta-endorphins

[Fessler et al., 1984; Rachlin et al., 1984; Dionne et al., 1984]. The cited authors used the contrast medium metrizamide in their studies.

Apart from these biochemical discrepancies between animal studies and clinical findings, there are also discrepancies at the behavioral level. A particularly striking observation is that in the animal, a profound analgesia can be observed — up to a 900% increase of the nociceptive threshold. A 200% increase of the nociceptive threshold is already equivalent to 3 mg/kg morphine [Fardin, 1982], whereas in man profound analgesia to acute experimental pain, to our knowledge, has not been observed [Gybels, 1979]. Usually, chronic pain relief is reported even when the threshold for acute pain is not influenced by the stimulation. The relationship between changes in chronic pain experience in patients and changes in acute pain thresholds in animals are not well known and it is possible that the mechanisms subserving acute and chronic pain are different [Wall, 1984]. Therefore, animal experiments which make use of models of chronic pain may help to elucidate pain-suppressive mechanisms in chronic pain conditions. In one such model it was shown that in arthritic rats scratching, which may be interpreted as a sign of chronic pain [De Castro-Costa et al., 1981, 1987], could be reduced by stimulation of nucleus paraventricularis thalami and that this response was not necessarily linked to increased tail-flick and hot-plate latencies [Kupers et al., 1988] (fig. 24/4).

The VPM-VPL Target

When the antinociceptive effect of VPM-VPL stimulation is studied with electrophysiological techniques the duration of the observed inhibition of 'nociceptive' neurons is very short and totally inadequate to explain long duration effects which can be observed when this stimulation is applied in patients with chronic pain. The mechanism by which the specific somatosensory system stimulation at the thalamic level relieves chronic pain, is not clear. Probably, it is not due to functional blocking of this system since lesions in it induce paresthesia, but do not stop the pain. Nor does activation of an endogenous opioid system seem to be the case, since the analgesic effect of the stimulation is always restricted to the side contralateral to the stimulation. Furthermore, the analgesic effect is not reversed by naloxone [Hosobuchi et al., 1977]. The issue of beta-endorphin levels in CSF following VP stimulation remains, however, a matter of debate [Mazars et al., 1979; Tsubokawa et al., 1984].

For a long time, two major neurophysiological concepts for the chronic pain following lesions in the nervous system have been proposed on clinical

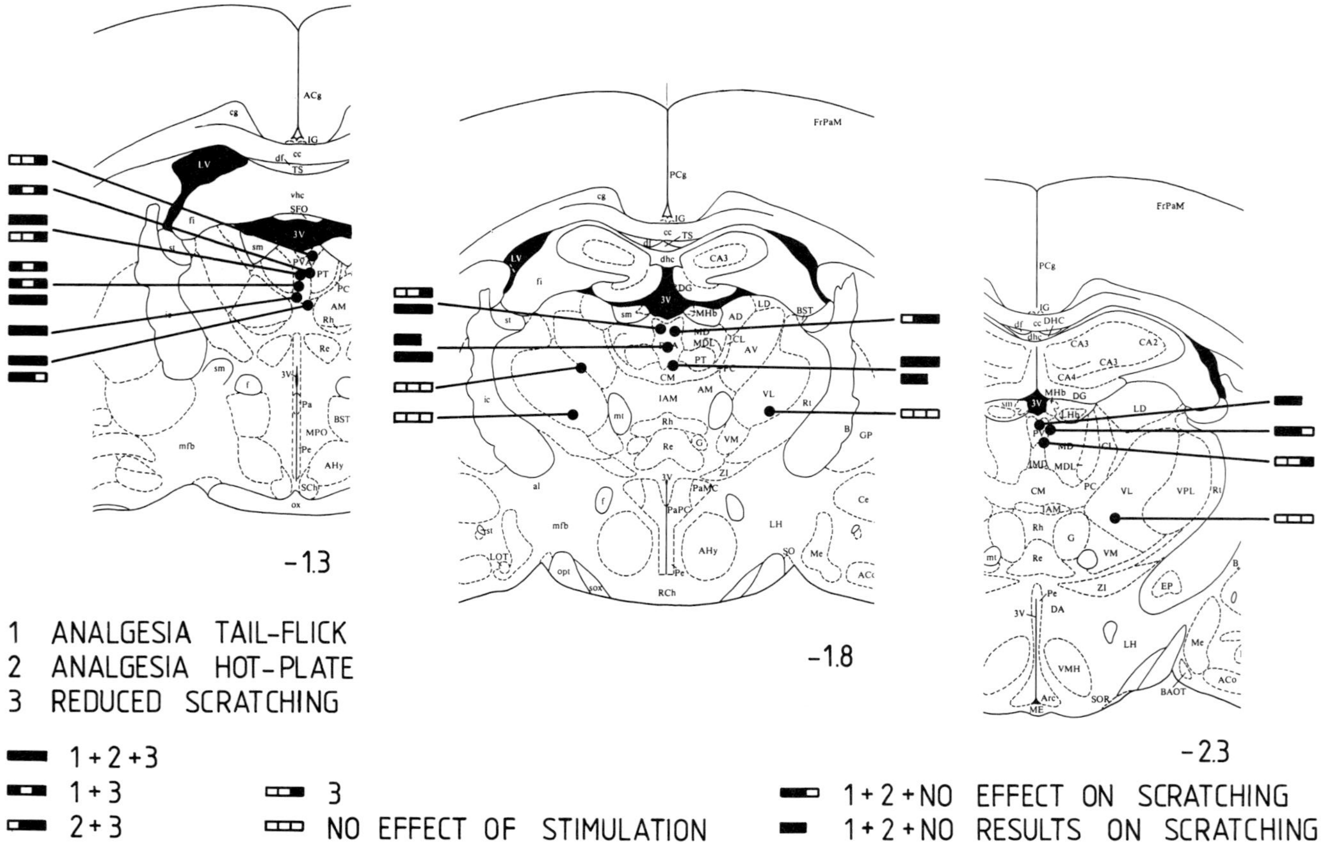

Fig. 24/4. Localization of electrodes in 24 initially normal rats. Responses to tail-flick and hot-plate upon stimulation were checked. The arthritis was induced by injection of killed *Mycobacterium butyricum* at base of tail with painful joints developing in 3 weeks. Such animals show severe spontaneous scratching strikingly inhibited by stimulation at electrodes in PV (paraventricular thalamic nucleus) but not in VL (ventrolateral thalamic nucleus). 20 electrodes were situated in PV, 4 in VL. For each animal, the effects of stimulation on tail-flick and hot-plate latencies in the normal condition and scratching during adjuvant-induced arthritis are indicated. From Kupers et al. [1988].

grounds; either a lack of inhibition resulting from the deafferentation, or a sensitization of central synapses which provokes hyperactivation of neurons resulting in 'quasi-epileptic foci'. Recent experiments on animals with nerve lesions have provided arguments for both views [Devor and Wall, 1981; Lombard and Larabi, 1983; Hylden et al., 1987]. The question arises whether activation of deafferented neurons, e.g. by electrical stimulation of the remaining afferents or by stimulation of the neurons directly, might interfere with these abnormal neurophysiological mechanisms underlying the painful state. This is not known, but it has been shown in the cat that hyperactivity in the trigeminal medullary subnucleus caudalis following retrogassserian trigeminal rhizotomy can be inhibited by VPM stimulation [Tsubokawa et al., 1985].

Complications and Side Effects

After implantation of an electrode in the PAG, there may be an oculomotor disorder, usually transient, and the development of tolerance has been stressed. Occasionally, an intracranial hemorrhage or an infection can occur. Erosion of the hardware through the scalp can be troublesome. Electrode migration and increased resistance of the electrode is very uncommon. In a few instances compulsive thalamic self-stimulation has been reported [Schmidt et al., 1981; Dieckmann and Witzmann, 1982; Portenoy et al., 1986].

Conclusions

There are many clinical indications that deep brain stimulation can be very valuable for treating chronic pain even in those conditions in which alternative treatments have failed. As in so many other therapies for chronic pain, it remains difficult to evaluate the functional worth of '50%' pain relief due to the electrical stimulation and hence the percentage of truly successful cases. Deep brain stimulation is not an established routine method and is mostly performed by those neurosurgeons who have a major interest in pain and its physiopathology; in their hands it is a very safe method. It is obvious that knowledge of how electrical stimulation of the brain has a suppressive effect on chronic pain remains fragmentary and that in explaining it one is on less firm ground than was initially thought.

Part III. Intraspinal and Intraventricular Administration of Neuropharmacological Drugs

Chapter 25. Intraspinal and Intraventricular Infusion of Opioids

Historical Note

The spinal fluid compartment has long been used for the administration of local anesthetics and neurolytic agents in the treatment of pain but a new and considerable interest in this and the ventricular compartment as well has been created by the discovery of opioid receptors in the spinal cord and in the brain. To the seminal publication of Yaksh and Rudy [1976] we owe our awareness of the fact that intrathecally injected morphine and other opiates produce 'potent analgesia' by direct action on the spinal cord. Indeed, spinal administration of opioids blocks the neural activity evoked by nociceptive input rather selectively, while leaving tactile and proprioceptive input and motor and sympathetic output relatively unchanged [Behar et al., 1979; Cousins et al., 1979a; Bromage et al., 1980; Yaksh, 1981].

The use of implantable systems, first reported by Pilon and Baker in 1976 for administration of a local anesthetic in patients with intractable pain or cancer, opened the way for the chronic administration of opioids in the CSF compartment. The efficacy of the method in the human was first reported in acute pain by Behar et al. [1979] and in chronic pain by Wang et al. [1979] who learned from Kerr of the Yaksh-Rudy experiments. Since these early publications there has been a rapid and widespread use of the method in a variety of clinical applications. In neurosurgical practice, most of the intraspinal and intraventricular administration of opioids has been long-term administration in chronic pain patients with carcinoma, and we shall lay emphasis on this type of pain problem and tactics of administration.

Route of Injection

After epidural administration of an opioid it can reach analgesic concentration in the CSF before such level is reached in the blood (fig. 25/1).

Opioids are administered to the CSF by epidural, intrathecal and intraventricular routes. Diffusion pathways after epidural administration of an opioid include blood vessels, root sleeves, arachnoidal villi, fat and the intact dura. The quantitative importance and the time course of the various diffusion pathways show differences according with the pharmacokinetic parameters distinctive for the specific opioid. Once the drug has entered the CSF by diffusion or direct application, as in the intrathecal and intraventricular route, it is not catabolized in the intrathecal space. Clearance routes for the opioids from the CSF are migration towards the opiate receptors, diffusion into CSF compartments including newly formed CSF, reabsorption by veins and villi, rediffusion through dura mater and neural sleeves and rostral spread. Both rostral spread and massive reuptake of the opioid in the blood stream present a danger of delayed respiratory depression. Highly lipid-soluble agents will spread from the CSF into the lipids of the neuraxis faster than poorly lipid-soluble agents. Therefore, high fat-soluble (lipophilic) opioids such as fentanyl will tend to have a rapid onset of action and the subsequent neural block will tend to be intense and limited to relatively few spinal segments. Hydrophilic and poorly lipid-soluble drugs may be expected to travel further in the subarachnoid space and to produce a less intense analgesia, but a greater degree of rostral spread, involving a larger number of spinal segments. The use of lipophilic opioids, reduced doses, dilution in a small volume, the concomitant administration of epinephrine (if epidural administration is used), the upright position of the patient (if intrathecal administration is used) and slow injection will reduce the intraspinal spread of opioids. Many of the different factors which have to do with the effects of intrathecal and epidural administration of opioids have been studied in great detail but many key issues regarding pharmacokinetics, pharmacodynamics and side effects still remain unanswered [Cousins and Mather, 1984].

Target Sites for Opioids in the CSF

The presence of opiate receptors in the spinal cord and their action on spinal cord nociceptive mechanisms has been the basis for the spinal use of narcotics. In behavioral tests, animal studies [Yaksh and Rudy, 1976; Yaksh

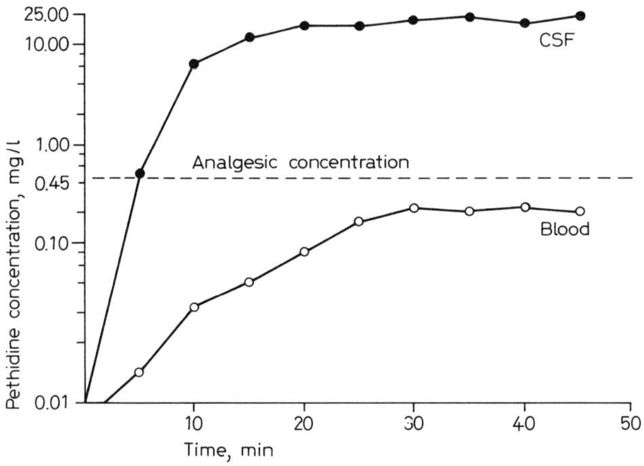

Fig. 25/1. Simultaneous blood and CSF pethidine concentrations after 100 mg pethidine by epidural injection. From Cousins et al. [1979a].

et al., 1980] show that analgesia occurs after such administration. The iontophoretic injection of opiates at the dorsal horn neurons reveals that the focal administration of these agents into the vicinity of the primary afferent terminals in the substantia gelatinosa will inhibit the discharge of wide dynamic range neurons in laminas IV and V and that this inhibition is reversed by naloxone [Duggan et al., 1977]. Opiate binding studies indicate that a significant proportion of this action in the spinal gray is in the substantia gelatinosa [Atweh and Kuhar, 1977] and it is in this area that the central terminations of cutaneous C-fibers have been directly traced [Sugiura et al., 1986].

Since the 1930s the depressant action of morphine on certain polysynaptic reflexes has been known and this effect has been verified in man in a study of paraplegics of traumatic origin in whom the neurological examination showed signs of a complete transverse lesion. In these subjects, morphine (0.1–0.3 mg/kg) provoked an intense and prolonged depression of polysynaptic nociceptive reflexes, without influencing the monosynaptic reflexes [Willer and Bussel, 1980]. Following the work of Martin et al. [1964], showing that the pharmacological profiles of various opiates in the chronic spinal dog differed from one another, the concept of a multiplicity of opioid receptors is now well established. It has been suggested that there are four — possibly five — distinct populations of opioid receptors in the spinal cord, the activation of which results in a selective modulation of the response of

Table 25/I. Opioid receptor-ligand relationship. From Yaksh [1987a, b][1]

Relative receptor selectivity	Endogenous ligand	Exogenous ligand	Antagonist
$\mu = \varepsilon = \delta >> K$	β-endorphin met-enkephalin	morphine sufentanyl morphiceptin/PLO17	naloxone β-funalnaltrexamine
		meptazinol	naloxonazine
$\delta >> \mu$ 10 to 20:1	met-enkephalin leucine-enkephalin	DADL $\delta > \mu$ 10–20:1	naloxone — $\mu > \delta$ 10–20:1 ICI 174864
		bispenicillamine — (D-pen^2-D-pen^5) Enk $\delta > \mu$ 10–20:1	
$K > \mu = \delta$	dynorphin 1–13	ethylketocyclazocine; U50488H	naloxone, MR-2266
σ	?	SKF 1004	none

[1] For identity of unusual chemicals indicated by letters and/or numbers, see table 1, Yaksh [1987a].

animals to noxious stimuli. In rats with chronically implanted intrathecal catheters, responses to cutaneous thermal stimulation are modulated by mu and delta receptors, whereas responses to visceral chemical tests (writhing) are modulated by mu and kappa receptors [Schmauss and Yaksh, 1984].

Table 25/I summarizes the opioid-receptor-ligand relationship while table 25/II shows the functional correlates of the different opioid receptor types, as they are recognized in 1987.

Besides these target sites for opioids at the spinal level, periventricular, periaqueductal and raphe nuclei are particularly rich in morphine receptors [Kuhar et al., 1973; Pert et al., 1975; Atweh and Kuhar, 1977].

Following the work of Tsou and Yang [1964] and Herz et al. [1970], many authors [see ref. in Yaksh and Rudy, 1978] have shown that injection of morphine in periventricular and periaqueductal structures in the rat can be followed by a profound analgesia, and this with a dose which is 200 times less than when, for instance, morphine is injected intraperitoneally [Jacquet and Lajtha, 1976].

The pharmacological identification of naturally occurring opiate-like substances [Hughes, 1975] and the physiology of stimulation-produced

Table 25/II. Functional correlates of multiple opioid receptor types. From Herz [1987].

Analgesia	
cerebral level	μ, ε (δ)
spinal level	μ, δ, κ
Sedation	κ
Respiratory depression	μ (not κ)
Cardiovascular control	δ, κ
Food intake	κ
Water balance	
diuresis	κ
antidiuresis	μ
Reinforcement	μ (not κ)
Euphoria	μ
Dysphoria	κ

analgesia (chapter 24) have led to the hypothesis of activation by morphine of these inhibitory controls originating from the region of the periaqueductal gray through the midline of the brain stem to the nucleus raphe magnus in the medulla, with subsequent relays via the dorsal lateral quadrant of the spinal cord to the spinal dorsal horn. This forms the basis for the direct intraventricular administration of morphine. However, the activation of these inhibitory controls by morphine has not been proven [for review, see Gebhart, 1982] and it has even been shown that morphine depresses the activity of these descending inhibitory controls [Duggan et al., 1980; Le Bars et al., 1980]. It has therefore been suggested that analgesia produced by intracerebro-ventricular morphine is due to a restoration of the somesthesic background activity in convergent dorsal horn neurons arising from diffuse noxious inhibitory controls (DNICS) [Bouhassira et al., 1986; Villanueva and Le Bars, 1986].

Choice of Drugs Used

Morphine has been the first and most widely used drug for administration in the CSF and can be considered as the classical reference opioid, but many opioids and opioid-agonist-antagonists are candidates for use for spinal and intraventricular administration. The opioid used should be available in aqueous solution, free of toxic preservatives and stabilizers, with a pH of the solution near 7.4, and it should be possible to administer the required dose in low volume. Criteria for the choice of a particular opioid have to take into consideration the therapeutic safety index, the rapidity, intensity and duration of action, the immediate and delayed side effects, the accumulation tendency and the likelihood of development of tolerance or dependency. As mentioned earlier, the two most important pharmacokinetic parameters are receptor binding affinity and liposolubility. There is a reverse relationship between receptor binding affinity and the dose necessary for efficient pain relief. In this respect sufentanyl and buprenorphine are superior to morphine, and this also holds for the rapidity of onset of the analgesia seen with these substances. A trend can be observed showing a growing interest for the high liposoluble opioids fentanyl, sufentanyl and buprenorphine whereas in earlier reports morphine was used almost exclusively. (For results with buprenorphine see Crawford et al. [1983] and Eriksen and Andersen [1984].) Pasqualucci et al. [1987] found this drug less satisfactory than morphine even though it entailed less risk of respiratory depression.

It has now been recognized that many nonopioid putative neurotransmitters are modulators of processing of nociceptive information at the dorsal horn neuron level. Some of those, such as glutamate, substance P and possibly CCK appear to have an excitatory effect on nociceptive transmission, while others, such as serotonin, noradrenaline, dopamine, calcitonin gene-related peptide, somatostatin, enkephalin and GABA, have at least at some sites an inhibitory effect on nociceptive transmission. With these new insights, somatostatin [Chrubasik et al., 1984], calcitonin [Fiore et al., 1983], and the alpha-2 adrenergic agonist, clonidine [Coombs et al., 1984; Tamsen and Gordh, 1984], have already been administered in the CSF for pain treatment, but the value of these agents in therapy has yet to be established and extreme care should always be taken to make sure that a given drug has no toxic effects on the nervous system. Yaksh et al. [1987] provide an excellent set of guidelines as to the minimum preclinical studies necessary prior to the use of a novel agent in the spinal canal of man.

Delivery of Opioids into the CSF

For repeated opioid administration into the CSF three types of injection sequences can be visualized: repeated bolus injection, continuous infusion, and continuous infusion with 'on demand' bolus. Different delivery systems will allow a variety of injection sequences. The types of delivery systems used can be categorized as follows: (1) percutaneous catheter; (2) percutaneous catheter with subcutaneous tunnelling; (3) totally implanted catheter with subcutaneous injection port; (4) totally implanted catheter with an implanted reservoir bag or port with a manual subcutaneous intermittent pump; (5) totally implanted catheter with an implanted reservoir bag or port with a stationary or portable infusion pump; (6) totally implanted catheter with an implanted infusion pump [Lazorthes et al., 1984b; Franetzki and Kollert, 1987].

The choice of the delivery system will depend on many factors, such as the life expectancy of the patient, cost-benefit analysis, safety, efficacy, etc., but ideally a drug-dispensing system should provide a way to turn the device on and off, give varying rates of flow, allow single or multiple bolus, allow a permanent infusion, have a large enough reservoir to administer drugs over many weeks or months, be easy to implant and refill, require no replacement during the life of the patients, give long-term reliable function and be as cheap as possible.

Bolus Intraspinal Morphine Injection in Cancer Pain

Clinical use was initiated in 1979 by Wang et al. who gave 0.5–1 mg of lumbar intrathecal morphine to 8 patients with pelvic cancer. Pain relief lasted 12–24 h without serious side effects (fig. 25/2). Ventafridda et al. [1979] described similar cancer pain relief in a group of 41 patients, in 10 of whom the needle was inserted through the C4–5 interspace. They noted a rapid development of tolerance. There was widespread corroboration that in man the intraspinal bolus administration of morphine could produce a profound analgesia of long duration in patients with cancer pain [Lazorthes et al., 1980; Müller et al., 1981]. In many clinics an initial trial period precedes implantation of a more permanent system. Shetter et al. [1986] found that 7 of 24 cancer patients elected not to continue treatment after the trial because of unacceptable side effects or inadequate relief.

In a Danish multicenter study 94 cancer patients were treated, the great majority by bolus epidural morphine injection, with a mean period of treatment of 65 days (range 7–283 days). The mean daily dose of morphine totaled approximately 12 mg (range 4–30 mg). Buprenorphine usually 1 mg twice a day was used in 12 patients and 3 alternated between morphine and buprenorphine to deal with the problem of tolerance. Satisfactory relief was achieved in 67% of the patients who were managed with these extradural

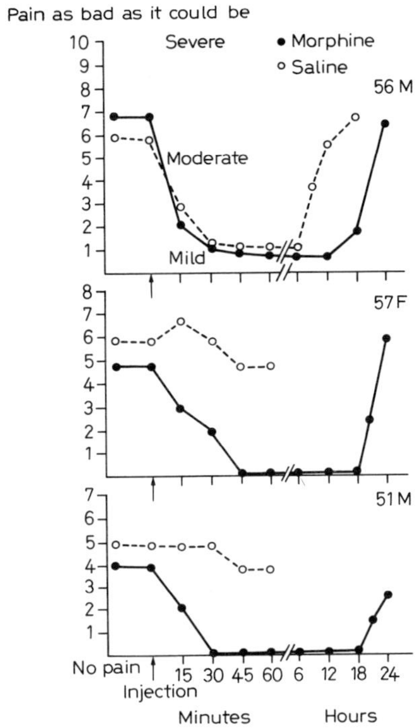

Fig. 25/2. Changes in intensity of pain after intrathecal injection of physiologic saline solution or morphine (0.5–1.0 mg) in 3 patients with pelvic cancer. From Wang et al. [1979].

opiates as the sole analgesic treatment. The incidence of side effects of long-term treatment was low compared to extradural opiates for postoperative pain. In 12 patients tachyphylaxis was suspected [Crawford et al., 1983].

In a study of 46 cancer patients by Wang [1985], 14 were treated by a single intrathecal injection with morphine and in 28 an intrathecal catheter was implanted for morphine bolus injection. Intrathecally low-dose morphine effectively relieved pain in 74% of the patients tested but with long-term application only 52% of the patients were successfully treated. The results of bolus injections usually once a day in nine other studies are summarized in table 25/III. When the pain is below mid-torso the tip of the catheter should lie opposite the middle of the cord segments T10 to S5 or roughly opposite T11 vertebral body and not in the lumbar region. Thus, when Moulin et al. [1986] gave the morphine at T9–10 they measured steady-

Table 25/III. Results of bolus intraspinal morphine injections for chronic pain (all cancer)

Author, year	Number of cases	Dose, mg/24 h		Follow-up, months		Pain relief	Tolerance	Respiratory depression	Side effects: confusion, somnolence	Site of injection
		range	av.	range	av.					
Davidson and Magora, 1983	53	2–8		usually circa 1 month		no other drugs needed at first in 81%	not in 1 month	0	0	epidural
Cioni et al., 1984	48	0.5–1				'satisfactory' in all			more side effects from epidural route	7 epidural 41 intrathecal
Eriksen and Andersen, 1984	526		16.4	up to 15	2	'excellent' 65%		0	0	epidural
Husebo, 1984	46	21		1/15–12		95% early relief	yes but relief on higher dose	0	0	epidural
Lazorthes et al., 1984a	30	0.5–5	1.5	1–14	3	'profound'	'limited'	0	'minimal'	intrathecal
Meyerson et al., 1984	21	up to 60		1/2–8	1 1/2	60% 'good' to death	distinguish from impaired delivery	0	0	epidural
Nobili et al., 1984	28	3–60	16	1/4–4	1 1/2	57% 'high degree'		0	0	epidural
Laugner et al., 1985	41	1.5 at first, 7 at end		1/4–16	2	decrease over time in quality of relief	45% increase by 1 mg each 19 days	0	mild	intrathecal
Meynadier et al., 1985	25		1	1–9		good in 96%		0	mild	intrathecal

state concentrations 3 times as high at that level as at L2–3. Several observers have found somatic pains more likely to be relieved than those classed as neurogenic, with continuous pains in the former category relieved at lower doses than pains coming in bursts [Arnér and Arnér, 1985; Meyerson et al., 1984].

Side Effects

Respiratory Depression

The major side effect of bolus intraspinal administration of morphine is respiratory depression. This complication has been reported with intrathecal morphine doses as small as 0.3 mg, and we have had one respiratory arrest circa 3 h after 0.15 mg into the CSF at about T11 superimposed on over 10 mg morphine s.c. A retrospective study of approximately 6,000–9,000 administrations of epidural morphine revealed an incidence of associated respiratory depression (requiring naloxone) in only 22 cases — in 9 within 1 h, in 7 after 6 h and in one of these not until 12 h. Repeated doses of i.v. naloxone may be required because of its much shorter duration of action than morphine [Gustafsson et al., 1982]. Respiratory depression after bolus intraspinal morphine can be seen as late as 16 h, thus providing a guide for the duration of surveillance. A so-called apnea monitor which sounds an alarm upon fall of respiratory rate to a predetermined level is useful until the safe dose is established for that person. In some patients the apnea appears only in sleep and the alarm wakens the patient who then resumes breathing. This syndrome seems to appear primarily in narcotic naive patients [Yaksh, 1981; Cousins and Mather, 1984]. Cancer pain patients have rarely developed respiratory complications, probably because of preexisting narcotic tolerance. Nevertheless, life-threatening respiratory depression is considered as the most significant untoward side effect of spinally administered opiates and probably linked to the CSF concentration of opioids. Respiration is controlled by neurons localized in the tractus solitarius and the nucleus ambiguous [Bertrand et al., 1973; Von Euler et al., 1973; Berger, 1977], and morphine administered into the fourth ventricle or into the bulbar subarachnoid space will produce a significant reduction in respiratory rate and an elevation in end tidal CO_2 [Florez et al., 1968].

Pruritus

Pruritus is seen in patients treated by epidural or intrathecal morphine both for short-term postoperative pain and for long-term cancer pain and appears coincident with or just after the development of the analgesia. The pruritus is not limited to segments of the spinal cord affected by the spinal opiate and the most severe itching is often observed in the palate and the face. Though systemic opiates, particularly morphine, are known to release histamine [Eckenhoff and Oech, 1960], it is not certain that the pruritus is in fact due to such release; some have reported that antihistamines will antagonize itching [Weddel and Ritter, 1980] while others deny this [Reiz and Westberg, 1980].

Urinary Retention

Urinary retention has been observed following spinal opiates both in patients with chronic pain [Magora et al., 1980; Müller et al., 1981] and in those with postoperative pain [Dirksen and Nijhuis, 1980; Scott et al., 1980], but it is reported to occur less frequently with continuous epidural than with bolus infusion. In a series of 1,200 postoperative patients receiving epidural morphine (10 mg), urinary retention was observed in approximately 15% of the patient population, and 70% of those showing retention were men [Reiz and Westberg, 1980]. The mechanism underlying such retention is not clear, though the involvement of parasympathetic outflow from the sacral cord seems probable.

Nausea and Vomiting

Nausea and vomiting occur in approximately 20% of chronic pain patients [Oyama et al., 1980; Müller et al., 1981]. Apparently this phenomenon wears off rapidly and vomiting is reduced with subsequent administration. An important structure in the mechanism of nausea and vomiting is the area postrema which lies superficially at the caudal end of the fourth ventricle [Borison and Wang, 1953].

Tolerance

In humans, the effect of repeated spinal administration of morphine has given rise to apparently differing observations. Ventafridda et al. [1979] noted a rapid development of tolerance in chronic cancer pain patients; the effectiveness of 1 mg morphine a day intrathecally diminished rapidly after 3–5 days of administration, while in the series reported by Müller et al. [1981], for instance, the level of pain relief produced by a fixed dose of opiates administered twice daily (2–5 mg of morphine intrathecally) was observed to be relatively stable for periods ranging from 14 to 30 days. After this period, the patients showed an increase in the dose of epidural opiate required to produce adequate pain relief. Usually, though, it is said that in acute pain treatment the problem is delayed respiratory depression, while the problem in chronic pain therapy is tolerance. The original studies of Yaksh [1983] in three species of macacca monkeys revealed a loss of responsiveness after 5–9 daily intrathecal doses of morphine with, however, significant recovery of opiate sensitivity after an opiate-free interval of 7 days. Happily, man is usually less prone to develop tolerance so promptly and at times efficacy to lower doses may partially reappear after 2 or 3 opiate-free days. Moreover, despite development of tolerance in every one of the 14 cases of Shetter et al. [1986], in 11 of them the original level of effectiveness of treatment was maintained by the higher doses. In the 17 cancer cases of Samuelsson et al. [1987b], the daily dose had to be increased from an average of 18 to 87 mg/day over the 3.5-month average period of treatment. When they measured CSF morphine levels in 8 patients, 2 of them showed decreased morphine concentrations despite increasing doses. This may be due to the development of a fibrous cocoon around the catheter in the epidural space along with focal thickening of the dura at the catheter, as was noted in 4 of 5 cases in the postmortem studies of Coombs et al. [1985a]. A significant fibrous mass requiring neurosurgical extirpation developed around the tip of one epidural catheter [Rodan et al., 1985]. However, in the three postmortem studies of Laugner et al. [1985] after chronic intrathecal catheters no abnormalities were seen in the cord, roots or meninges. The catheter may shift to a less favorable ventral extradural position, as occurred in one of our patients, causing a marked abrupt decrease in the pain relief. Radiographic checks and/or catheter replacements should perhaps be standard practice when 'tolerance' comes on apace. Samuelsson et al. [1987a] placed 39 epidural catheters in 14 patients. In general, this group finds that the dura presents a more variable barrier to epidural morphine than the blood vessel walls since plasma but not CSF levels of morphine can be predicted from the epidural dose. Meyerson et al. [1984] had one patient whose failing effects of up to 300 mg/24 h was related to rapid absorption into the epidural vessels.

It has been suggested [Yaksh, 1981] that the rate of development of tolerance is proportional to the concentration of the agonist at the receptor, and thus the lower the necessary dose of opiate, the slower the onset of tolerance. Bolus injection favors initially excessive receptor activation, because of the need to maintain sufficient levels of the opiate for periods sufficient to avoid repeated administration at short intervals, and therefore may lead to a more rapid onset of tolerance. For this reason, it has been contended that continuous administration of the agent in such a way that infusion rate matches clearance is favorable to combat tolerance. However, the pump alone is not the final answer; for example, Erickson et al. [1984] found that most of their cancer patients 'had early demand for increased dosage and less adequate pain control even with continuous intrathecal doses up to 100 mg daily'. Moreover, while tolerance develops rapidly after epidural administration of morphine in rats [Yaksh et al., 1977; Tung et al., 1981], cats [Tung and Yaksh, 1981] and primates [Yaksh and Reddy, 1981], there are indications that in animals under conditions of chronic pain no significant tolerance develops to systemically administered opiates [Colpaert, 1979; Colpaert et al., 1980]. Finally, there seems to be a relative lack of cross-tolerance between the mu and delta agonists [for review, see Yaksh, 1981], respectively morphine and DADL, and this offers the possibility of changing to another effective agent as soon as tolerance to the first one appears. Moulin et al. [1984] found in 10 patients no longer relieved by systemic opiates that a dose of intrathecal DADL one fourth that of intrathecal morphine gave pain relief usually lasting over twice as long and usually of greater degree than that with morphine. Onofrio and Yaksh [1983] had already demonstrated in a patient no longer relieved by large doses of continuous intrathecal and systemic morphine that almost complete relief was recouped by 1 mg DADL intrathecally per day. However, Moulin et al. [1986] have a patient in whom such high infusion rates of intrathecal morphine were given 'as to result in opioid tolerance at both mu and delta receptor sites so that the analgesic selectivity expected of DADL was lost'. Coombs et al. [1985b] have recorded a similar experience. Other strategies that theoretically might be employed to delay tolerance include the use of nonopioid analgesics like alpha-adrenergic amines, such as clonidine, nonopioid neuropeptides, such as somatostatin and calcitonin, and enkephalinase inhibitors, such as bestatin and thiorphan.

Route of Bolus Administration: Epidural versus Intrathecal

The main advantage of intrathecal (IT) over epidural (ED) administration is that in the former morphine is placed close to the opiate receptors and that correspondingly lesser doses are needed, resulting in fewer systemic side effects. Yaksh [1987a] states that up to 10 times higher doses are required via the epidural route to equal the analgesic effect of the intrathecal placement. When a chronic placement of the catheter is the goal, other advantages of the intrathecal route include the absence of a dural reaction surrounding the catheter as is the case with an epidural placement, the possibility of sampling spinal fluid for the purpose of culture, diagnosis or determination of drug levels, as well as the possibility of administration of other drugs such as peptides, antibiotics and radiographic contrast agents. Disadvantages of the intrathecal route are the possibility of headache, infection in the form of meningitis and of arachnoiditis. Delayed respiratory depression seems to be somewhat more common with intrathecal administration than with epidural administration.

Continuous Intraspinal Infusion

Besides the possible important advantage of postponing tolerance that was discussed earlier, continuous intraspinal opioid delivery has some obvious practical advantages over parenteral therapy and bolus delivery. Among these, stable spinal analgesic levels, improved patient comfort and low infection risk seem particularly important.

The initial clinical trials of continuous intraspinal morphine were accomplished in 1981 with the first reliable implanted infusion reservoir [Onofrio et al., 1981; Coombs et al., 1981]. This pump delivers morphine at a continuous preset rate of 2–3 ml/day from a 50-ml reservoir (fig. 25/3). It consists of a hollow titanium and silicone cylinder with two internal chambers separated by a metal bellows. A two-phase (gas-liquid) fluorocarbon charging fluid is sealed between the metal bellows internal chamber and the wall of the titanium cylinder. The internal drug chamber within the metal bellows is percutaneously filled via a resealable septum. Refilling the drug reservoir compresses the fluorocarbon charging fluid which then goes into the fluid state. The patient's body temperature warms the charging fluid, generating a vapor pressure which exerts continuous pressure on the metal bellows drug chamber. This pressure forces the drug out of the drug chamber through an outlet filter and a capillary flow restrictor tube. The drug then flows from the restrictor tube through a silicone rubber catheter to either the epidural or intrathecal implantation site. Flow rate is constant and preset by the characteristics of the individual restrictor and filter. An auxiliary sideport connects directly with the reservoir catheter, permitting supplementary bolus narcotic

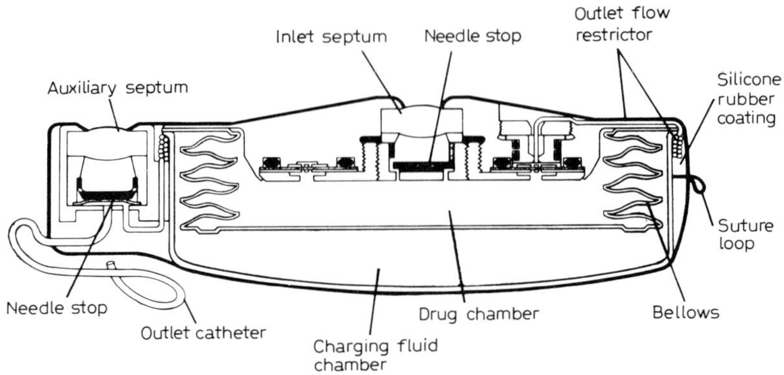

Fig. 25/3. Cross-sectional view of the Infusaid® model 400 implantable infusion reservoir. The representation is from documentation material of the maker of the reservoir.

injections, as well as other therapeutic and diagnostic measures. Because of its principle, the rate of this type of pump is dependent on external factors and can change unintentionally by up to 50% and drug concentrations will affect flow rates [Rippe et al., 1984].

Quick adaptations to the changing needs of the patient are difficult and therefore electrically controlled devices have been developed. One such device [Penn et al., 1984] consists of a battery, an RF receiver and transmitter, a microprocessor, a reservoir, a bacteriostatic filter and a rotary pump (fig. 25/4). To control the implanted pump a programming device with an RF link and a printer is used. The programming device can detect the pump's functional status (on, off, drug delivery program), how much fluid is in the reservoir, if the battery has adequate capacity, and if the alarm system is functioning. The programmer can modify the flow profile and set the pump's regime. An emergency instruction to turn the pump off is available. An audible alarm can be set to warn when the calculated reservoir is below a given amount, the battery is low or the device is not functioning properly. The reservoir is filled via a self-sealing port. The goal of this computer-controlled electrically driven rotary pump is to give maximum flexibility as to dose and timing of medication delivery. The drug can be given continuously or in single or intermittent bolus form. This flexibility is an obvious advantage, but since the capacity of the battery is limited, the device's expected life is also limited. Changing the program of the pump also requires the presence of a physician experienced in its use.

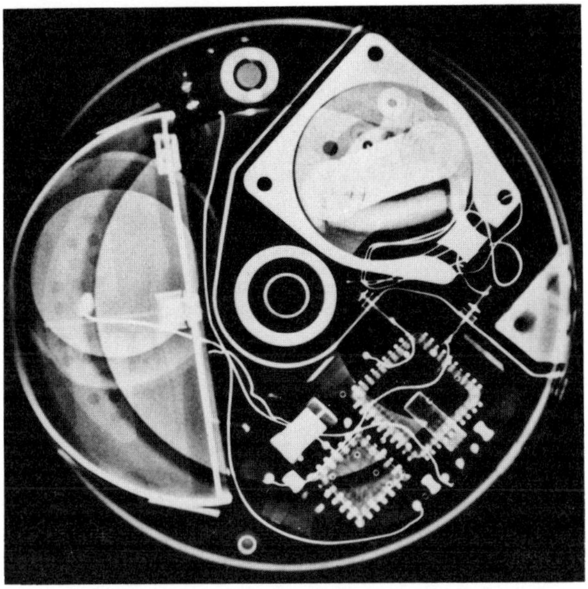

Fig. 25/4. The Medtronic® drug administration implantable system. The photograph was provided by the maker of the device.

The results of continuous intraspinal morphine infusion with implanted devices in patients with chronic pain, mainly of malignant origin, are summarized in table 25/IV. A recent collation gives the results of 3,443 intrathecal chronic morphine infusions by 19 doctors in 163 patients — nearly all with cancer pain [Yaksh and Onofrio, 1987]. In this group the mean and median infusion doses required increased by 3- and 5-fold over a 3- and 6-month period, respectively. However, there was great variation with about half of the patients showing less than a 2-fold increase. At the other end of the scale those with rapid development of tolerance need other therapy.

From this evolving experience, no firm conclusions can be drawn. However, there is an indication that the majority of cancer patients treated with continuous epidural or intrathecal morphine by means of an implanted pump with chronic infusion have obtained a pain control which was better than their pre-implant conventional narcotic regimen. Continuous intraspinal morphine produced less sedative side effects, an improved sense of well-being and increased activities of daily living in many of the treated patients.

Table 25/IV. Results of continuous intraspinal morphine infusion with implanted devices in chronic pain (mostly cancer)

Author, year	n	Doses, mg/24 h, min.–max.	Follow-up, months		Analgesia	Tolerance	Side effects	
			range	av.			resp.	drowsiness
Onofrio et al., 1981	1	0.62–1.8 IT	4		good	–	–	–
Greenberg et al., 1982	1	1–150 IT	1		modest	++	–	–
Harbaugh et al., 1982	2	1–30 ED	6		good	1	–	–
Coombs and Saunders, 1985	16	1.5–50 IT + ED	6 weeks to 8 months		good in cancer 11; usually severe after 1–3 months; bad in benign 6	+	–	–
Penn et al., 1984	14	initial dose × 4 IT + ED	1–13	5	excellent in 8; good in 3; poor in 1	1	–	–
Auld et al., 1985	26	–7 ED		24	excellent + good 21; fair + poor 5 (all nonmalignant)	1		
Krames et al., 1985	17	1.75–6.8 IT + ED	1–18	5	good in 16; bad in 1 (nonmalignant)	6	–	–
Shetter et al., 1986	9	1.5–40.3 IT + ED	1–23	3	excellent 6; good 1; fair 2	+		
Penn and Paice, 1987	43	av. increase dose × 2.5 IT	–46	8.4	excellent + good 28 (of 35 cancer patients) excellent + good 8 (of 8 nonmalignant)	(in 2 of 43 patients)	–	–

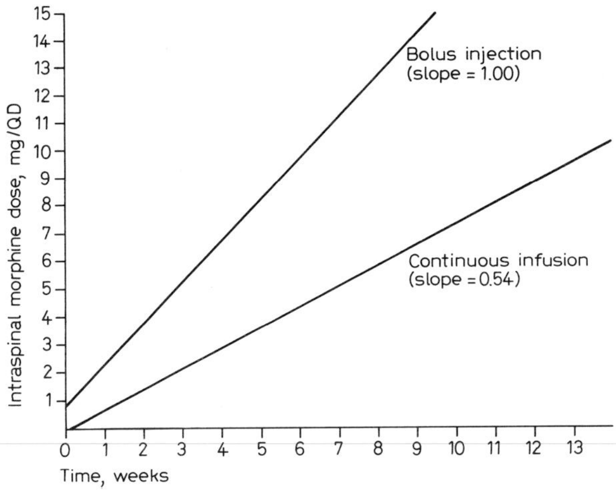

Fig. 25/5. Comparison of cumulative curves (bolus versus continuous infusion). The y-intercept, slope, and r value for bolus injection were –1.64, 1.00 and 0.81 (5 patients) and for continuous infusion were 0.49, 0.54 and 0.95 (8 patients). The difference in the rate of tolerance development between the two groups is statistically significant (χ^2 4.429; $p<0.05$). From Shetter et al. [1986].

Analgesia was sustained for at least 3 months and this with few side effects but at a cost of progressive increases in the intraspinal dosage. This may be due to many factors, such as progression and extension of the cancer process, decreased drug delivery due to pump failure, plugged spinal catheter, etc., and true opiate receptor tachyphylaxis. This tolerance seems to develop more rapidly with bolus administration than with continuous infusion [Shetter et al., 1986] (fig. 25/5), and such tolerance is not a major deterrent to effective pain control in patients who have been preoperatively screened with intraspinal bolus injection and with survival times projected at less than 4–6 months. As observed earlier, several strategies have been described to circumvent tolerance.

When tolerance does develop, an early resort to open surgery should be considered. Thus, when this occurred in a patient of Penn and Paice [1987] they performed a percutaneous cordotomy, recouping excellent relief until the patient's death with one fifth the (unsatisfactory) preoperative dose of morphine. Laugner et al. [1985] reported similar experiences in 2 patients. Astonishingly high doses of morphine have been given by Jansen [1984] with 'about normal circadian rhythms and no neurological sequelae' in one

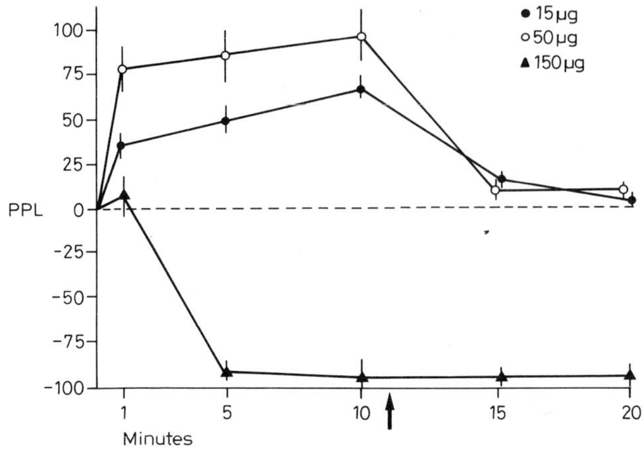

Fig. 25/6. The effect of intrathecal morphine on the response latency of rats to the hot water (49 °C) tail immersion test. Pretrial latencies were found for each animal before the experiment. The animals were then injected intrathecally with morphine (10 µl over 1 min) and then exposed to the tail immersion test at 1, 5, 10, 15 and 20 min. Results are expressed as percentage changes from the pretrial latencies (PPL), each animal acting as its own control. Naloxone (7.5 µg in 5 µl) was injected intrathecally at 11 min after the morphine injections (indicated by the arrow). n = 5 for the 15- and 50-µg doses; n = 8 for the 150-µg dose. Results shown are the means ± SEM. From Woolf [1981].

patient in whom 235 mg morphine epidurally/day yielded morphine levels of 48 mg/ml in CSF and 2.8 mg/ml in serum, or 140,000 times the 0.02-µg/ml effective plasma level for analgesia in opioid-naive postoperative patients [Dahlström et al., 1982].

It is also not without interest to note that high concentrations of intrathecal morphine in rats can provoke hyperalgesia which is not naloxone-reversible, possibly due to the principal morphine glucuronide metabolite which inhibits the inhibitory neurotransmitter glycine [Woolf, 1981] (fig. 25/6).

Occasional reports of patients with severe pain of benign origin who have been satisfactorily managed with chronic intraspinal continuous morphine for periods of 6 months or longer are intriguing. Thus, Auld et al. [1985] implanted epidurally 32 continuous delivery (Infusaid) systems in the great majority for the failed back syndrome. Although two thirds had 'good to excellent' relief of their pain, the longest follow-up was for only 2 years. Also using a continuous delivery system but usually with an intrathecal catheter, Penn and Paice [1987] achieved significant decreases in pain and increases in activity in 4 of 8 patients with noncancerous pain. That careful selection is imperative is indicated by the failure to relieve pain of nonmalignant origin described by Arnér and Arnér [1985] in every one of 10 consecutive cases who also had cancer pain. Coombs et al.. [1983] found such a poor response to continuous epidural morphine in 5 patients with failure of much low back surgery that they have confined their use of this therapy to patients with cancer in their subsequent detailed reports. After extensive neurological and psychological appraisal and favorable results with temporary catheters, we implanted permanent epidural catheters in 3 patients between August 1981 and May 1982. Failed low back surgery with arachnoiditis was the problem in 2 and phantom pain in an upper limb in the third. The first 2 maintain relief at 68 and 76 months. One has required gradually increasing doses which have reached 17 mg/day; the other has needed decreased doses down to none in the last 6 months. All 3 have had relief enabling them to work. The catheter of the man with the painful phantom became blocked because he needed to use it so infrequently and it now requires replacement. The foregoing type of results has led us and others to continue further exploration of this approach. Valid conclusions must wait for large series of these patients who have been followed for many years.

Intraventricular Administration

Intraventricular administration of drugs is not a new procedure. In 1965 Obrador described intraventricular encephalo-pharmaco-therapy for which he had constructed a special device which permitted frequent intraventricular injections of drugs through a percutaneous puncture. He examined the actions of several drugs in cases of cerebral coma, parkinsonism, intractable facial pain, epilepsy and psychosis. He commented that Cushing [1932] had already studied the autonomic effects induced by the injection of pituitrin and pilocarpine into the lateral ventricles in man.

Leavens et al. [1982] reported an initial study in which 6 patients with intractable pain due to cancer were selected for a trial of intrathecal morphine, and in whom the catheter tip was placed in the lumbar subarachnoid space or lateral ventricle (in 4 patients). These authors did not specify why the intraventricular route was chosen. They found that the minimum effective initial dose of morphine in adults was 1 mg in the lumbar region and 2.5–4 mg intraventricularly — in the latter area much higher than subsequent observers. Pain relief ranged from 80 to 100%. They did not observe severe respiratory depression. Lobato et al. [1983] initiated chronic intraventricular morphine in patients with intractable pain caused by facial and disseminated cancer because they had found that, when producing chronic spinal opiate analgesia, low-dose morphine injected into the cisterna magna can suppress pain in any anatomical location without producing concomitant respiratory depression. They placed their catheter in the right lateral ventricle at the level of the foramen of Monro. Good to excellent analgesia lasting for 12–52 h was achieved with morphine doses varying from 0.25 to 1 mg. The onset of analgesia occurred within 2–30 min of drug installation. In 11 of their 17 patients some degree of tolerance to morphine occurred with the passage of time, while the duration of treatment ranged from 2 weeks to 4 months. They used an initial single low dose of morphine 0.25 or 0.5 mg into the cistern in 49 patients as a satisfactory prognosticator of the analgesia subsequently achieved by chronic intraventricular injections [Madrid et al., 1984]. They commented that probably intraventricular morphine acts at a supraspinal level and that the short latency until the onset of analgesia observed in their patients was consistent with this hypothesis. In the one patient who developed respiratory depression this was easily reversed by a dose of i.v. naloxone which did not interfere with the analgesic effect — an observation confirmed by Lazorthes et al. [1985].

Indications for the intraventricular route have been the necessity of stopping peridural administration because of local problems or mechanical disturbance of the device [Roquefeuil et al., 1983, 1984], the desire to evaluate the efficacy of intraspinal versus intraventricular routes of administration and as well to define the clinical indications for each route [Nurchi, 1984; Thiébaut et al., 1985; Lazorthes et al., 1985; Lobato et al., 1985].

For ventricular administration, usually a subcutaneous access port is connected to a ventricular catheter placed in the frontal horn of the lateral ventricle near the foramen of Monro and sometimes in the third ventricle. The first morphine doses are of the order of 0.1 mg and are progressively increased over successive days. During this titration period the patients are closely monitored.

Table 25/V, taken from a study of Lazorthes et al. [in press], summarizes the present results of intraventricular administration of morphine in cancer pain. Out of a total of 281 cases, 60 patients presented with diffuse metastases, 138 with cervico-facial, 35 with thoracic and 48 with abdomino-pelvic cancer pains.

From this limited experience it appears that in patients who have become tolerant to large doses of parenterally administered morphine, intraventricu-

Table 25/V. Daily doses of intraventricular morphine for relief of cancer pain. From Lazorthes et al. [in press].

Author, year	n	Doses, mg/day, min.–max.	Follow-up days		Analgesia, %	Tolerance	Side effects	
			range	av.			respiration	dysphagia, disorientation confusion, somnolence
Leavens et al., 1982	4	0.5–7	2–90	85	75	1	–	–
Lobato et al., 1983, 1985	44	0.25–16	6–150	55	97	–	3	5
Roquefeuil et al., 1983, 1984, 1985	8	0.4–7	8–120	73	80	1	–	2
Nurchi, 1984	5	2–4	8–48		100	–	1	–
Thiebaut et al., 1985	32	0.10–15	4–230	50	90	9	1	6
Lenzi et al., 1985	38	0.5–2	4–292	65	95	–	1	5
Obbens et al., 1987	20	3–60	7–510	98	>50	+++	–	3
Blond et al., 1988	79	0.05–3	3–132	65	94	–	2	–
Lazorthes et al., in press	51	0.10–20	12–230	115	88	2	2	7

lar injection of morphine can produce fast and complete analgesia with low doses (0.3 mg/24 h) [Lazorthes et al., in press]. There is a progressive increase in morphine consumption with time, but this seems to be modest, infrequently exceeding a level 4 times the initial daily requirement [Lazorthes et al., 1985; Lenzi et al., 1985]. Major tolerance is rare, but the occasional patient's pain is untouched even by large doses of greater than 16 mg/day [Coombs et al., 1985b; Lobato et al., 1983; Lenzi et al., 1985]. Analgesia usually takes effect in 5–30 min depending partly on the position of the distal end of the ventricular catheter with respect to the foramen of Monro. In these patients, the incidence of central respiratory depression is low and drowsiness rare; dysphoria and hallucinations have occurred while side effects such as nausea, vomiting, constipation and urinary retention, although common in the first few days, are likely to disappear. Some of the reports are a little too optimistic in their grading system. Thus, we should not classify relief at 40–80% as good [Lenzi et al., 1985]; however, 63% of their 38 patients had a 'final evaluation' of 80–100% or excellent relief — a laudable result indeed. The best results have occurred in those in good condition who were not previously treated with opiates or other potent analgetics. A reduction in anxiety and a feeling of well-being were often described. The group from the M.D. Anderson Tumor Institute have noted faster relief of pain in the abdomen or legs from intraventricular than from intrathecal injections. Nor have multiple punctures of reservoirs leading to the ventricle presented major infection problems to that group [Obbens et al., 1987]. Only 15 of their 332 patients given intraventricular chemotherapy developed meningitis; this was controlled by antibiotics without removal of the reservoir in all but 4.

We have, in collaboration with Hitchcock, treated one patient with pain in the right lower limb persisting for 12 years and many operations after a left cerebral stroke. The almost unbelievably low dose of 0.05 mg of morphine in a catheter he placed in the right lateral ventricle produced complete relief of pain for one to 2 days at the price of severe bilateral weakness of the legs! Half this dose gives a half day of relief without the weakness. Satisfactory relief continued for 7 months; then a major left cerebral infarct produced a right hemiplegia and complete relief of her pain.

Conclusions

Most of the authors are of the opinion that the intraspinal administration of morphine is indicated for intractable cancer pain limited to the lower part of the body, but that after failure of intraspinal analgesia and as well for either diffuse pains or those above the diaphragm, the intraventricular route is indicated. Tentatively we can say the treatment seems encouraging enough so that one should promptly resort to a trial of it for cancer pain. A few of us are finding long sustained relief in some carefully selected patients whose lasting intense pain is unrelated to cancer. The relative values of continuous infusion pumps versus intermittent, often patient-controlled devices are still under assessment.

References

Abbe, R.: A contribution to the surgery of the spine. Med. Rec. *35:* 149–152 (1889).

Adams, C.B.T.; Kaye, A.H.; Teddy, P.J.: The treatment of trigeminal neuralgia by posterior fossa microsurgery. J. Neurol. Neurosurg. Psychiat. *45:* 1020–1026 (1982a).

Adams, J.E.; Hosobuchi, Y.: Technique and technical problems. Neurosurgery *1:* 196–199 (1977).

Adams, J.E.; Hosobuchi, Y.; Fields, H.L.: Stimulation of internal capsule for relief of chronic pain. J. Neurosurg. *41:* 740–747 (1974).

Adams, J.E.; Lippert, R.; Hosobuchi, Y.: Commissural myelotomy; in Schmidek, Sweet, Operative neurosurgical techniques: indications, methods and results, pp. 1155–1161 (Grune & Stratton, New York 1982b).

Adams, J.E.; Rutkin, B.B.: Lesions of the centrum medianum in the treatment of movement disorders. Confinia neurol. *26:* 231–236 (1965).

Adams R.D.; Kubik, C.S.: The morbid anatomy of the demyelinating diseases. Am. J. Med. *12:* 510–546 (1952).

Adar, R.: Iatrogenic brachial plexus injuries. Mayo Clin. Proc. *54:* 277 (1979).

Akaike, A.; Shibata, T.; Satoh, M.; Takagi, H.: Analgesia induced by microinjection of morphine into, and electrical stimulation of, the nucleus reticularis paragigantocellularis of rat medulla oblongata. Neuropharmacology *17:* 775–778 (1978).

Akil, H.; Richardson, D.E.; Barchas, J.D.; Li, C.H.: Appearance of beta-endorphin-like immunoreactivity in human ventricular cerebrospinal fluid upon analgesic electrical stimulation. Proc. natn. Acad. Sci. USA *75:* 5170–5172 (1978).

Albe-Fessard, D.; Berkley, K.J.; Kruger, L.; Ralston, H.J.; Willis, W.D.: Diencephalic mechanisms of pain sensation. Brain Res. Rev. *9:* 217–296 (1985).

Albe-Fessard, D.; Dondey, M.; Nocilaidis, S.; Le Beau, J.: Remarks concerning the effect of diencephalic lesions on pain and sensitivity with special reference to lemniscally mediated control of noxious afferences. Confinia neurol. *32:* 174–184 (1970).

Alvarez-Garijo, J.A.; Valls, C.B.; Mengual, M.V.: Tratamiento quirúrgico de la cefalea facial vegetativa. Rev. Esp. Oto-Neuro-Oftalm. *33:* 7–11 (1975).

Amano, K.; Kawamura, H.; Tanikawa, T.; Kawabatake, H.; Notani, M.; Iseki, H.; Shiwaku, T.; Nagao, T.; Iwata, Y.; Taira, T.; Umezawa, Y.; Simizu, T.; Kitamura, K.: Long-term follow-up study of rostral mesencephalic reticulotomy for pain relief — report of 34 cases. Appl. Neurophysiol. *49:* 105–111 (1986).

Amano, K.; Kitamura, K.; Kawamura, H.; Tanikawa, T.; Kawabatake, H.; Notani, M.; Iseki, H.; Shiwaku, T.; Suda, T.; Demura, H.: Alterations of immunoreactive beta-endorphin in the third ventricular fluid in response to electrical stimulation of the human periaqueductal gray matter. Appl. Neurophysiol. *43:* 150–158 (1980).

Amano, K.; Tanikawa, T.; Iseki, H.; Kawabatake, H.; Notani, M.; Kawamura, H.; Kitamura, K.: Single neuron analysis of the human midbrain tegmentum. Appl. Neurophysiol. *41:* 66–78 (1978).

Amano, K.; Tanikawa, T.; Kawamura, H.; Iseki, H.; Notani, M.; Kawabatake, H.; Shiwaku, T.; Suda, T.; Demura, H.; Kitamura, K.: Endorphins and pain relief. Further observations on electrical stimulation of the lateral part of the periaqueductal gray matter during rostral mesencephalic reticulotomy for pain relief. Appl. Neurophysiol. *45:* 123–135 (1982).

Andersen, E.; Dafny, N.: An ascending serotonergic pain modulation pathway from the dorsal raphe nucleus to the parafascicularis of the thalamus. Brain Res. *269:* 57–67 (1983).

André, N.A.: Observations pratiques sur les maladies de l'urètre et sur plusieurs faits convulsifs, et la guérison de plusieurs maladies chirurgicales. Imprimeur de Collège et de l'Acad. Roy. de Chir., pp. 320–367 (Olivier, Paris 1756).

Andrew, J.; Watkins, E.S.: A stereotactic atlas of the human thalamus and adjacent structures (Williams & Wilkins, Baltimore 1969).

Andy, O.J.: Successful treatment of long-standing hysterical pain and visceral disturbances by unilateral anterior thalamotomy. Case report. J. Neurosurg. *39:* 252–254 (1973).

Apfelbaum, R.I.: A comparison of percutaneous radiofrequency trigeminal neurolysis and microvascular decompression of the trigeminal nerve for the treatment of tic douloureux. Neurosurgery *1:* 16–21 (1977).

Apfelbaum, R.I.: Technical considerations for facilitation of selective percutaneous radiofrequency neurolysis of the trigeminal nerve. Neurosurgery *3:* 396–399 (1978).

Apfelbaum, R.I.: Surgical management of disorders of the lower cranial nerves; in Schmidek, Sweet, Operative neurosurgical techniques: indications, methods and results, vol. 2, pp. 1063–1082 (Grune & Stratton, New York 1982).

Apfelbaum, R.I.: Personal communication (1983).

Arias, M.J.: Percutaneous retrogasserian glycerol rhizotomy for trigeminal neuralgia. A prospective study of 100 cases. J. Neurosurg. *65:* 32–36 (1986).

Arieff, A.J.; Bell, J.L.; Tigay, E.L.: Reflex physiopathic disturbances. Surgery Gynec. Obstet. *118:* 1029–1034 (1964).

Armour, D.: Surgery of the spinal cord and its membranes. Lancet *i:* 691–697 (1927).

Arnér, S.; Arnér, B.: Differential effects of epidural morphine in the treatment of cancer-related pain. Acta anesth. scand. *29:* 32–36 (1985).

Arnér, S.; Lindblom, U.; Meyerson, B.: Letters to the editor. Pain *24:* 117–118 (1986).

Arnot, R.E.; Clinical indications for pre-frontal lobotomy. J. nerv. ment. Dis. *109:* 267–269 (1949).

Arnulf, G.: La chirurgie du sympathique dans la douleur de R. Leriche à nos jours. Bull. Acad. natn. méd. 163: 928–934 (1979).

Aronoff, G.: Personal communication (1987).

Arutjunov, A.I.: Khirurgicheskoje lechenije njekotorykh form njeutolimykh bolej komissurotomiej. Vrach Delo *2:* 117–122 (1952).

Ascherl, R.; Blümel, G.: Zum Krankheitsbild der Sudeck'schen Dystrophie. Fortschr. Med. *99:* 712–720 (1981).

Atkins, H.J.B.: Sympathectomy by the axillary approach. Lancet *i:* 538–539 (1954).

Atkinson, J.R.: Cingulotomy and mesencephalotomy at the BNI. Material presented to the American College of Surgeons, Miami 1973.

Atweh, S.F.; Dajani, B.M.; Saadé, N.E.; Jabbur, S.J.: Supraspinal inhibition of trigeminal input into subnucleus caudalis by dorsal column stimulation. Brain Res. *348:* 401–404 (1985).

Atweh, S.F.; Kuhar, M.J.: Autoradiographic localization of opiate receptors in rat brain. I. Spinal cord and lower medulla. Brain Res. *124:* 53–67 (1977).

Augustinsson, L.E.; Carlsson, C.A.; Holm, J.; Jivegärd, L.: Epidural electrical stimulation in severe limb ischemia. Ann. Surg. *202:* 104–110 (1985).

Auld, A.W.; Maki Hokela, A.; Murdoch, D.M.: Intraspinal narcotic analgesia in the treatment of chronic pain. Spine *10:* 777–781 (1985).

Azerad, J.; Hunt, C.C.; Laporte, Y.; Pollin, B.; Thiesson, D.: Afferent fibers in cat ventral roots: electrophysiological and histological evidence. J. Physiol. *379:* 229–243 (1986).

Baddeley, R.M.: The place of upper dorsal sympathectomy in the treatment of primary Raynaud's disease. Br. J. Surg. *52:* 426–430 (1965).

Ballantine, H.T.; Bouckoms, A.J.; Thomas, E.K.; Giriunas, I.E.: Treatment of psychiatric illness by stereotactic cingulotomy. Biol. Psychiat. *22:* 807–819 (1987).

Bantli, H.; Bloedel, J.R.; Thienprasit, P.: Supraspinal interactions from dorsal column stimulation. J. Neurosurg. *42:* 296–300 (1975).

Barba, D.; Alksne, J.F.: Success of microvascular decompression with and without prior surgical therapy for trigeminal neuralgia. J. Neurosurg. *60:* 104–107 (1984).

Barber, R.P.; Vaughn, J.E.; Slemmon, J.R.; Salvaterra, P.M.; Roberts, E.; Leeman, S.E.: The origin, distribution and synaptic relationships of substance P axons in rat spinal cord. J. comp. Neurol. *184:* 331–352 (1979).

Barbera, J.; Barcia-Salorio, J.L.; Broseta, J.: Stereotaxic pontine spinothalamic tractotomy. Surg. Neurol. *11:* 111–114 (1979).

Barbut, D.; Polak, J.M.; Wall, P.D.: Substance P in spinal cord dorsal horn decreases following peripheral nerve injury. Brain Res. *205:* 289–298 (1981).

Barcia-Salorio, J.L.; Broseta, J.; Roldán, P.; Masbout, G.; García-March, G.; Joanes, V.; Vanaclocha, V.; Piquer, J.; Cerda, M.: Lesión de la zona de entrada de las raíces posteriores (DREZ) en el dolor por afectación traumática o neoplásica del plexo braquial; in Arjuna, Combined Meeting Reunión Conjunta, Society of British Neurological Surgeons, Society of Neurosurgeons of South Africa, Sociedad Luso-Española de Neurocirugía, Granada 1985, pp. 149–159 (Gráficos Arte, Granada 1985).

Barnes, R.: Causalgia: A review of 48 cases; in Seddon, Peripheral nerve injuries, pp. 156–185 (HMSO, London 1954).

Barrash, J.M.; Leavens, M.E.: Dorsal rhizotomy for the relief of intractable pain of malignant tumor origin. J. Neurosurg. *38:* 755–757 (1973).

Bartlett, J.R.; Bridges, P.K.: The extended subcaudate tractotomy lesion; in Sweet, Obrador, Martin-Rodriguez, Neurosurgical treatment in psychiatry, pain and epilepsy, pp. 387–398 (University Park Press, Baltimore 1977).

Basbaum, A.I.: Conduction of the effects of noxious stimulation by short-fiber multisynaptic systems in the spinal cord of the rat. Expl. Neurol. *40:* 699–716 (1973).

Basbaum, A.I.; Fields, H.L.: Endogenous pain control mechanisms: review and hypothesis. Ann. Neurol. *4:* 451–462 (1978).

Basbaum, A.I.; Fields, H.L.: The origin of descending pathways in the dorso-lateral funiculus of the spinal cord of the cat and rat: further studies on the anatomy of pain modulation. J. comp. Neurol. *187:* 513–532 (1979).

Basbaum, A.I.; Wall, P.D.: Chronic changes in the response of cells in adult cat dorsal horn following partial deafferentation: the appearance of responding cells in a previously nonresponsive region. Brain Res. *116:* 181–204 (1976).

Baskin, D.S.; Mehler, W.R.; Hosobuchi, Y.; Richardson, D.E.; Adams, J.E.; Flitter, M.A.: Autopsy analysis of the safety, efficacy and cartography of electrical stimulation of the central gray in humans. Brain Res. *371:* 231–236 (1986).

Baxter, A.D.; O'Kafo, B.A.: Ejaculatory failure after chemical sympathectomy. Anesth. Analg. *63:* 770–771 (1984).

Beaver, D.L.: Electron microscopy of the Gasserian ganglion in trigeminal neuralgia. J. Neurosurg. *26:* 138–150 (1967).

Beck, D.W.; Olson, J.J.; Urig, E.J.: Percutaneous retrogasserian glycerol rhizotomy for treatment of trigeminal neuralgia. J. Neurosurg. *65:* 28–31 (1986).

Behar, M.; Magora, F.; Olshwang, D.; Davidson, J.T.: Epidural morphine in treatment of pain. Lancet *i:* 527–529 (1979).

Belber, C.J.; Rak, R.A.: Balloon compression rhizolysis in the surgical management of trigeminal neuralgia. Neurosurgery *20:* 908–913 (1987).

Bell, C.: Idea of a new anatomy of the brain (Strahan & Preston, London 1811).

Belmusto, L.; Brown, E.; Owens, G.: Clinical observations on respiratory and vasomotor disturbance as related to cervical cordotomies. J. Neurosurg. *20:* 225–232 (1963).

Benabid, A.L.; Henriksen, S.J.; McGinty, J.F.; Bloom, F.E.: Thalamic nucleus ventro-postero-lateralis inhibits nucleus parafascicularis response to noxious stimuli through a nonopioid pathway. Brain Res. *280:* 217–231 (1983).

Benabid, A.L.; Schaerer, R.; De Rougemont, J.; Pallo, D.; Barge, M.; Chirossel, J.P.; Clamadieu, M.H.: Clinical evaluation of stereotactic isotope hypophysectomy in advanced breast cancer. Rev. Endocrine-Rel. Cancers, suppl. April, pp. 111–117 (1978).

Benassy, J.: A propos du procès-verbal. Au sujet de la communication de MM. Motta et Afanassieff: Traitement des moignons douloureux et causalgies. Chirurgie *103:* 926–927 (1977).

Bennett, W.H.; A case in which acute spasmodic pain in the left lower extremity was completely relieved by sub-dural division of the posterior roots of certain spinal nerves. Med. chir. Trans., Lond. *72:* 329–348 (1889).

Benoist, J.M.; Kayser, V.; Gautron, M.; Guilbaud, G.: Low dose of morphine strongly depresses responses of specific nociceptive neurones in the ventro-basal complex of the rat. Pain *15:* 333–344 (1983).

Berger, A.J.: Dorsal respiratory group neurons in the medulla of cat: spinal projections, responses to lung inflation and superior laryngeal nerve stimulation. Brain Res. *135:* 213–254 (1977).

Berguer, R.; Smit, R.: Transaxillary sympathectomy (T2 to T4) for relief of vasospastic/sympathetic pain of upper extremities. Surgery *89:* 764–769 (1981).

Bernard, E.J.; Nashold, B.S.; Caputi, F.; Moossy, J.J.: Nucleus caudalis DREZ lesions for facial pain. Br. J. Neurosurg. *1:* 81–92 (1987a).

Bernard, J.F.; Besson, M.A.W.; Besson, J.M.; Peschanski, M.: A spino-ponto-amygdalian pathway for pain. Pain, suppl. 4, p. S242 (1987b).

Bertrand, F.; Hugelin, A.; Vibert, J.-F.: Quantitative study of anatomical distribution of respiratory related neurons in the pons. Exp. Brain Res. *16:* 383–399 (1973).

Besson, J.M.; Chaouch, A.: Peripheral and spinal mechanisms of nociception. Physiol. Rev. *67:* 67–185 (1987).

Besson, J.M.; Guilbaud, G.; Abdelmoumene, M.; Chaouch, A.: Physiologie de la nociception. J. Physiol., Paris *78:* 7–107 (1982).

Bettag, W.; Yoshida, T.: Über stereotaktische Schmerzoperationen. Acta neurochir. *8:* 299–317 (1960).

Birkenfeld, R.; Fisher, R.G.: Successful treatment of causalgia of upper extremity with medullary spinothalamic tractotomy. J. Neurosurg. *20:* 303–311 (1963).

Bischoff, E.P.E.: Microscopic analysis of the anastomoses between the cranial nerves (1865). Translated and edited by Sachs, Valtin (University Press of New England, Hanover 1977).

Bishop, G.H.: The relation between nerve fiber size and sensory modality: phylogenetic implication of the afferent innervation of cortex. J. nerv. ment. Dis. *128:* 89–114 (1959).

Black R.G.: A laboratory model for trigeminal neuralgia. Adv. Neurol. *4:* 651–658 (1974).

Bleasel, K.; Lazarus, L.: Cryogenic hypophysectomy. Med. J. Aust. *ii:* 148–156 (1965).

Blond, S.; Meynadier, J.; Dupard, T.; Hurtevent, J.F.; Assaker, R.; Brichard, C.; Guieu, J.D.; Christiaens, J.L.; Demaille, A.: La morphinothérapie intra-cérébroventriculaire: indications et résultats à propos de 79 patients. Neuro-Chirurgie (1988).

Bloom, F.; Battenberg, E.; Rossier, J.; Ling, N.; Leppaluoto, T.M.; Vargo, T.M.; Guillemin, R.: Endorphins are located in the intermediate and anterior lobes of the pituitary gland, not in the neurohypophysis. Life Sci. *20:* 43–48 (1977).

Blumberg, H.; Jänig, W.: Changes in unmyelinated fibers including sympathetic postganglionic fibers of a skin nerve after peripheral neuroma formation. J. autonom. nerv. Syst. *6:* 173–183 (1982).

Blumberg, H.; Jänig, W.: Discharge pattern of afferent fibers from a neuroma. Pain *20:* 335–353 (1984).

Blume, H.G.: Radiofrequency denaturation in occipital pain: a new approach in 114 cases. Adv. Pain Res. Ther. *1:* 691–698 (1976).

Blume, H.; Richardson, R.; Rojas, C.: Epidural nerve stimulation of the lower spinal cord and cauda equina for the relief of intractable pain in failed low back surgery. Appl. Neurophysiol. *45:* 456–460 (1982).

Bogduk, N.; Long, D.M.: The anatomy of the so-called 'articular nerves' and their relationship to facet denervation in the treatment of low-back pain. J. Neurosurg. *51:* 172–177 (1979).

Bogduk, N.; Long, D.M.: Percutaneous lumbar medial branch neurotomy. A modification of facet denervation. Spine *5:* 193–200 (1980).

Bogduk, N.; Macintosh, J.; Marsland, A.: Technical limitations to the efficacy of radiofrequency neurotomy for spinal pain. Neurosurgery *20:* 529–535 (1987).

Bohm, E.; Hojeberg, S.: Late results of decompression operation for trigeminal neuralgia. A follow-up study of 110 cases. Acta chir. scand. *120:* 233–236 (1960).

Bohm, E.; Strang, R.R.: Glossopharyngeal neuralgia. Brain *85:* 371–388 (1962).

Boivie, J.; Meyerson, B.A.: A correlative anatomical and clinical study of pain suppression by deep brain stimulation. Pain *13:* 113–126 (1982).

Bonica, J.J.: Causalgia and other reflex sympathetic dystrophies. Adv. Pain Res. Ther. *3:* 141–166 (1979).

Borges, L.F.; Silverberg, R.A.; Ogilvy, C.S.: Axonal transport of stilbamidine (in preparation, 1988).

Borison, H.L.; Wang, S.C.: Physiology and pharmacology of vomiting. Pharmacol. Rev. *5:* 193–230 (1953).

Botterell, E.H.; Callaghan, J.C.; Jousse, A.T.: Pain in paraplegia. Clinical management and surgical treatment. Proc. R. Soc. Med. *47:* 281–288 (1954).

Bouchard, G.; Mayanagi, Y.; Martins, L.F.: Advantages and limits of intracerebral stereotactic operations for pain; in Sweet, Obrador, Martin-Rodriguez, Neurosurgical treatment in psychiatry, pain and epilepsy, pp. 693–696 (University Park Press, Baltimore 1977).

Bouckoms, A.J.: Psychosurgery; in Wall, Melzack, Textbook of pain, pp. 666–676 (Churchill-Livingstone, Edinburgh 1984).

Bouckoms, A.M.: Non-malignant pain treated with long-term oral narcotics. Pain (1989) (to be published).

Bouhassira, D.; Villanueva, L.; Le Bars, D.: Effects of intraventricular (i.c.v.) morphine upon diffuse noxious inhibitory controls (DNIC) in the rat. Neurosci. Lett., suppl. 26, p. S410 (1986).

Bowsher, D.: Termination of the central pain pathway in man: the conscious appreciation of pain. Brain *80:* 606–622 (1957).

Boyd, A.M.; Ratcliffe, A.H.; Jepson, R.P.; James, G.W.H.: Intermittent claudication: a clinical study. J. Bone Jt Surg. *31B:* 325–355 (1949).

Brandt, F.; Wittkamp, P.: Spätresultate der Thermokoagulation im Ganglion Gasseri beim Tic Douloureux. Neurochirurgia *26:* 133–135 (1983).

Breeze, R.; Ignelzi, R.J.: Microvascular decompression for trigeminal neuralgia. Results with special reference to the late recurrence rate. J. Neurosurg. *57:* 487–490 (1982).

Brenner, H.; Pendl, G.: Ipsilateraler Chordotomieeffekt — ein seltener Fall einer ungekreuzten Schmerzbahn. Wien med. Wschr. *116:* 1041–1042 (1966).

Brett, D.C.; Ferguson, G.C.; Ebers, G.C.; Paty, D.W.: Percutaneous trigeminal rhizotomy. Treatment of trigeminal neuralgia secondary to multiple sclerosis. Archs Neurol. *39:* 219–221 (1982).

Bricolo, A.; Dalle Ore, G.: Percutaneous microcompression of the Gasserian ganglion for trigeminal neuralgia: preliminary results. Acta neurochir. *69:* 102 (1983).

Brihaye, J.; Thiry, S.; Leclercq, R.: Le traitement chirurgical de la douleur. Acta chir. belg., suppl. 11 (1962).

Brihaye, J.; Violon, A.: La douleur causalgique. Acta chir. belg. *77:* 195–200 (1978).

Brisman, R.: Trigeminal neuralgia and multiple sclerosis. Archs Neurol. *44:* 379–381 (1987a).

Brisman, R.: Bilateral trigeminal neuralgia. J. Neurosurg. *67:* 44–48 (1987b).

Broager, B.: Commissural myelotomy. Surg. Neurol. *2:* 71–74 (1974).

Broggi, G.: Thermorhizotomy in trigeminal neuralgia: preliminary considerations on 46 cases. Adv. Neurosurg. *3:* 297–300 (1975).

Broggi, G.; Franzini, A.; Giorgi, C.; Lasio, G.; Servello, D.: Radiofrequency percutaneous trigeminal rhizotomy. Considerations in 1,000 consecutive cases of essential trigeminal neuralgia. J. Neurosurg. Sci. *29:* 165 (1985).

Broggi, G.; Siegfried, J.: The effect of graded thermocoagulation on trigeminal evoked potentials in the cat. Acta neurochir., suppl. 24, pp. 175–178 (1977).

Broggi, G.; Siegfried, J.: Percutaneous differential radiofrequency rhizotomy of glossopharyngeal nerve in facial pain due to cancer. Adv. Pain Res. Ther. *2:* 469–473 (1979).

Bromage, P.R.; Camporesi, E.; Leslie, J.: Epidural narcotics in volunteers: sensitivity to pain and to carbon dioxide. Pain *9:* 145–160 (1980).

Bronec, P.R.; Saris, S.C.; Nashold, B.S.: Dorsal root entry zone coagulation; in Symon, Operative surgery: fundamentals in international techniques. Neurosurgery (in press).

Broseta, J.; Barbera, J.; De Vera, J.A.; Barcia-Salorio, J.L.; Garcia-March, G.; Bonzalez-Darder, J.; Ravaina, F.; Joanes, V.: Spinal cord stimulation in peripheral arterial disease. J. Neurosurg. *64:* 71–80 (1986).

Browne, L.: Radiofrequency lesioning of the trigeminal ganglion for the treatment of trigeminal neuralgia. Ir. med. J. *78:* 68–71 (1985).

Brummer, S.B.; Turner, M.J.: Electrical stimulation with Pt electrodes. I. A method for determination of 'real' electrode areas. IEEE Trans. biomed. Engng *24:* 436–439 (1977a).

Brummer, S.B.; Turner, M.J.: Electrical stimulation with Pt electrodes. II. Estimation of maximum surface redox (theoretical non-gassing) limits. IEEE Trans. biomed. Engng *24:* 440–443 (1977b).

Brummer, S.B.; Turner, M.J.: Electrochemical considerations for safe electrical stimulation of the nervous system with platinum electrodes. IEEE Trans. biomed. Engng *24:* 59–63 (1977c).

Bruyn, G.W.: Nervus intermedius neuralgia (Hunt). Cephalalgia *4:* 71–78 (1984).

Bues, E.: Die vordere Ohrzone in Diagnostik und Therapie der Glossopharyngicus-Neuralgie. Dt. Z. NervHeilk. *185:* 471–487 (1963).

Buker, R.H.; Cox, W.A.; Scully, T.J.; Seitter, G.; Pauling, F.W.: Causalgia and transthoracic sympathectomy. Am. J. Surg. *124:* 724–727 (1972).

Bullitt, E.; Friedman, A.: Material presented to the DREZ Symposium, Duke University, Durham 1987.

Burchiel, K.J.: Abnormal impulse generation in focally demyelinated trigeminal roots. J. Neurosurg. *53:* 674–683 (1980).

Burchiel, K.J.: Personal communication (1987).

Burchiel, K.J.; Russell, L.C.: Spontaneous activity of ventral root axons following peripheral nerve injury. J. Neurosurg. *62:* 408–413 (1985).

Burchiel, K.J.; Russell, L.C.: Has the amount of spontaneous electrical activity in experimental neuromas been overestimated?; in Pubols, Sessle, Effects of injury on trigeminal and spinal somatosensory systems, pp. 77–83 (Liss, New York 1987).

Burchiel, K.J.; Steege, T.D.; Howe, J.F.; Loeser, J.D.: Comparison of percutaneous radiofrequency gangliolysis and microvascular decompression for the surgical management of tic douloureux. Neurosurgery *9:* 111–119 (1981).

Burchiel, K.J.; Wyler, A.R.; Harris, A.B.: Epileptogenic agents applied to trigeminal ganglia: absence of neuronal hyperexcitability. Epilepsia *19:* 567–579 (1978).

Burstein, R.; Cliffer, K.D.; Giesler, G.J.: The spinohypothalamic tract: a direct nociceptive projection from the spinal cord to the hypothalamus. Pain, suppl. 4, p. S241 (1987).

Burton, C.: Seminar on dorsal column stimulation: summary of proceedings. Surg. Neurol. *1:* 285–289 (1973).

Burton, C.: Dorsal column stimulation: optimization of application. Surg. Neurol. *4:* 171–179 (1975).

Burton, C.V.: Percutaneous radiofrequency facet denervation. Appl. Neurophysiol. *39:* 80–86 (1976/77).

Cain, D.P.: Sensory kindling: implications for development of sensory prostheses. Neurology *29:* 1595–1599 (1979).

Calvin, W.H.; Devor, M.; Howe, J.F.: Can neuralgias arise from minor demyelination? Spontaneous firing, mechanosensitivity and afterdischarge from conducting axons. Expl. Neurol. *75:* 755–763 (1982).

Calvin, W.H.; Loeser, J.D.; Howe, J.F.: A neurophysiological theory for the pain mechanism of tic douloureux. Pain *3:* 147–154 (1977).

Campbell, J.A.; Lipton, S.: Somatosensory evoked potentials recorded from within the anterolateral quadrant of the human spinal cord. Adv. Pain Res. Ther. *5:* 193–196 (1983).

Campbell, J.K.: Cluster headache: The treatment-resistant patients; in Ninan, Cluster headache, chap. 14, pp. 127–133 (SP Medical & Scientific Books, New York 1984).

Campbell, J.N.: Examination of possible mechanisms by which stimulation of the spinal cord in man relieves pain. Appl. Neurophysiol. *44:* 181–186 (1981).

Campbell, J.N.; Long, D.M.: Peripheral nerve stimulation in the treatment of intractable pain. J. Neurosurg. *45:* 692–699 (1976).

Campbell, J.N.; Miles, J.: Evoked potentials as an aid to lesion making in the dorsal root entry zone. Neurosurgery *15:* 951–959 (1984).

Campbell, J.N.; Raja, S.N.; Meyer, R.A.: Painful sequelae of nerve injury; in Dubner, Gebhart, Bond, Pain Research and Clinical Management, vol. 3, pp. 135–143 (Elsevier, Amsterdam 1988).

Campbell, J.N.; Taub, A.: Local analgesia from percutaneous electrical stimulation. A peripheral mechanism. Archs Neurol., Chicago *28:* 347–350 (1973).

Campos, M.; Medina, E.; Ribeiro, A.: Coagulation of the ganglion of Gasser with radiofrequency for trigeminal neuralgia (to be published).

Cannon, J.T.; Prieto, G.J.; Lee, A.; Liebeskind, J.C.: Evidence for opioid and non-opioid forms of stimulation-produced analgesia in the rat. Brain Res. *243:* 315–321 (1982).

Carayon, A.; Bourrel, P.: Indications et résultats du traitement chirurgical précoce de 150 causalgies. Ann. Chir. *17:* 554–560 (1963).

Cassinari, V.; Infuso, L.; Pagni, C.A.: Some experiences with stereotactic surgery of pain. Excerpta Medica Int. Congr. Ser., No. *60:* 121–123 (1963).

Cassinari, V.; Pagni, C.A.: Central pain: a neurosurgical survey (Harvard University Press, Cambridge 1969).

Chapman, W.P.; Rose, A.; Solomon, H.C.: Measurements of heat stimulus producing motor withdrawal reaction in patients following frontal lobotomy. ARNMD *XXVII:* 754–768 (1948).

Chorobski, J.; Penfield, W.: Cerebral vasodilator nerves and their pathway from the medulla oblongata, with observations on the pial and intracerebral vascular plexus. Archs Neurol. Psychiat. *28:* 1257–1289 (1932).

Chouké, K.S.; Hodes, P.J.: The pterygo-alar bar and its recognition by roentgen methods in trigeminal neuralgia. Am. J. Roentg. *65:* 180–182 (1951).

Chrubasik, J.; Meynadier, J.; Blond, S.; Scherpereel, P.; Ackerman, E.; Weinstock, M.; Bonath, K.; Cramer, H.; Wunsch, E.: Somatostatin, a potent analgesic. Lancet *ii:* 1208–1209 (1984).

Chung, J.M.; Fang, Z.R.; Hori, Y.; Lee, K.H.; Willis, W.D.: Prolonged inhibition of primate spinothalamic tract cells by peripheral nerve stimulation. Pain *19:* 259–275 (1984a).

Chung, J.M.; Lee, K.H.; Hori, Y.; Endo, K.; Willis, W.D.: Factors influencing peripheral nerve stimulation produced inhibition of primate spinothalamic tract cells. Pain *19:* 277–293 (1984b).

Chung, K.; Langford, L.A.; Applebaum, A.E.; Coggeshall, R.E.: Primary afferent fibers in the tract of Lissauer in the rat. J. comp. Neurol. *184:* 587–598 (1979).

Cioni, B.; D'Annunzio, V.; Meglio, M.; Rossi, G.F.: Personal experience with intrathecal morphine in the treatment of cancer pain. Pain, suppl. 2, p. S343 (1984).

Clifton, G.L.; Coggeshall, R.E.; Vance, W.H.; Willis, W.D.: Receptive fields of unmyelinated ventral root afferent fibres in the cat. J. Physiol. *256:* 573–600 (1976).

Cline, M.; Ochoa, J.; Torebjörk, H.E.: Chronically sensitized C nociceptors in skin; patient with hyperalgesia and ongoing pain. Electroenceph. clin. Neurophysiol. *66:* S20–S21 (1987).

Cloward, R.B.: Cervical chordotomy by the anterior approach. Technique and advantages. J. Neurosurg. *21:* 19–25 (1964).

Coderre, T.J.; Grimes, R.W.; Melzack R.: Deafferentation and chronic pain in animals: an evaluation of evidence suggesting autotomy is related to pain. Pain *26:* 61–84 (1986).

Coggeshall, R.E.: An overview of dorsal root axon branching and ventral root afferent fibers; in Rowe, Willis, Development, organization and processing in somatosensory pathways, pp. 105–110 (Liss, New York 1985).

Coggeshall, R.E.; Coulter, J.D.; Willis, W.D.: Unmyelinated axons in the ventral roots of the cat lumbosacral enlargement. J. comp. Neurol. *153:* 39–58 (1974).

Coggeshall, R.E.; Ito, H.: Sensory fibers in ventral root L7 and S1 in the cat. J. Physiol. *267:* 215–235 (1977).

Colombo, F.: Somatosensory-evoked potentials after mesencephalic tractotomy for pain syndromes. Neuroradiologic and clinical correlations. Surg. Neurol. *21:* 453–458 (1984).

Colpaert, F.C.: Can chronic pain be suppressed despite purported tolerance to narcotic analgesia? Life Sci. *24:* 1201–1210 (1979).

Colpaert, F.C.: Evidence that adjuvant arthritis in the rat is associated with chronic pain. Pain *28:* 201–222 (1987).

Colpaert, F.C.; Niemegeers, C.J.E.; Jansen, P.A.J.; Maroli, A.N.: The effects of prior fentanyl administration and of pain on fentanyl analgesia: tolerance to and enhancement of narcotic analgesia. J. Pharmac. exp. Ther. *213:* 418–424 (1980).

Comte, P.: Monopolar versus bipolar stimulation. Appl. Neurophysiol. *45:* 156–159 (1982).

Cook, A.W.; Kawakami, Y.: Commissural myelotomy. J. Neurosurg. *47:* 1–6 (1977).

Cook, A.W.; Nathan, P.W.; Smith, M.C.: Sensory consequences of commissural myelotomy. Brain *107:* 547–568 (1984).

Cook, A.W.; Oygar, A.; Baggenstos, P.; Pacheco, S.; Kleriga, E.: Vascular disease of extremities. Electrical stimulation of spinal cord and posterior roots. N.Y. State J. Med. *76:* 366–368 (1976).

Coombs, D.W.; Fratkin, J.D.; Meier, F.A.; Nierenberg, D.W.; Saunders, R.L.: Neuropathologic lesions and CSF morphine concentrations during chronic intraspinal morphine infusion. A clinical and post-mortem study. Pain *22:* 337–351 (1985a).

Coombs, D.W.; Saunders, R.L.: Intraspinal infusion of narcotic drugs; in Wilkins, Rengachary, Neurosurgery, vol. 3, pp. 2390–2397 (McGraw-Hill, New York 1985).

Coombs, D.W.; Saunders, R.L.; Gaylor, M.S.; Block, A.R.; Colton, T.; Harbaugh, R.; Pageau, M.G.; Mroz, W.: Relief of continuous chronic pain by intraspinal narcotics infusion via an implanted reservoir. J. Am. med. Ass. *17:* 2336–2339 (1983).

Coombs, D.W.; Saunders, R.L.; Gaylor, M.S.; Pageau, M.G.; Leith, M.G.; Schaiberger, C.: Continuous epidural analgesia via implanted morphine reservoir. Lancet *ii:* 425–426 (1981).

Coombs, D.W.; Saunders, R.L.; LaChance, D.; Savage, S.; Ragnarsson, T.S.; Jensen, L.E.: Intrathecal morphine tolerance: use of intrathecal clonidine, DADLE, and intraventricular morphine. Anesthesiology *62:* 358–363 (1985b).

Coombs, D.W.; Savage, S.; LaChance, D.; Saunders, R.L.; Jensen, L.E.; Gaylor, M.S.: Intrathecal clonidine control of cancer pain when spinal morphine tolerance develops. Pain, suppl. 2, p. S21 (1984).

Cooper, I.S.: Clinical and physiologic implications of thalamic surgery for disorders of sensory communication. I. Thalamic surgery for intractable pain. J. neurol. Sci. *2:* 493–519 (1965).

Cooper, I.S.; Amin, I.; Candra, R.; Waltz, J.M.: A surgical investigation of the clinical physiology of the LP-pulvinar complex in man. J. neurol. Sci. *18:* 89–110 (1973).

Corkin, S.: A prospective study of cingulotomy; in Valenstein, The psychosurgery debate, pp. 164–204 (Freeman, San Francisco 1980).

Cosman, E.R.; Nashold, B.S.; Levitt, J.O.: Theoretical aspects of radiofrequency lesion in the dorsal root entry zone. Neurosurgery *15:* 945–950 (1984).

Cotton, L.T.; Cross, F.W.: Lumbar sympathectomy for arterial disease. Review. Br. J. Surg. *72:* 678–683 (1985).

Cousins, M.J.; Bridenbaugh, P.O.: Neural blockade in clinical anesthesia and management of pain (Lippincott, Philadelphia 1980).

Cousins, M.J.; Mather, L.E.: Intrathecal and epidural administration of opioids. Anesthesiology *61:* 276–310 (1984).

Cousins, M.J.; Mather, L.E.; Glynn, C.J.; Wilson, P.R.; Graham, J.R.: Selective spinal analgesia. Lancet *i:* 1141–1142 (1979a).

Cousins, M.J.; Reeve, T.S.; Glynn, C.J.; Walsh, J.A.; Cherry, D.A.: Neurolytic lumbar sympathetic blockade: duration of denervation and relief of rest pain. Anaesth. intensive Care *7:* 121–135 (1979b).

Cowie, R.A.; Hitchcock, E.R.: The late results of antero-lateral cordotomy for pain relief. Acta neurochir. *64:* 39–50 (1982).

Crawford, M.E.; Andersen, H.B.; Augustenborg, G.; Bay, J.; Beck, O.; Benveniste, D.; Larsen, L.B.; Carl, P.; Djernes, M.; Eriksen, J.; Grell, A.M.; Henriksen, H.; Johansen, S.H.; Jorgensen, H.O.K.; Moller, I.W.; Pedersen, J.E.P.; Ravlo, O.: Pain treatment on outpatient bases utilizing extradural opiates. A Danish multicentre study comprising 105 patients. Pain *16:* 41–47 (1983).

Crock, H.V.; Yoshizawa, H.: The blood supply of the vertebral column and spinal cord in man (Springer, Wien 1977).

Cross, F.W.; Cotton, L.T.: Chemical lumbar sympathectomy for ischemic rest pain. A randomized, prospective controlled clinical trial. Am. J. Surg. *150:* 341–345 (1985).

Crue, B.L.; Todd, E.M.: A simplified technique of sacral rhizotomy for pelvic pain. J. Neurosurg. *21:* 835–837 (1964).

Crue, B.L.; Todd, E.M.; Carregal, J.A.: Posterior approach for high cervical percutaneous radiofrequency cordotomy. Confinia neurol. *30:* 41–52 (1968).

Crue, B.L.; Todd, E.M.; Carregal, E.J.A.: Percutaneous radiofrequency stereotaxic trigeminal tractotomy; in Crue, Pain and suffering, pp. 69–80 (Thomas, Springfield 1970).

Cushing, H.: The major trigeminal neuralgias and their surgical treatment based on experiences with 332 Gasserian operations. I. Varieties of facial neuralgia. Am. J. med. Sci. *160:* 157–184 (1920).

Cushing, H.: Papers relating to the pituitary body, hypothalamus and parasympathetic nervous system (Thomas, Springfield 1932).

Dahlstrom, B.; Tamsen, A.; Paalzow, L.; Hartvig, P.: Patient-controlled analgesic therapy. IV. Pharmacokinetics and analgesic plasma concentrations of morphine. Clin. Pharmacokinet. *7:* 266–279 (1982).

Dale, W.A.; Lewis, M.R.: Management of ischemia of the hand and fingers. Surgery *67:* 62–79 (1970).

Dan, N.G.: Personal communication (1988).

Dandy, W.E.: Glossopharyngeal neuralgia (tic douloureux). Its diagnosis and treatment. Archs Surg. *15:* 198–214 (1927).

Dandy, W.E.: An operation for the cure of tic douloureux. Partial section of the sensory root at the pons. Archs Surg. *18:* 687–734 (1929).

Dandy, W.E.: Treatment of trigeminal neuralgia by the cerebellar route. Ann. Surg. *96:* 787–795 (1932a).

Dandy, W.E.: Certain functions of the roots and ganglia of the cranial sensory nerves. Archs Neurol. Psychiat. *27:* 22–29 (1932b).

Dandy, W.E.: Concerning cause of trigeminal neuralgia. Am. J. Surg. *24:* 447–455 (1934).

Dargent, M.; Mansuy, L.; Cohen, J.; De Rougemont, J.: Les problèmes posés par la douleur dans l'évolution des cancers gynécologiques. Lyon chirurg. *59:* 62–83 (1963).

Daum, S.; Vogein-Rappoport; Gruner, J.; Foncin, J.F.: Sclérose en plaques révélée à l'âge de 64 ans par une névralgie trigéminale. Etude anatomo-clinique. Revue neurol. *102:* 500–503 (1960).

Davidson, J.T.; Magora, F.: Intrathecal and epidural opiates: background and assessment; in Lipton, Miles, Persistent pain: modern methods of treatment, vol. 4, pp. 43–61 (Grune & Stratton, New York 1983).

Davis, L.; Hart, J.T.; Crain, R.C.: The pathway for visceral afferent impulses within the spinal cord. Surgery Gynec. Obstet. *48:* 647–651 (1929).

Davis, L.; Martin, J.: Studies upon spinal cord injuries. II. The nature and treatment of pain. J. Neurosurg. *4:* 483–491 (1947).

Davis, R.; Gray, E.: Technical factors important to dorsal column stimulation. Appl. Neurophysiol. *44:* 160–170 (1981).

De Castro-Costa, M.; De Sutter, P.; Gybels, J.; Van Hees, J.: Adjuvant-induced arthritis in rats: a possible animal model of chronic pain. Pain *10:* 173–185 (1981).

De Castro-Costa, M.; Gybels, J.; Kupers, R.; Van Hees, J.: Scratching behaviour in arthritic rats: a sign of chronic pain or itch? Pain *29:* 123–131 (1987).

De la Porte, C.; Siegfried, J.: Lumbrosacral spinal fibrosis (spinal arachnoiditis). Its diagnosis and treatment by spinal cord stimulation. Spine *8:* 593–603 (1983).

Denecke, H.J.: Zur Chirurgie des N. petrosus major bei langjährigem Gesichts- und Kopfschmerz. (Greater petrosal nerve surgery in long-term cluster headache). HNO *25:* 48–50 (1977).

Denny-Brown, D.; Kirk, E.J.; Yanagisawa, N.: The tract of Lissauer in relation to sensory transmission in the dorsal horn of spinal cord in the macaque monkey. J. comp. Neurol. *151:* 175–200 (1973).

De Rougemont, J.: Personal communication (1973).

Deshpande, N.; Moricca, G.; Saullo, F.; Di Martino, L.; Kwa, G.: Some aspects of pituitary function after neuroadenolysis in patients with metastatic cancer. Tumori *67:* 355–359 (1981).

Devor, M.: Potassium channels moderate ectopic excitability of nerve-end neuromas in rats. Neurosci. Lett. *40:* 181–186 (1983).

Devor, M.; Wall, P.D.: Plasticity in the spinal cord sensory map following peripheral nerve injury in rats. J. Neurosci. *1:* 679–684 (1981).

Dickenson, A.: The inhibitory effects of thalamic stimulation on the spinal transmission of nociceptive information in the rat. Pain *17:* 213–224 (1983).

Dieckmann, G.; Krainick, J.-U.; Thoden, U.: Stereotaxic induction stimulation for pain; in Schaltenbrand, Walker, Stereotaxy of the human brain; 2nd revised and enlarged edition, pp. 498–502 (Thieme, Stuttgart 1982).

Dieckmann, G.; Veras, G.: II. Plexus avulsion pain (neurogenic pain). High frequency coagulation of dorsal root entry zone in patients with deafferentation pain. Acta neurochir. suppl. 33, pp. 445–450 (1984).

Dieckmann, G.; Veras, G.; Sogabe, K.: Retrogasserian glycerol injection or percutaneous stimulation in the treatment of typical and atypical trigeminal pain. 8th Int. Congr. Neurological Surgery, Abstract 227 (1985).

Dieckmann, G.; Witzmann, A.: Initial and long-term results of deep brain stimulation for chronic intractable pain. Appl. Neurophysiol. *45:* 167–172 (1982).

Dionne, R.A.; Mueler, G.P.; Young, R.F.; Greenberg, R.P.; Hargreaves, K.M.; Gracely, R.; Dubner, R.: Contrast medium causes the apparent increase in beta-endorphin levels in human cerebrospinal fluid following brain stimulation. Pain *20:* 313–321 (1984).

Dirksen, R.; Nijhuis, G.M.M.: Epidural opiate and perioperative analgesia. Acta anaesth. scand. *24:* 367–374 (1980).

Doerr, M.; Krainick, J.-U.; Thoden, U.: Pain perception in man after long-term spinal cord stimulation. J. Neurol. *217:* 261–270 (1978).

Dogliotti, M.: First surgical sections, in man, of the lemniscal lateralis (pain-temperature path) at the brain stem, for the treatment of diffuse rebellious pain. Anesth. Analg. *17:* 143–145 (1938).

Dondelinger, R.; Kurdziel, J.C.: Percutaneous phenol neurolysis of the lumbar sympathetic chain with computed tomography control. Ann. Radiol. *27:* 376–379 (1984).

Dornhorst, A.C.: Hyperaemia induced by exercise and ischaemia. Br. med. Bull. *19:* 137–140 (1963).

Dornhorst, A.C.; Sharpey-Schafer, E.P.: Collateral resistance in limbs with arterial obstruction: spontaneous changes and effects of sympathectomy. Clin. Sci. *10:* 371–381 (1951).

Dott, N.: [Facial pain]. Proc. R. Soc. Med. *44:* 1034–1037 (1951).

Doupe, J.; Cullen, C.H.; Chance, G.Q.: Post-traumatic pain and the causalgic syndrome. J. Neurol. Neurosurg. Psychiat. *7:* 33–48 (1944).

Drake, C.G.; McKenzie, K.G.: Mesencephalic tractotomy for pain. Experience with six cases. J. Neurosurg. *10:* 457–462 (1953).

Druckman, R.; Lende, R.: Central pain of spinal cord origin. Neurology *15:* 518–522 (1965).

Drummond, P.D.; Gonski, A.; Lance, J.W.: Facial flushing after thermocoagulation of the Gasserian ganglion. J. Neurol. Neurosurg. Psychiat. *46:* 611–616 (1983).

Dubner, R.; Sharav, Y.; Gracely, R.H.; Price, D.D.: Idiopathic trigeminal neuralgia: sensory features and pain mechanisms. Pain *31:* 23–33 (1987).

Duff, R.S.: Circulatory changes in the forearm following sympathectomy. Clin. Sci. *10:* 529–540 (1951).

Duggan, A.W.; Griersmith, H.T.; North, R.A.: Morphine and supraspinal inhibition of spinal neurones: evidence that morphine decreases tonic descending inhibition in the anaesthetized cat. Br. J. Pharmacol. *69:* 461–466 (1980).

Duggan, A.W.; Hall, J.G.; Headley, P.M.: Suppression of transmission of nociceptive impulses by morphine: selective effects of morphine administered in the region of the substantia gelatinosa. Br. J. Pharmacol. *61:* 65–76 (1977).

Durán-Obiols, F.: Neurectomy of the greater superficial petrosal nerve and posterior cervical rhizotomy in the treatment of certain localized forms of cephalgia. 2nd Int. Congr. Neurological Surgery, Washington 1961, abstr. 39, pp. 79–80.

Durward, Q.J.; Rice, G.P.; Ball, M.J.; Gilbert, J.J.; Kaufmann, J.C.E.: Selective spinal cordectomy: clinicopathological correlation. J. Neurosurg. *56:* 359–367 (1982).

Dykes, R.W.; Terzis, J.K.: Spinal nerve distributions in the upper limb: the organization of the dermatome and afferent myotome. Phil. Trans. R. Soc. Lond. B *293:* 509–554 (1981).

Earle, K.M.: The tract of Lissauer and its possible relations to the pain pathway. J. comp. Neurol. *96:* 93–111 (1952).

Echols, D.H.: Sensory rhizotomy following operation for ruptured intervertebral disc. A review of 62 cases. J. Neurosurg. *31:* 335–338 (1969).

Echols, D.H.: The effectiveness of thoracic rhizotomy for chronic pain. Neurochirurgia *13:* 69–74 (1970).

Eckenhoff, J.E.; Oech, S.R.: The effects of narcotics and antagonists upon respiration and circulation in man. Clin. Pharmacol. Ther. *1:* 483–524 (1960).

Ehni, G.; Eckles, N.E.: Interruption of the pituitary stalk in the patient with mammary cancer. J. Neurosurg. *16:* 628–652 (1959).

Eiras, J.; Garcia, J.; Gomez, J.; Carcavilla, L.I.; Ucar, S.: First results with extralemniscal myelotomy. Acta neurochir., suppl. 30, pp. 377–381 (1980).

Ekbom, K.: Nitroglycerin as a provocative agent in cluster headache. Archs Neurol. *19:* 487–493 (1968).

Ekbom, K.: A clinical comparison of cluster headache and migraine. Acta neurol. scand. *46:* suppl. 41 (1970).

Ekbom, K.; Lindgren, L.; Nilsson, B.Y.; Hardebo, J.E.; Waldenlind, E.: Chronic migrainous neuralgia treated by retrogasserian injection of glycerol. Presented to the 5th Int. Migraine Symp., London 1984.

Ekbom, K.; Olivarius, B.: Chronic migrainous neuralgia — diagnostic and therapeutic aspects. Headache *11:* 97–101 (1971).

Elithorn, A.; Glithero, E.; Slater, E.: Leucotomy for pain. J. Neurol. Neurosurg. Psychiat. *21:* 249–261 (1958).

Emmers, R.; Tasker, R.R.: The human somesthetic thalamus (Raven Press, New York 1975).

Endroczi, E.; Babichev, V.; Hartman, G.; Koranyi, L.: Changes in evoked potentials of the hypothalamus to brain stem stimulation in female rats. Endocrinol. exp. *2:* 1–10 (1968).

Erdemir, H.; Gelman, S.; Galbraith, J.G.: Prediction of the needed level of sympathectomy for posttraumatic reflex sympathetic dystrophy. Surg. Neurol. *17:* 353–354 (1982).

Erickson, D.L.; Lo, J.; Michaelson, M.: Intrathecal morphine for treatment of pain due to malignancy. Pain, suppl. 2, p. S19 (1984).

Eriksen, J.; Andersen, H.B.: Pain treatment on long term basis, using extradural opiates. Pain, suppl. 2, p. S335 (1984).

Ervin, F.R.; Mark, V.H.: Stereotactic thalamotomy in the human. II. Physiologic observations on the human thalamus. Archs Neurol. *3:* 368–380 (1960).

Esposito, S.; Bruni, P.; Delitala, A.; Canova, A.; Hernandez, R.; Collovini, G.M.: Therapeutic approach to the Pancoast pain syndrome. Appl. Neurophysiol. *48:* 262–266 (1985).

Fairman, D.: Unilateral thalamic tractotomy for the relief of bilateral pain in malignant tumors. Confinia neurol. *29:* 146–152 (1967).

Fairman, D.: Neurophysiological basis for the hypothalamic lesion and stimulation by chronic implanted electrodes for the relief of intractable pain in cancer. Adv. Pain Res. Ther. *1:* 843–847 (1976).

Fairman, D.; Llavallol, M.A.: Thalamic tractotomy for the alleviation of intractable pain in cancer. Cancer *31:* 700–707 (1973).

Falconer, M.A.: Relief of phantom pain by cordotomy; in Knighton, Dumke, Pain, p. 273 (Little, Brown, Boston 1966).

Fardin, V.: Réévaluation des effets analgésiques induits par stimulation électrique de la substance grise périaqueductale et implication du groupe B3 (noyaux raphe magnus et paragigantocellularis) dans la modulation de la nociception chez le rat; thèse, Paris (1982).

Fascendini, A.; Biroli, F.; Cassinari, V.: Critical evaluation of commissural myelotomy in the treatment of intractable pain. J. neurosurg. Sci. *23:* 265–272 (1979).

Feldman, R.A.: Patterned response of lamina V cells: cutaneous and dorsal funicular stimulation. Physiol. Behav. *15:* 79–84 (1975).

Fessler, R.G.; Brown, F.D.; Rachlin, J.R.; Mullan, S.: Elevated beta-endorphin in cerebrospinal fluid after electrical brain stimulation: artifact of contrast infusion? Science *224:* 1017–1019 (1984).

Fields, H.L. Pain (McGraw-Hill, New York 1987).

Fiore, C.E.; Castorina, F.; Malatino, L.S.; Tamburino, C.: Antalgic activity of calcitonin: effectiveness of the epidural and subarachnoid routes in man. Int. J. clin. Pharm. Res. *3:* 257–260 (1983).

Fischer, E.G.: Personal communication (1985).

Fitzgerald, M.: Alterations in the ipsi- and contralateral afferent inputs of dorsal horn cells produced by capsaicin treatment of one sciatic nerve in the rat. Brain Res. *248:* 97–107 (1982).

Flanigan, D.P.; Kraft, R.O.: Continuing experience with palliative chemical splanchnicectomy. Archs Surg. *113:* 509–511 (1978).

Florez, M.; McCarty, L.E.; Borison, H.L.: A comparative study in the cat of the respiratory effects of morphine injected intravenously and into the cerebrospinal fluid. J. Pharmac. exp. Ther. *163:* 448–455 (1968).

Flothow, P.G.: Relief of pain from a neurologic viewpoint. NW. Med. *29:* 69–76 (1930).

Foerster, O.: Vorderseitenstrangdurchschneidung im Rückenmark zur Beseitigung von Schmerzen. Berl. klin. Wschr. *50:* 1499 (1913).

Foerster, O.: The dermatomes in man. Brain *56:* 1–39 (1933).

Foerster, O.: Symptomatologie der Erkrankungen des Grosshirns. Bumke Foersters Hand. Neurol. *6:* 32–54 (1936).

Foerster, O.; Altenburger, H.; Krill, F.W.: Über die Beziehungen des vegetativen Nervensystems zur Sensibilität. Z. ges. Neurol. Psychiat. *121:* 139–185 (1929).

Foerster, O.; Gagel, O.: Die Vorderseitenstrangdurchschneidung beim Menschen. Eine klinisch-patho-physiologisch-anatomische Studie. Z. ges. Neurol. Psychiat. *138:* 1–92 (1932).

Foltz, E.L.; White, L.E.: Pain 'relief' by frontal cingulumotomy. J. Neurosurg. *19:* 89–100 (1962).

Foltz, E.L.; White, L.E.: Rostral cingulumotomy and pain 'relief'; in Knighton, Dumke, Pain, pp. 469–491 (Little, Brown, Boston 1966).

Fordyce, W.E.; Roberts, A.H.; Sternbach, R.A.: The behavioral management of chronic pain: a response to critics. Pain *22:* 113–125 (1985).

Foreman, R.D.; Beall, J.E.; Applebaum, A.E.; Coulter, J.D.; Willis, W.D.: Effects of dorsal column stimulation on primate spinothalamic tract neurons. J. Neurophysiol. *39:* 534–546 (1976).

Fox, J.L.; Rizzoli, H.V.: Identification of radiologic coordinates for the posterior articular nerve of Luschka in the lumbar spine. Surg. Neurol. *1:* 343–346 (1973).

Fraioli, B.; Cantore, G.: Personal communication (1985).

Fraioli, B.; Esposito, V.; Santoro, A.: Treatment of trigeminal neuralgia by percutaneous techniques: therapeutic protocol. Pain, suppl. 4, p. S126 (1987).

Fraioli, B.; Ferrante, L.; Santoro, A.; DiGiugno, G.: Recent progress in the treatment of trigeminal neuralgia: glycerol into the trigeminal cistern and percutaneous Gasserian compression by means of Fogarty's catheter. Acta neurochir., suppl. 33, pp. 507–510 (1984).

Franetzki, M.; Kollert, D.: Externally portable and implantable devices for continuous delivery of analgetics. Acta neurochir., suppl. 38, pp. 76–79 (1987).

Frank, F.; Gaist, T.; Fabrizi, A.; Cohadon, F.; LaPorte, A.; Sedan, R.; Peragut, J.C.; Sethian, M.; Sturiale, C.: Résultats de la thermo-coagulation percutanée sélective du ganglion de Gasser dans la névralgie faciale essentielle. Synthèse des résultats obtenus chez 939 patients traités. Neurochirurgie *31:* 179–182 (1985a).

Frank, F.; Sturiale, C.; Gaist, G.; Fabrizi, A.P.; Frank-Ricci, R.: Stereotactic mesencephalic tractotomy in the treatment of Pancoast syndrome. Appl. Neurophysiol. *48:* 274–276 (1985b).

Frank, F.; Tognetti, F.; Gaist, G.; Frank, G.; Galassi, E.; Sturiale, C.: Stereotaxic rostral mesencephalotomy in treatment of malignant faciothoracobrachial pain syndromes. J. Neurosurg. *56:* 807–811 (1982).

Franz, D.N.; Iggo, A.: Dorsal root potentials and ventral root reflexes evoked by nonmyelinated fibers. Science *162:* 1140–1142 (1968).

Fraser, I.; Windle, R.; Smart, J.G.; Barrie, W.W.: Ureteric injury following chemical sympathectomy. Br. J. Surg. *71:* 349 (1984).

Freeman, L.W.; Heimburger, R.F.: Surgical relief of pain in paraplegic patients. Archs Surg. *55:* 433–440 (1947).

Freeman, W.; Watts, J.W.: Psychosurgery: intelligence, emotional and social behavior following prefrontal lobotomy for mental disorders (Thomas, Springfield 1942).

Freeman, W.; Watts, J.W.: Psychosurgery: intelligence, emotional and social behavior following prefrontal lobotomy for mental disorders; 2nd ed. (Thomas, Springfield 1950).

French, L.A.: High cervical tractotomy: technique and results. Clin. Neurosurg. *21:* 239–245 (1974).

French, L.A.; Peyton, W.T.: Ipsilateral sensory loss following cordotomy. J. Neurosurg. *5:* 403–404 (1948).

Friedman, A.H.; Nashold, B.S.; Ovelmen-Levitt, J.: Dorsal root entry zone lesions for the treatment of post-herpetic neuralgia. J. Neurosurg. *60:* 1258–1262 (1984).

Frigyesi, T.L.; Siegfried, J.; Broggi, G.: The selective vulnerability of evoked potentials in the trigeminal sensory root to graded thermocoagulation. Expl. Neurol. *49:* 11–21 (1975).

Fromm, G.H.; Chatta, A.S.; Terrence, C.F.; Glass, J.D.: Role of inhibitory mechanisms in trigeminal neuralgia. Neurology *31:* 683–687 (1981).

Fromm, G.H.; Terrence, C.F.; Maroon, J.C.: Trigeminal neuralgia. Current concepts regarding etiology and pathogenesis. Archs Neurol. *41:* 1204–1207 (1984).

Fulton, J.F.; Jacobsen, C.F.: The functions of the frontal lobes, a comparative study in monkeys, chimpanzees and man. Abstr. 2nd Int. Neurol. Congr., pp. 70–71 (1935); see also Adv. Mod. Biol., Moscow *4:* 113–123 (1935).

Fyfe, T.; Quin, R.O.: Phenol sympathectomy in the treatment of intermittent claudication: a controlled clinical trial. Br. J. Surg. *62:* 68–71 (1975).

Ganz, E.; Mullan, S.: Percutaneous cordotomy; in Lipton, Persistent pain: modern methods of treatment, vol. 1, pp. 21–33 (Academic Press, London/Grune & Stratton, New York 1977).

Gardner, A.M.N.; Solomou, G.: Relief of the pain of unresectable carcinoma of pancreas by chemical splanchnicectomy during laparotomy. Ann. R. Coll. Surg. Engl. *66:* 409–411 (1984).

Gardner, W.J.: Personal communication (1951).

Gardner, W.J.: The mechanism of tic douloureux. Trans. Am. neurol. Ass. *78:* 168–173 (1953).

Gardner, W.J.: Concerning the mechanism of trigeminal neuralgia and hemifacial spasm. J. Neurosurg. *19:* 947–958 (1962).

Gardner, W.J.: Trigeminal neuralgia. Clin. Neurosurg. *15:* 1–56 (1968).

Gardner, W.J.; Miklos, M.V.: Response of trigeminal neuralgia to 'decompression' of sensory root. J. Am. med. Ass. 170: 1773–1776 (1959).

Gardner, W.J.; Stowell, A.; Dutlinger, R.: Resection of the greater superficial petrosal nerve in the treatment of unilateral headache. J. Neurosurg. *4:* 105–114 (1947).

Gebhart, G.F.: Opiate and opioid peptide effects on brain stem neurons: relevance to nociception and antinociceptive mechanisms. Pain *12:* 93–140 (1982).

Gerhart, K.D.; Yezierski, R.P.; Fang, Z.R.; Willis, W.D.: Inhibition of primate spinothalamic tract neurons by stimulation in ventral posterior lateral (VPLc) thalamic nucleus: possible mechanisms. J. Neurophysiol. *49:* 406–423 (1983).

Gerhart, K.D.; Yezierski, R.P.; Wilcox, T.K.; Grossman, A.E.; Willis, W.D.: Inhibition of primate spinothalamic tract neurons by stimulation in ipsilateral or contralateral ventral posterior lateral (VPL) thalamic nucleus. Brain Res. *229:* 514–519 (1981).

Ghostine, S.Y.; Comair, Y.G.; Turner, D.M.; Kassell, N.F.; Azar, C.G.: Phenoxybenzamine in the treatment of causalgia. Report of 40 cases. J. Neurosurg. *60:* 1263–1268 (1984).

Gianasi, G.: Neuroadenolysis of the pituitary gland (NALP) in treatment of widespread cancer pain; in Rizzi, Visentin, Pain, pp. 473–484 (Piccin/Butterworth, London 1984).

Gibson, S.J.; Polak, J.M.; Bloom, S.R.; Wall, P.D.: The distribution of nine peptides in rat spinal cord with special emphasis on the substantia gelatinosa and on the area around the central canal (lamina X). J. comp. Neurol. *201:* 65–79 (1981).

Gildenberg, P.L.: Percutaneous cervical cordotomy. Appl. Neurophysiol. *39:* 97–113 (1976/77).

Gildenberg, P.L.: Spinal stereotaxic procedures; in Schaltenbrand, Walker, Stereotaxy of the human brain; 2nd ed., pp. 469–474 (Thieme, Stuttgart 1982).
Gildenberg, P.L.; De Vaul, R.A.: The chronic pain patient: evaluation and management; in Gildenberg, Pain and headache, vol. 7, pp. 1–148 (Karger, Basel 1985).
Gildenberg, P.L.; Hirschberg, R.M.: Limited myelotomy for the treatment of intractable cancer pain. J. Neurol. Neurosurg. Psychiat. *47:* 94–96 (1984).
Gildenberg, P.L.; Lin, P.M.; Polakoff, P.P.; Flitter, M.A.: Anterior percutaneous cervical cordotomy: determination of target point and calculation of angle of insertion. J. Neurosurg. *28:* 173–177 (1968).
Gildenberg, P.L.; Murthy, K.S.K.: Influence of dorsal column stimulation upon human thalamic somatosensory-evoked potentials. Appl. Neurophysiol. *43:* 8–17 (1980).
Gildenberg, P.L.; Zanes, C.; Flitter, M.; Lin, P.M.; Lautsch, E.V.; Truex, R.C.: Impedance measuring device for detection of penetration of the spinal cord in anterior percutaneous cervical cordotomy. Technical note. J. Neurosurg. *30:* 87–92 (1969).
Gilman, A.G.; Goodman, L.S.; Gilman, A.: Pharmacological basis of therapeutics; 6th ed. (Macmillan, New York 1980).
Giorgi, C.; Broggi, G.: Surgical treatment of glossopharyngeal neuralgia and pain from cancer of nasopharynx. A 20-year experience. J. Neurosurg. *61:* 952–955 (1984).
Glees, P.; Bailey, E.A.: Schichtung und Fasergrösse des Tractus spinothalamicus des Menschen. Mschr. Psychiat. Neurol. *122:* 129–141 (1951).
Goddard, G.V.: Development of epileptic seizures through brain stimulation at low intensity. Nature, Lond. *214:* 1020–1021 (1967).
Goedhart, Z.D.; Francaviglia, N.; Feirabend, H.K.P.; Voogd, J.: Median commissural myelotomy for malignant sacral pain. 1st Int. Symp., Pain Clinic, Delft 1984.
Goktepe, E.O.; Young, L.B.; Bridges, P.K.: A further review of the results of stereotactic subcaudate tractotomy. Br. J. Psychiat. *126:* 270–280 (1975).
Gol, A.: Relief of pain by electrical stimulation of the septal area. J. neurol. Sci. *5:* 115–120 (1967).
Goldstein, A.: Opioid peptides (endorphins) in pituitary and brain. Science *193:* 1081–1086 (1976).
Goldstein, M.; Ectors, P.; Dereume, J.P.; Van der Stricht, J.: Les complications de la sympathectomie lombaire. Etude rétrospective de 791 malades. Acta chir. belg. *76:* 73–79 (1977).
Goldthwait, J.E.: The lumbo-sacral articulation. An explanation of many cases of 'lumbago', 'sciatica', and paraplegia. Boston med. J. *64:* 365–372 (1911).
Gordon, S.: Causalgia. A case report. Plast. reconstr. Surg. *28:* 417–419 (1961).
Gorecki, J.P.; Tasker, R.R.; Hirayama, T.: Chronic gasserian ganglion stimulation in the management of central and deafferentation pain. Transplantation/Implantation Today *4:* 42–47 (1987).
Graf, C.J.: Trigeminal compression for tic douloureux. An evaluation. J. Neurosurg. *20:* 1029–1032 (1963).
Granit, R.; Leksell, L.; Skoglund, C.R.: Fibre interaction in injured or compressed region of nerve. Brain *67:* 125–140 (1944).
Grant, F.C.; Weinberger, L.M.: Experiences with intramedullary tractotomy. I. Relief of facial pain and summary of operative results. Archs Surg. *42:* 681–692 (1941a).
Grant, F.C.; Weinberger, L.M.: Experiences with intramedullary tractotomy. IV. Surgery of the brainstem and its operative complications. Surgery Gynec. Obstet. *72:* 747–754 (1941b).

Grant, F.C.; Wood, F.A.: Experiences with cordotomy. Clin. Neurosurg. *5:* 38–65 (1958).

Gray, H.: Anatomy, descriptive and surgical. Revised American edition from 15th English edition of 1901 (Bounty Books, New York 1977).

Graziussi, G.; Terracciano, S.; Cacace, R.: La termocoagulazione percutanea selettiva con radiofrequenze nella nevralgia essenziale del trigemino. Osservazioni su 205 casi personali. Riv. Neurobiol., Arezzo *28:* 280–286 (1982).

Greco, T.: L'alcolizzazione delle ipofisi nel trattamento dei tumori maligni. Vantaggi di questo metodo e consideratione conclusive. Osped. Ital. Chir. *12:* 439–448 (1965).

Greco, T.; Sbaragli, F.; Cammilli, L.: L'alcolizzazione della ipofisi per via transfenoidale nella terapia di particoloari tumori maligni. Settim. med. *45:* 355–356 (1957).

Greenberg, H.S.; Taren, J.; Ensminger, W.D.; Doan, K.: Benefit from and tolerance to continuous intrathecal infusion of morphine for intractable cancer pain. J. Neurosurg. *57:* 360–364 (1982).

Gregor, M.; Zimmermann, M.: Dorsal root potentials produced by afferent volleys in cutaneous group III fibers. J. Physiol. *232:* 413–425 (1973).

Gros, C.; Frèrebeau, P.; Privat, J.M.; Benezech, J.: Place of hypophysectomy in the neurosurgical treatment of pain. Adv. Neurosurg. *3:* 264–272 (1975).

Groth, K.; Adams, J.; Richardson, D.; Hosobuchi, Y.; Ray, C.; Turnbull, I.; Long, D.: Deep brain stimulation for chronic intractable pain (Medtronic, Minneapolis 1982).

Grunert, V.; Kraus, H.; Sunder-Plassmann, M.; Gestring, G.F.: Die kommissurale Myelotomie: Indikation und Ergebnis. Wien klin. Wschr. *82:* 865–868 (1970).

Gudmundsson, K.; Rhoton, A.L.; Rushton, J.G.: Detailed anatomy of the intracranial portion of the trigeminal nerve. J. Neurosurg. *35:* 592–600 (1971).

Guilbaud, G.; Iggo, A.; Tegner, R.: Sensory receptors in ankle joint capsules of normal and arthritic rats. Exp. Brain Res. *58:* 29–40 (1985).

Guillaume, J.; Mazars, G.; Valleteau de Mouillac: La myélotomie commissurale. Presse méd. *53:* 666–667 (1945).

Gustafsson, L.L.; Schildt, B.; Jacobsen, K.: Adverse effects of extradural and intrathecal opiates: report of a nationwide survey in Sweden. Br. J. Anaesth. *54:* 479–486 (1982).

Gutierrez-Lara, F.: Stereotactic cingulotomy, a rational and effective approach for causalgia (report of 14 cases). Excerpta Med. Int. Congr. Ser., No. 293, p. 38 (1973).

Gybels, J.M.: Electrical stimulation of the central gray for pain relief in humans: a critical review. Adv. Pain Res. Ther. *3:* 499–509 (1979).

Gybels, J.: The suggested mechanisms of chronic pain and the rationale of neurosurgical treatment. Acta neurochir., suppl. 33, pp. 397–406 (1984).

Gybels, J.; Cosyns, P.: Modulation of clinical and experimental pain in man by electrical stimulation of thalamic periventricular gray; in Zotterman, Sensory functions of the skin. Wenner-Gren, vol. 27, pp. 521–530 (Pergamon Press, Oxford 1976).

Gybels, J.; Dom, R.; Cosyns, P.: Electrical stimulation of the central gray for pain relief in human: autopsy data. Acta neurochir., suppl. 30, pp. 259–268 (1980).

Gybels, J.; Kupers, R.: Central and peripheral electrical stimulation of the nervous system in the treatment of chronic pain. Acta neurochir., suppl. 38, pp. 64–75 (1987).

Gybels, J.; Van Hees, J.; Peluso, F.: Modulation of experimentally produced pain in man by electrical stimulation of some cortical, thalamic and basal ganglia structures. Adv. Pain Res. Ther. *1:* 475–478 (1976).

Haines, S.J.: Comments. Neurosurgery *19:* 538–539 (1986).

Haines, S.J.; Jannetta, P.J.; Zorub, D.S.: Microvascular relations of the trigeminal nerve. An anatomical study with clinical correlation. J. Neurosurg. *52:* 381–386 (1980).

Håkanson, S.: Trigeminal neuralgia treated by the injection of glycerol into the trigeminal cistern. Neurosurgery *9:* 638–646 (1981).

Håkanson, S.: Trigeminal neuralgia treated by retrogasserian injection of glycerol; thesis, Stockholm (1982).

Håkanson, S.: Retrogasserian glycerol injection as a treatment of tic douloureux. Adv. Pain Res. Ther. *5:* 927–933 (1983).

Håkanson, S.; Leksell, L.: Stereotactic radiosurgery in trigeminal neuralgia; in Pauser, Gerstenbrand, Gross, Gesichtsschmerz: Schmerzstudien 2 (Fischer, New York 1979).

Håkanson, S.; Pearson, L.A.: The effect of pure glycerol on rat sciatic nerve. An experimental model for treatment of trigeminal neuralgia with glycerol injections. Neurosurgery *10:* 1–6 (1982).

Halliday, A.M.; Loque, V.: Painful sensations evoked by electrical stimulation in the thalamus; in Somjen, Neurophysiology studied in man, pp. 221–230 (Excerpta Medica, Amsterdam 1972).

Hamada, S.; Asahara, H.; Fukushima, T.: Comparison of percutaneous Gasserian-ganglion glycerol injection and microvascular decompression for the management of trigeminal neuralgia. Jap. J. Anesthesiol. *34:* 1668–1672 (1985).

Hambrecht, F.T.; Reswick, J.B.: Functional electrical stimulation: application in neural prostheses (Dekker, New York 1977).

Hamby, W.B.: Effectiveness of various operations for trigeminal neuralgia. J. Neurosurg. *17:* 1039–1044 (1960).

Hammond, D.L.: Control systems for nociceptive afferent processing. The descending inhibitory pathways; in Yaksh, Spinal afferent processing, pp. 363–390 (Plenum Press, New York 1986).

Handwerker, H.O.; Iggo, A.; Zimmermann, M.: Segmental and supraspinal actions on dorsal horn neurons responding to noxious and non-noxious skin stimuli. Pain *1:* 147–165 (1975).

Hannington-Kiff, J.G.: Intravenous regional sympathetic block with guanethidine. Lancet *i:* 1019–1020 (1974).

Hannington-Kiff, J.G.: Relief of Sudeck's atrophy by regional intravenous guanethidine. Lancet *i:* 1132–1133 (1977).

Hannington-Kiff, J.G.: Relief of causalgia in limbs by regional intravenous guanethidine. Br. med. J. *ii:* 367–368 (1979).

Hannington-Kiff, J.G.: 'In limbo': a dissertation on the relief of dystrophic, inflammatory, ischaemic and spastic conditions of limbs by the local deposition of high doses of drugs administered during regional circulatory occlusion with a tourniquet. Jacksonian Prize manuscript (unpublished, 1980).

Hannington-Kiff, J.G.: Hyperadrenergic-effected limb causalgia: relief by i.v. pharmacologic norepinephrine blockade (Letter). Am. Heart J. *103:* 152–153 (1982).

Hannington-Kiff, J.G.: Antisympathetic drugs in limbs; in Wall, Melzack, Textbook of pain, pp. 566–573 (Churchill-Livinstone, London 1984).

Hannington-Kiff, J.G.: Antisympathetic drugs in limbs; in Wall, Melzack, Textbook of pain (Churchill-Livingstone, London 1988).

Harbaugh, R.E.; Coombs, D.W.; Saunders, R.L.; Gaylor, M.; Pageau, M.: Implanted continuous epidural morphine infusion system. Preliminary report. J. Neurosurg. *56:* 803–806 (1982).

Hardy, D.G.; Rhoton, A.L.: Microsurgical relationships of the superior cerebellar artery and the trigeminal nerve. J. Neurosurg. *49:* 669–678 (1978).

Hardy, J.D.; Wolff, H.G.; Goodell, H.: Pain sensations and reactions (Williams & Wilkins, Baltimore 1952).

Hardy, T.L.; Bertrand, G.; Thompson, C.J.: Position and organization of thalamic cellular activity during diencephalic recording. II. Joint- and muscle-evoked activity. Appl. Neurophysiol. *43:* 28–36 (1980).

Hardy, T.L.; Bertrand, G.; Thompson, C.J.: Touch-evoked thalamic cellular activity. The variable position of the anterior border of somesthetic SI thalamus and somatotopography. Appl. Neurophysiol. *44:* 302–313 (1981).

Harris, W.: Alcohol injection of the Gasserian ganglion for trigeminal neuralgia. Lancet *i:* 218–221 (1912).

Harris, W.: Persistent pain in lesions of the peripheral and central nervous system. Br. med. J. *ii:* 896–900 (1921a).

Harris, W.: Glossopharyngeal neuralgia. Brain *44:* 557–571 (1921b).

Harris, W.: Neuritis and Neuralgia (Oxford University Press, London 1926).

Harris, W.: Alcohol injection of the Gasserian ganglion for migrainous neuralgia. Lancet *ii:* 481–482 (1940).

Hassler, R.: Über die Thalamus-Stirnhirnverbindungen beim Menschen. Nervenarzt *19:* 9–12 (1948).

Hassler, R.: The division of pain conduction into systems of pain sensation and pain awareness; in Janzen, Keidel, Herz, Steichele, Pain: basic principles — pharmacology — therapy, pp. 98–112 (Thieme, Stuttgart 1972).

Hassler, R.; Riechert, T.: Klinische und anatomische Befunde bei stereotaktischen Schmerzoperationen im Thalamus. Arch. Psychiat. Z. ges. Neurol. *200:* 93–122 (1959).

Hatangdi, V.S.; Boas, R.A.: Lumbar sympathectomy: a single needle technique. Br. J. Anaesth. *57:* 285–289 (1985).

Haxton, H.A.: Chemical sympathectomy. Br. med. J. *i:* 1026–1028 (1949).

Hayashi, H.: Morphology of terminations of small and large myelinated trigeminal primary afferent fibers in the cat. J. comp. Neurol. *240:* 71–89 (1985).

Head, H.; Holmes, G.: Sensory disturbances from cerebral lesions. Brain *34:* 102–254 (1911).

Head H.; Thompson, T.: The grouping of afferent impulses within the spinal cord. Brain *29:* 537–541 (1906).

Heath, R.G.; Mickle, W.A.: Evaluation of seven years experience with depth electrode studies in human patients; in Ramey, O'Doherty, Electrical studies on the unanesthetized brain, p. 214 (Hoeber, New York 1960).

Hécaen, H.; Talairach, T.; David, M.; Dell, M.B.: Mémoires originaux. Coagulations limitées du thalamus dans les algies du syndrome thalamique. Rev. neurol. *81:* 917–931 (1949).

Hekmatpanah, J.: Techniques and results of percutaneous cordotomy. Med. Clins N. Am. *52:* 189–201 (1968).

Helfant, M.H.; Leksell, L.; Strang, R.R.: Experiences with intractable pain treated by stereotaxic mesencephalotomy. Acta chir. scand. *129:* 573–580 (1965).

Henderson, W.R.: The anatomy of the gasserian ganglion and the distribution of pain in relation to injections and operations for trigeminal neuralgia. Ann. R. Coll. Surg. *37:* 346–373 (1965).

Herz, A.: Opiates, opioids and their receptors in the modulation of pain. Acta neurochir., suppl. 38, pp. 36–40 (1987).

Herz, A.; Albus, K.; Metys, J.; Schubert, P.; Teschemacher, H.J.: On the central sites for the antinociceptive action of morphine and fentanyl. Neuropharmacology *9:* 539–551 (1970).

Hillman, P.; Wall, P.D.: Inhibitory and excitatory factors influencing the receptive fields of lamina V spinal cord cells. Exp. Brain Res. *9:* 284–306 (1969).

Hitchcock, E.: Stereotaxic spinal surgery. A preliminary report. J. Neurosurg. *31:* 386–392 (1969).

Hitchcock, E.: Stereotactic trigeminal tractotomy. Ann. clin. Res. *2:* 131–135 (1970a).

Hitchcock, E.: Stereotactic cervical myelotomy. J. Neurol. Neurosurg. Psychiat. *33:* 224–230 (1970b).

Hitchcock, E.: Progress in neurosurgical treatment of intractable pain from Simpson's day. J. R. Coll. Surg. Edinb. *16:* 24–37 (1971).

Hitchcock, E.: Stereotaxic pontine spinothalamic tractotomy. J. Neurosurg. *39:* 746–752 (1973).

Hitchcock, E.: Stereotactic myelotomy. Proc. R. Soc. Med. *67:* 771–772 (1974).

Hitchcock, E.: Stereotactic spinal surgery. Neurol. Surg. *433:* 271–280 (1977).

Hitchcock, E.; Kim, M.C.; Sotelo, M.: Further experience in stereotactic pontine tractotomy. Appl. Neurophysiol. *48:* 242–246 (1985a).

Hitchcock, E.; Leece, B.: Somatotopic representation of the respiratory pathways in the cervical cord of man. J. Neurosurg. *27:* 320–329 (1967).

Hitchcock, E.; Sotelo, M.G.; Kim, M.C.: Analgesic levels and technical method in stereotactic pontine spinothalamic tractotomy. Acta neurochir. *77:* 29–36 (1985b).

Hitchcock, E.R.; Schvarcz, J.R.: Stereotaxic trigeminal tractotomy for post-herpetic facial pain. J. Neurosurg. *37:* 412–417 (1972).

Hitchcock, E.R.; Teixeira, M.J.: A comparison of results from center-median and basal thalamotomies for pain. Surg. Neurol. *15:* 341–351 (1981).

Hitchcock, E.R.; Teixeira, M.; Pinto, J.: Percutaneous trigeminal radiofrequency rhizotomy. J. R. Coll. Surg. Edinb. *28:* 74–79 (1983).

Hodge, C.J.; King, R.B.: Medical modification of sensation. J. Neurosurg. *44:* 21–28 (1976).

Hökfelt, T.; Elde, R.; Johansson, O.; Terenius, L.; Stein, L.: The distribution of enkephalin-immunoreactive cell bodies in the rat central nervous system. Neurosci. Lett. *5:* 25–31 (1977).

Honda, C.N.; Perl, E.R.: Functional and morphological features of neurons in the midline dorsal horn of the caudal spinal cord in the cat. Brain Res. *340:* 285–295 (1985).

Hood, T.W.; Siegfried, J.: Epidural versus thalamic stimulation for the management of brachial plexus lesion pain. Acta neurochir., suppl. 33, pp. 451–457 (1984).

Horch, K.W.; Lisney, S.J.W.: Changes in primary afferent depolarization of sensory neurones during peripheral nerve regeneration in the cat. J. Physiol. *313:* 287–299 (1981).

Horowitz, S.H.: Iatrogenic causalgia. Classification, clinical findings, and legal ramifications. Archs Neurol. *41:* 821–824 (1984).

Horsley, V.; Taylor, J.; Colman, W.S.: Remarks on the various surgical procedures devised for the relief or cure of trigeminal neuralgia (tic douloureux). Br. med. J. *ii:* 1139–1143, 1191–1193, 1249–1252 (1891).

Hosobuchi, Y.: Tryptophan reversal of tolerance to analgesia induced by central grey stimulation. Lancet *ii:* 47 (1978).

Hosobuchi, Y.: The current status of analgesic brain stimulation. Acta neurochir., suppl. 30, 219–227 (1980a).

Hosobuchi, Y.: The majority of unmyelinated afferent axons in human ventral roots probably conduct pain. Pain *8:* 167–180 (1980b).

Hosobuchi, Y.: Analgesia induced by brain stimulation with chronically implanted electrodes; in Schmidek, Sweet, Operative neurosurgical techniques: indications, methods and results, vol. 2, pp. 981–991 (Grune & Stratton, New York 1982a).

Hosobuchi, Y.: Fine afferent pathways into the central nervous system. Presented to the Am. Pain Society 3rd Gen. Meet., Miami (1982b).

Hosobuchi, Y.: Subcortical electrical stimulation for control of intractable pain in humans. Report of 122 cases (1970–1984). J. Neurosurg. *64:* 543–553 (1986).

Hosobuchi, Y.; Adams, J.E.; Linchitz, R.: Pain relief by electrical stimulation of the central gray matter in humans and its reversal by naloxone. Science *197:* 183–185 (1977).

Hosobuchi, Y.; Adams, J.E.; Rutkin, B.: Chronic thalamic stimulation for the control of facial anesthesia dolorosa. Archs Neurol. *29:* 158–161 (1973).

Hosobuchi, Y.; Adams, J.E.; Weinstein, P.R.: Preliminary percutaneous dorsal column stimulation prior to permanent implantation. J. Neurosurg. *37:* 242–245 (1972).

Hosobuchi, Y.; Rossier, J.; Bloom, F.E.; Guillemin, R.: Stimulation of human periaqueductal gray for pain relief increases immunoreactive beta-endorphin in ventricular fluid. Science *203:* 279–281 (1979).

Hosobuchi, Y.; Wemmer, J.: Disulfiram inhibition of development of tolerance to analgesia induced by central gray stimulation in humans. Eur. J. Pharmacol. *43:* 385–387 (1977).

Hovelacque, A.: Anatomie des nerfs craniens et rachidiens et du système grand sympathique chez l'homme (Doin, Paris 1927).

Howe, J.F.; Loeser, J.D.; Calvin, W.H.: Mechanosensitivity of dorsal root ganglia and chronically injured axons. A physiological basis for the radicular pain of nerve root compression. Pain *3:* 25–41 (1977).

Hu, J.W.; Ball, G.J.; Sessle, B.J.: Comparison of responses of rostral and caudal trigeminal brain stem neurons to electrical and thermal stimulation of tooth pulp in cats. Neurosci. Abstr. *7:* 532 (1987).

Hughes, J.: Isolation of an endogenous compound from the brain with pharmacological properties similar to morphine. Brain Res. *88:* 295–308 (1975).

Hughes-Davies, D.I., Redman, L.R.: Chemical lumbar sympathectomy. Anesthesia *31:* 1068–1075 (1976).

Hun, H.: Analgesia, thermic anaesthesia, and ataxia resulting from loci of softening in medulla oblongata etc. N.Y. Med. J. *65:* 513, 581, 613 (1897).

Hunt, J.M.: Geniculate neuralgia (neuralgia of the nervus facialis). Arch. Neurol. Psychiat. *37:* 253–285 (1937).

Hunt, J.R.: The sensory field of the facial nerve. A further contribution to the symptomatology of the geniculate ganglion. Brain *38:* 418–446 (1915).

Hunt, W.E.; Goodman, J.H.; Bingham, W.G.: Stimulation of the dorsal spinal cord for treatment of intractable pain: a preliminary report. Surg. Neurol. *4:* 153–156 (1975).

Hurt, R.W.; Ballantine, H.T.: Stereotactic anterior cingulate lesions for persistent pain. A report on 68 cases. Clin. Neurosurg. *21:* 334–351 (1974).

Husebo, S.: Treatment of severe cancer pain with epidural morphine. Pain, suppl. 2, p. S336 (1984).

Hylden, J.L.K.; Nahin, R.L.; Dubner, R.: Altered responses of nociceptive cat lamina I spinal dorsal horn neurons after chronic sciatic neuroma formation. Brain Res. *411:* 341–350 (1987).

Hyndman, O.R.: Lissauer's tract section. A contribution to chordotomy for the relief of pain (preliminary report). J. int. Coll. Surg. *5:* 394–400 (1942).

Hyndman, O.R.; Van Epps, C.: Possibility of differential section of the spinothalamic tract. A clinical and histologic study. Archs Surg. *38:* 1036–1053 (1939).

Hyndman, O.R.; Wolkin, J.: Anterior chordotomy. Further observations on physiologic results and optimum manner of performance. Archs Neurol. Psychiat. *50:* 129–148 (1943).

Iacono, R.P.: Mesencephalotomy for pain relief. J. Neurosurg. *57:* 582 (1982).

Igarashi, S.; Suzuki, F.; Iwasaki, K.; Koyama, T.; Umeda, S.: Glycerol injection method for trigeminal neuralgia. No. Shinkei Geka *13:* 267–273 (1985).

Ignelzi, R.J.; Nyquist, J.: Direct effect of electrical stimulation in post-amputation pain. Surg. Neurol. *4:* 167–171 (1976).

Ignelzi, R.J.; Nyquist, J.K.: Excitability changes in peripheral nerve fibers after repetitive electrical stimulation. Implications in pain modulation. J. Neurosurg. *51:* 824–833 (1979).

Isamat, F.; Ferran, E.; Acebes, J.J.: Selective percutaneous thermocoagulation rhizotomy in essential glossopharyngeal neuralgia. J. Neurosurg. *55:* 575–580 (1981).

Ischia, S.; Luzzani, A.; Maffezzoli, G.F.; Pacini, L.; Nicolini, F.: Percutaneous cervical cordotomy: technical considerations and results in 400 treated cases; in Rizzi, Visentin, Pain therapy, pp. 367–379 (Elsevier, Amsterdam 1983).

Ishijima, B.: Presented at the DREZ Symp., Durham 1987.

Isler, H.: Independent historical development of the concepts of cluster headache and trigeminal neuralgia. Func. Neurol. *2:* 141–148 (1987).

Jacquet, Y.F.; Lajtha, A.: The periaqueductal gray site of morphine analgesia and tolerance as shown by 2-way cross-tolerance between systemic and intracerebral injection. Brain Res. *103:* 501–513 (1976).

Jannetta, P.J.: Gross (mesoscopic) description of the human trigeminal nerve and ganglion. J. Neurosurg. *26:* 109–111 (1967a).

Jannetta, P.J.: Arterial compression of the trigeminal nerve at the pons in patients with trigeminal neuralgia. J. Neurosurg. *26:* 159–162 (1967b).

Jannetta, P.J.: Microsurgical approach to the trigeminal nerve for tic douloureux. Prog. neurol. Surg., vol. 7, pp. 180–200 (Karger, Basel 1976).

Jannetta, P.J.: Neurovascular compression in cranial nerve and systemic disease. Ann. Surg. *192:* 518–523 (1980).

Jannetta, P.J.: Vascular decompression in trigeminal neuralgia; in Samii, Jannetta, The cranial nerves, pp. 331–340 (Springer, Berlin 1981a).

Jannetta, P.J.: Cranial nerve vascular compression syndromes (other than tic douloureux and hemifacial spasm). Clin. neurosurg. *28:* 445–456 (1981b).

Jannetta, P.J.: Microsurgical management of trigeminal neuralgia. Archs Neurol. *42:* 800 (1985).

Jannetta, P.J.; Rand, R.W.: Transtentorial subtemporal retrogasserian neurectomy in trigeminal neuralgia by microsurgical technique. Bull. Los Angeles Neurol. Soc. *31:* 93–99 (1966).

Jansen, E.C.: Epidural morphine administered by portable pumps in the treatment of severe cancer pain. Pain, suppl. 2, p. S20 (1984).

Jefferson, A.: Cordectomy for intractable pain in paraplegia; in Lipton, Miles, Persistent pain: modern methods for treatment, vol. 4, pp. 115–132 (Grune & Stratton, London 1983).

Jefferson, A.: Personal communication (1987).

Jensen, T.S.; Rasmussen, P.: Amputation; in Wall, Melzack, Textbook of pain, pp. 402–412 (Churchill-Livingstone, Edinburgh 1984).

Jensen, T.S.; Rasmussen, P.; Reske-Nielsen, E.: Association of trigeminal neuralgia with multiple sclerosis: clinical and pathological features. Acta neurol. scand. *65:* 182–189 (1982).

Jones, E.G.: The thalamus (Plenum Press, New York 1985).

Jones, M.W.; Hodge, C.J.; Apkarian, A.V.; Stevens, R.T.: A dorsal spinothalamic pathway in cat. Brain Res. *335:* 188–193 (1985).

Kadowaki, M.H.; Levett, J.M.: Sympathectomy in the treatment of angina and arrhythmias. Ann. thor. Surg. *41:* 572–578 (1986).

Kahn, E.A.; Peet, M.M.: The technique of anterolateral cordotomy. J. Neurosurg. *5:* 276–283 (1948).

Kahn, E.A.; Rand, R.W.: On the anatomy of anterolateral cordotomy. J. Neurosurg. *9:* 611–619 (1952).

Kallio, K.E.: Permanency of results obtained by sympathetic surgery in the treatment of phantom pain. Acta orthop. scand. *19:* 391–397 (1950).

Kane, K.; Taub, A.: A history of local electrical analgesia. Pain *1:* 125–138 (1975).

Kanpolat, Y.; Onol, B.: Experimental percutaneous approach to the trigeminal ganglion in dogs with histopathological evaluation of radiofrequency lesions. Acta neurochir., suppl. 30, pp. 363–366 (1980).

Kanpolat, Y.; Tümer, B.; Selcuki, M.: Trigeminal nevralji tedavisinde Gasser ganglionu radyofrekans termokoacülasyonu. Ank. Tip. Bul. *4:* 71–78 (1982).

Kapur, T.R.; Dalton, G.A.: Transsphenoidal hypophysectomy for metastatic carcinoma of the breast. Br. J. Surg. *56:* 332–337 (1969).

Karplus, J.P.; Kreidl, A.: Ein Beitrag zur Kenntnis der Schmerzleitung im Rückenmark. Pflügers Arch. ges. Physiol. *158:* 275–287 (1914).

Karplus, J.P.; Kreidl, A.: Ein Beitrag zur Kenntnis der Schmerzleitung im Rückenmark. II. Mitteilung. Pflügers Arch. ges. Physiol. *207:* 134–139 (1925).

Katz, J.; Levin, A.B.: Treatment of diffuse metastatic cancer pain by instillation of alcohol into the sella tursica. Anesthesiology *46:* 115–121 (1977).

Kawakami, M.; Terasawa, E.: Differential control of sex hormone and oxytocin upon evoked potentials in the hypothalamus and midbrain reticular formation. Jap. J. Physiol. *17:* 65–93 (1967).

Kayser, V.; Guilbaud, G.: Dose-dependent analgesic and hyperalgesic effects of systemic naloxone in arthritic rats. Brain Res. *226:* 344–348 (1981).

Kerr, F.W.L.: Structural relations of the trigeminal spinal tract to uper cervical roots and solitary nucleus in cat. Expl Neurol. *4:* 134–148 (1961).

Kerr, F.W.L.: Spinal V nucleolysis: intractable craniofacial pain. Surg. Forum *17:* 419–421 (1966).

Kerr, F.W.L.: Pathology of trigeminal neuralgia: light and electron microscopic observations. J. Neurosurg. *26:* 151–156 (1967a).

Kerr, F.W.L.: Evidence for a peripheral etiology of trigeminal neuralgia. J. Neurosurg. *26:* 168–174 (1967b).

Kerr, F.W.L.: Neuroanatomical substrates of nociception in the spinal cord. Pain *1:* 325–356 (1975a).

Kerr, F.W.L.: The ventral spinothalamic tract and other ascending systems of the ventral funiculus of the spinal cord. J. comp. Neurol. *159:* 335–356 (1975b).

Kerr, F.W.L.: Central nervous system changes and deafferentation pain: the role of reorganization and gliosis. Adv. Pain Res. Ther. *5:* 663–675 (1983).

Kerr. F.W.L.; Olafson, R.A.: Trigeminal and cervical volleys: convergence on single units in spinal gray at C-1 and C-2. Archs Neurol. *54:* 161–178 (1961).

Kevetter, G.A.; Haber, L.H.; Yezierski, R.P.; Chung, J.M.; Martin, R.F.; Willis, W.D.: Cells of origin of the spinoreticular tract in the monkey. J. comp. Neurol. *207:* 61–74 (1982).

King, J.S.: Randomized trial of the Rees and Shealy methods for the treatment of low back pain; in Morley, Current controversies in neurosurgery, pp. 80–94 (Saunders, Philadelphia 1976).

King, R.B.: Evidence for a central etiology of tic douloureux. J. Neurosurg. *26:* 175–180 (1967).

King, R.B.: Anterior commissurotomy for intractable pain. J. Neurosurg. *47:* 7–11 (1977).

King, R.B.; Barnett, J.C.: Studies of trigeminal nerve potentials: over-reaction to tactile facial stimulation in acute laboratory preparations. J. Neurosurg. *14:* 617–627 (1957).

King, R.B.; Meagher, J.N.; Barnett, J.C.: Studies of trigeminal nerve potentials in normal compared to abnormal preparations. J. Neurosurg. *13:* 176–183 (1956).

Kircher, C.; Hongchien, H.A.: The nucleus cervicalis lateralis in primates, including man. Anat. Rec. *160:* 376 (1968).

Kirk, E.J.; Denny-Brown, D.: Functional variation in dermatomes in the Macaque monkey following dorsal root lesions. J. comp. Neurol. *139:* 307–320 (1970).

Kirklin, J.W.; Chenoweth, A.I.; Murphey, F.: Causalgia; review of its characteristics, diagnosis, and treatment. Surgery *21:* 321–342 (1947).

Kirsch, W.M.; Lewis, J.A.; Simon, R.H.: Experiences with electrical stimulation devices for the control of chronic pain. Med. Instrum. *9:* 217–220 (1975).

Kirschner, M.: Zur Electrochirurgie. Arch. klin. Chir. *161:* 761–768 (1931).

Kirschner, M.: Die Behandlung der Trigeminusneuralgie (nach Erfahrungen an 1113 Kranken). Münch. med. Wschr. *89:* 235–239 (1942).

Klar, E.: Über die Erfahrungen mit der Electrokoagulation bei der Trigeminusnevralgie an der Heidelberger Chirurgischen Universitätsklinik. Arch. klin. Chir. *294:* 713–723 (1960).

Klumpp, D.; Zimmermann, M.: Irreversible differential block of A- and C-fibres following local nerve heating in the cat. J. Physiol. *298:* 471–482 (1980).

Klun, B.; Prestor, B.: Microvascular relations of the trigeminal nerve: An anatomical study. Neurosurgery *19:* 535–539 (1986).

Knight, G.: Stereotactic tractotomy in the surgical treatment of mental illness. J. Neurol. Neurosurg. Psychiat. *28:* 304–310 (1965).

Knyihar-Csillik, E.; Szucs, A.; Csillik, B.: Iontophoretically applied microtubule inhibitors induce transganglionic degenerative atrophy of primary central nociceptive terminals and abolish chronic autochtonous pain. Acta neurol. scand. *66:* 401–412 (1982).

Kolluri, S.; Heros, R.C.: Microvascular decompression for trigeminal neuralgia. A five-year follow-up study. Surg. Neurol. *22:* 235–240 (1984).

Korenman, E.M.D.; Devor, M.: Ectopic adrenergic sensitivity in damaged peripheral nerve axons in the rat. Expl Neurol. *72:* 63–81 (1981).

Krainick, J.-U.; Thoden, U.; Riechert, T.: Spinal cord stimulation in post-amputation pain. Surg. Neurol. *4:* 167–170 (1975).

Krainick, J.-U.; Thoden, U.; Riechert, T.: Pain reduction in amputees by long-term spinal cord stimulation. Long-term follow-up study over 5 years. J. Neurosurg. *52:* 346–350 (1980).

Krames, E.S.; Gershow, J.; Glassberg, A.; Kenefick, T.; Lyons, A.; Taylor, P.; Wilkie, D.: Continuous infusion of spinally administered narcotics for the relief of pain due to malignant disorders. Cancer *56:* 696–702 (1985).

Krause, F.: Die Neuralgie des Trigeminus nebst der Anatomie und Physiologie der Nerven (Vogel, Leipzig 1896).

Krieg, W.J.S.: Functional neuroanatomy; 1st ed. (Blakiston, New York 1942).

Kruger, L.; Young, R.F.: Specialized features of the trigeminal nerve and its central connections; in Samii, Jannetta, The cranial nerves — anatomy — pathology — pathophysiology — diagnosis — treatment, pp. 273–302 (Springer, Berlin 1981).

Kudo, T.; Yoshii, N.; Shimizu, S.; Aikawa, S.; Nakahama, H.: Effects of stereotaxic thalamotomy to intractable pain and numbness. Preliminary report. Keio J. Med. *15:* 191–194 (1966).

Kudo, T.; Yoshii, N.; Shimizu, S.; Aikawa, S.; Nishioka, S.; Nakahama, H.: Stereotaxic thalamotomy for pain relief. Tohoku J. exp. Med. *96:* 219–234 (1968).

Kugelberg, E.; Lindblom, U.: The mechanism of the pain in trigeminal neuralgia. J. Neurol. Neurosurg. Psychiat. *22:* 36–43 (1959).

Kuhar, M.J.; Pert, C.B.; Snyder, S.H.: Regional distribution of opiate receptor binding in monkey and human brain. Nature, Lond. *245:* 447–450 (1973).

Kumar, K.; Wyant, G.M.: Deep brain stimulation for alleviating chronic intractable pain. Can. J. Surg. *28:* 20–22 (1985).

Kunc, Z.: La localisation des trajects de la douleur des nerfs IX, X et VII dans la moelle allongée et la possibilité de leur tractotomie sélective. Acta neurochir. *8:* 327–334 (1960).

Kunc, Z.: Significant factors pertaining to the results of trigeminal tractotomy; in Hassler, Walker, Trigeminal neuralgia, pp. 90–100 (Thieme, Stuttgart 1970).

Kunc, Z.; Fuchsova, M.; Novak, M.: Excision of the spinal trigeminal tract. Acta neurochir. *41:* 233–241 (1978).

Kunkel, R.S.; Dohn, D.F.: Surgical treatment of chronic migrainous neuralgia. Clevel. Clin. Q. *41:* 189–192 (1974).

Kunkle, E.C.; Pfeiffer, J.B.; Wilhoit, W.M.; Hamrick, L.W.: Recurrent brief headache in 'cluster' pattern. Trans. Am. neurol. Ass. *77:* 240–243 (1952).

Kupers, R.C.; Vos, B.P.J.; Gybels, J.M.: Stimulation of the nucleus paraventricularis thalami suppresses scratching and biting behaviour of arthritic rats and exerts a powerful effect on tests for acute pain. Pain *32:* 115–125 (1988).

Kux, M.: Thoracic endoscopic sympathectomy for treatment of upper-limb hyperhidrosis. Lancet *i:* 1320 (1977).

Lahuerta, J.; Lipton, S.; Miles, J.: Percutaneous radiofrequency gangliolysis in the treatment of trigeminal neuralgia. Eur. Neurol. *24:* 272–275 (1985).

Laitinen, L.V.: Personal communication (1985).

LaMotte, C.: Distribution of the tract of Lissauer and the dorsal root fibers in the primate spinal cord. J. comp. Neurol. *172:* 529–562 (1977).

LaMotte, C.C.; Johns, D.R.; Lanerolle, N.C.: Immunohistochemical evidence of indolamine neurons in monkey spinal cord. J. comp. Neurol. *206:* 359–370 (1982).

LaMotte, C.; Pert, C.B.; Snyder, S.H.: Opiate receptor binding in primate spinal cord: distribution and changes after dorsal root section. Brain Res. *112:* 407–412 (1976).

LaRossa, J.T.; Strong, M.S.; Melby, J.C.: Endocrinologically incomplete transethmoidal transsphenoidal hypophysectomy with relief of bone pain in breast cancer. New Engl. J. Med. *298:* 1332–1335 (1978).

Larson, S.J.; Sances, A.; Riegel, D.H.; Meyer, G.A.; Dallmann, D.E.; Swiontek, T.: Neurophysiological effects of dorsal column stimulation in man and monkey. J. Neurosurg. *41:* 217–223 (1974).

Lasjaunias, P.; Berenstein, A.: Surgical neuroangiography. I. Functional anatomy of craniofacial arteries (Springer, Berlin 1987).

Laugner, B.; Muller, A.; Thiébaut, J.-B.; Farcot, J.B.: Analgésie par site implantable pour injections intrathécales itératives de morphine. Ann. Fr. Anesth. Réanim. *4:* 511–520 (1985).

Lauterborn, J.C.; Chang, P.S.; Gall, C.M.: Colocalization of enkephalin and CCK in a portion of the spinothalamic tract. Neurosci. Abstr. *13:* 1701 (1987).

Law, J.D.: Spinal stimulation: statistical superiority of monophasic stimulation of narrowly separated longitudinal bipoles having rostral cathodes. Appl. Neurophysiol. *46:* 129–137 (1983).

Law, J.D.: The 'failed back syndrome' treated by percutaneous spinal stimulation. 2nd Ann. Meet., San Diego 1986.

Law, J.D.; Swett, J.; Kirsch, W.M.: Retrospective analysis of 22 patients with chronic pain treated by peripheral nerve stimulation. J. Neurosurg. *52:* 482–485 (1980).

Lazorthes, G.; Gaubert, J.: Le syndrome de la branche postérieure des nerfs rachidiens. Presse méd. *87:* 2022 (1956).

Lazorthes, G.; Gouaze, A.; Zadeh, J.O.; Santini, J.J.; Lazorthes, Y.; Burdin, P.: Arterial vascularization of the spinal cord. Recent studies of the anastomotic substitution pathways. J. Neurosurg. *35:* 253–262 (1971).

Lazorthes, Y.: European study on deep brain stimulation. Resumé 3rd Eur. Workshop on Electrical Neurostimulation (in mimeo). (Medtronic, Paris 1979).

Lazorthes, Y.; Bastide, R.; Cros, J.; Verdie, J.C.: Bolus and continuous chronic infusion of spinal intrathecal morphine for cancer pain. Pain, suppl. 2, p. S19 (1984a).

Lazorthes, Y.; Gouarderes, C.; Verdie, J.C.; Monsarrat, B.; Bastide, R.; Campan, L.; Alwan, A.; Cros, J.: Analgésie par injection intrathécale de morphine. Etude pharmacocinétique et application aux douleurs irréductibles. Neuro-chirurgie *26:* 159–164 (1980).

Lazorthes, Y.; Siegfried, J.; Gouarderes, C.; Bastide, R.; Cros, J.; Verdie, J.C.: Periventricular gray matter stimulation versus chronic intrathecal morphine in cancer pain. Adv. Pain Res. Ther. *5:* 467–475 (1983).

Lazorthes, Y.; Verdie, J.C.: Traitement par thermocoagulation percutanée des névralgies trigéminales et glosso-pharyngiennes. Bull. Group. int. Rech. sc. Stomat. Odont. *20:* 297–309 (1977).

Lazorthes, Y.; Verdie, J.C.; Bastide, R.; Caute, B.; Clemente, G.: Les systèmes implantables pour administration épidurale et intrathécale chronique d'opioides; in Spinal opioids and the relief of pain. INSERM *127:* 391–416 (1984b).

Lazorthes, Y.; Verdie, J.C.; Bastide, R.; Lavados, A.; Descouens, D.: Spinal versus intraventricular chronic opiate administration with implantable drug delivery devices for cancer pain. Appl. Neurophysiol. *48:* 234–241 (1985).

Lazorthes, Y.; Verdie, J.C.; Caute, B.; Maranhao, R.; Tafani, M.: Intra-cerebro-ventricular morphinotherapy for control of chronic cancer pain (in press).

Lazorthes, Y.; Verdie, J.C.; Lagarrigue, J.: Thermocoagulation percutanée des nerfs rachidiens à visée analgésique. Neuro-chirurgie *22:* 445–453 (1976).

Leavens, M.E.; Hill, C.S.; Cech, D.A.; Weyland, J.B.; Weston, J.S.: Intrathecal and intraventricular morphine for pain in cancer patients: initial study. J. Neurosurg. *56:* 241–245 (1982).

Le Bars, D.; Guilbaud, G.; Chitour, D.; Besson, J.-M.: Does systemic morphine increase descending inhibitory controls of dorsal horn neurones involved in nociception? Brain Res. *202:* 223–228 (1980).

LeBeau, G.; Bouvet, M.; Feld, M.: Traitement des états d'agitation anxieuse par la topectomie. Sem. Hôp. Paris *25:* 1932–1947 (1948).

LeBeau, J.: Psycho-chirurgie et fonctions mentales (Masson, Paris 1954).

Leclercq, T.A.: Electrode migration in epidural stimulation. Pain, suppl. 2, p. S78 (1984).

Lee, F.C.: Trigeminal neuralgia. J. med. Ass. Ga. *26:* 431–436 (1937).

Leksell, L.: Trigeminusneuralgi. Nagra neurofysiologiska aspekter och en ny behandlinsmethod. Läkartidningen *68:* 5145–5158 (1971).

Lembcke, W.: Über die mediolongitudinale Chordotomie im Halsmarkbereich. Zentbl. Chir. *89:* 439–443 (1964).

Lende, R.A.; Kirsh, W.M.; Druckman, R.: Relief of facial pain after combined removal of precentral and postcentral cortex. J. Neurosurg. *34:* 537–543 (1971).

Lenzi, A.; Galli, G.; Gandolfini, M.; Marini, G.: Intraventricular morphine in paraneoplastic painful syndrome of the cervicofacial region: experience in thirty-eight cases. Neurosurgery *17:* 6–11 (1985).

Leriche, R.: Du traitement de la douleur dans les cancers abdominaux et pelviens inopérables ou récidivés. Gaz. Hôpit. civils milit. *109:* 917–922 (1936).

Leriche, R.: The surgery of pain (Baillière, Tindall & Cox, London 1939).

Le Roy, P.L.: Stimulation of the spinal neuraxis by biocompatible electrical current in the human. Appl. Neurophysiol. *44:* 187–193 (1981).

Letcher, F.S.; Goldring, S.: The effect of radiofrequency current and heat on peripheral nerve action potential in the cat. J. Neurosurg. *24:* 42–47 (1968).

Levin, A.B.; Cosman, E.R.: Thermocouple-monitored cordotomy electrode. Technical note. J. Neurosurg. *53:* 266–268 (1980).

Levin, A.B.; Katz, J.; Benson, R.C.; Jones, A.G.: Treatment of pain of diffuse metastatic cancer by stereotactic chemical hypophysectomy: long-term results and observations on mechanism of action. Neurosurgery *6:* 258–262 (1980).

Levin, A.B.; Ramirez, L.F.; Katz, J.: The use of stereotaxic chemical hypophysectomy in the treatment of thalamic pain syndrome. J. Neurosurg. *59:* 1002–1006 (1983).

Levin, B.E.; Hubschmann, O.R.: Dorsal column stimulation: effect on human cerebrospinal fluid and plasma catecholamines. Neurology *30:* 65–71 (1980).

Levine, J.D.; Gordon, N.C.; Fields, H.: Naloxone dose dependently produces analgesia and hyperalgesia in postoperative pain. Nature, Lond. *278:* 740–741 (1979).

Levitt, M.: Dysesthesias and self-mutilation in humans and subhumans: a review of clinical and experimental studies. Brain Res. Rev. *10:* 247–290 (1985).

Levitt, M.; Levitt, J.H.: The deafferentation syndrome in monkeys: dysesthesias of spinal origin. Pain *10:* 129–147 (1981).

Levy, R.M.; Lamb, S.; Adams, J.E.: Deep brain stimulation for chronic pain: long-term follow-up in 145 patients from 1972–1984. Pain, suppl. 2, p. S115 (1984).

Levy, W.J.; Nutkiewicz, A.; Ditmore, Q.M.; Watts, C.: Laser-induced dorsal root entry zone lesions for pain control. Report of three cases. J. Neurosurg. *59:* 884–886 (1983).

Lewin, W.: Observations on selective leucotomy. J. Neurol. Neurosurg. Psychiat. *24:* 37–44 (1961).
Lewin, W.; Phillips, C.G.: Observations on partial removal of the post central gyrus for pain. J. Neurol. Neurosurg. Psychiat. *15:* 143–147 (1952).
Liberson, W.T.; Voris, H.C.; Uematsu, S.: Recording of somatosensory evoked potentials during mesencephalotomy for intractable pain. Confinia neurol. *32:* 185–194 (1970).
Lidz, T.; Payne, R.L.: Causalgia: report of recovery following relief of emotional stress. Archs Neurol. Psychiat. *53:* 222–225 (1945).
Light, A.R.: Spinal projections of physiologically identified axons from the rostral medulla of cats. Adv. Pain Res. Ther. *5:* 373–379 (1983).
Light, A.R.: The normal anatomy and physiology of the spinal cord dorsal horn. Appl. Neurophysiol. *51:* 78–88 (1988).
Lilly, J.C.: Injury and excitation by electric current. A. The balanced pulse-paire waveform; in Sheer, Electrical stimulation of the brain, p. 60 (University of Texas Press, Austin 1961).
Lin, P.M.; Gildenberg, P.L.; Polakoff, P.P.: An anterior approach to percutaneous lower cervical cordotomy. J. Neurosurg. *25:* 553–560 (1966).
Lippert, R.G.; Hosobuchi, Y.; Nielsen, S.L.: Spinal commissurotomy. Surg. Neurol. *2:* 373–377 (1974).
Lipton, S.: Percutaneous cervical cordotomy and pituitary injection of alcohol; in Swerdlow, Relief of intractable pain, pp. 269–304 (Elsevier, Amsterdam 1983).
Lipton, S.; McLennan, J.E.: Percutaneous spinothalamic tractotomy: the prototype of neurosurgical pain control; in Cousins, Bridenbaugh, Neural blockade, pp. 679–690 (Lippincott, Philadelphia 1980).
Lipton, S.; Miles, J.B.; Williams, N.E.: Pituitary injection of alcohol for inoperable and intractable cancer pain. Adv. Pain Res. Ther. *3:* 905–909 (1979).
Lipton, S.; Miles, J.; Williams, N.; Bark-Jones, N.: Pituitary injection of alcohol for widespread cancer pain. Pain *5:* 73–82 (1978).
Lissauer, H.: Beitrag zur pathologischen Anatomie der Tabes dorsalis und zum Faserverlauf im menschlichen Rückenmark. Neur. Zentbl. *4:* 245–246 (1885).
Litwin, M.S.: Postsympathectomy neuralgia. Archs. Surg. *84:* 591–595 (1962).
Livingston, W.K.: Pain mechanisms. A physiologic interpretation of causalgia and its related states, pp. 83–99 (Macmillan, New York 1943).
Lobato, R.D.; Madrid, J.L.; Fatela, L.V.; Gozalo, A.; Rivas, J.J.; Sarabia, R.: Analgesia elicited by low-dose intraventricular morphine in terminal cancer patients. Adv. Pain Res. Ther. *9:* 673–681 (1985).
Lobato, R.D.; Madrid, J.L.; Fatela, L.V.; Rivas, J.J.; Reig, E.; Lamas, E.: Intraventricular morphine for control of pain in terminal cancer patients. J. Neurosurg. *59:* 627–633 (1983).
Lobato, R.D.; Rivas, J.J.; Sarabia, R.; Madrid, J.L.: Percutaneous compression of the Gasserian ganglion for trigeminal neuralgia. Pain, suppl. 4, p. S129 (1987).
Loeser, J.D.: Dorsal rhizotomy for the relief of chronic pain. J. Neurosurg. *36:* 745–755 (1972).
Loeser, J.D.: Dorsal rhizotomy; in Youmans, Neurological surgery, vol. 6, pp. 3664–3671 (Saunders, Philadelphia 1982).
Loeser, J.D.; Ward, A.A.; White, L.E.: Chronic deafferentation of human spinal cord neurons. J. Neurosurg. *29:* 48–50 (1968).

Löfström, J.B.; Lloyd, J.W.; Cousins, M.J.: Sympathetic neural blockade of upper and lower extremity; in Cousins, Bridenbaugh, Neural blockade in clinical anesthesia and management of pain, pp. 355–382 (Lippincott, Philadelphia 1980).

Loh, L.; Nathan, P.W.: Painful peripheral states and sympathetic blocks. J. Neurol. Neurosurg. Psychiat. *41:* 664–671 (1978).

Lombard, M.C.; Larabi, Y.: Electrophysiological study of cervical dorsal horn cells in partially deafferented rats. Adv. Pain Res. Ther. *5:* 147–154 (1983).

Long, D.M.: Electrical stimulation for relief of pain from chronic nerve injury. J. Neurosurg. *39:* 718–722 (1973).

Long, D.M.: Stimulation of peripheral nerves, spinal cord and brain for pain relief; in Swerdlow, Relief of intractable pain, pp. 239–267 (Elsevier, Amsterdam 1983).

Long, D.M.; Erickson, D.L.: Stimulation of the posterior columns of the spinal cord for relief of intractable pain. Surg. Neurol. *4:* 134–141 (1975).

Long, D.M.; Erickson, D.L.; Campbell, J.N.; North, R.B.; Electrical stimulation of the spinal cord and peripheral nerves for pain control. A 10-year experience. Appl. Neurophysiol. *44:* 207–217 (1981).

Long, D.M.; Hagfors, N.: Electrical stimulation in the nervous system: the current status of electrical stimulation of the nervous system for relief of pain. Pain *1:* 109–123 (1975).

Longoni, F.; Romagnoli, G.; Albonico, C.; Montorsi, M.; Marastoni, F.: La neuralgia postsimpatectomia lumbar. Nuestra experience. Angiologia *33:* 118–122 (1981).

Lora, J.; Long, D.: So-called facet denervation in the management of intractable back pain. Spine *1:* 121–126 (1976).

Lorenz, R.: Methods of percutaneous spinothalamic tract section; in Krayenbühl, Advances and technical standards in neurosurgery, vol. 3, pp. 123–145 (Springer, Wien 1976).

Luft, R.; Olivecrona, H.: Experiences with hypophysectomy in man. J. Neurosurg. *10:* 301–316 (1953).

Lunsford, L.D.: Trigeminal neuralgia: treatment by glycerol rhizotomy; in Wilkins, Rengachary, Neurosurgery, pp. 2351–2356 (McGraw-Hill, New York 1985).

Lunsford, L.D.; Apfelbaum, R.I.: Choice of surgical therapeutic modalities for treatment of trigeminal neuralgia: microvascular decompression, percutaneous retrogasserian thermal or glycerol rhizotomy. Clin. Neurosurg. *32:* 319–333 (1985).

Lunsford, L.D.; Bennett, M.H.: Percutaneous retrogasserian glycerol rhizotomy for tic douloureux: part I. Neurosurgery *14:* 424–429 (1984).

Lunsford, L.D.; Bennett, M.H.; Martinez, A.J.: Experimental trigeminal glycerol injection. Electrophysiologic and morphologic effects. Archs Neurol. *42:* 146–149 (1985).

MacCarty, C.S.: The treatment of spastic paraplegia by selective spinal cordectomy. J. Neurosurg. *11:* 539–545 (1954).

MacLean, P.D.: Psychosomatic disease and the 'visceral brain'; recent developments bearing on the Papez theory of emotion. Psychosom. Med. *11:* 338–353 (1949).

Macon, J.B.; Poletti, C.E.; Sweet, W.H.: Human trigeminal root evoked potentials during differential thermal and chemical trigeminal rhizotomy. Surg. Forum *32:* 486–488 (1981).

Maddy, J.A.; Winternitz, W.W.; Norrell, H.: Cryohypophysectomy in the management of advanced prostatic cancer. Cancer *28:* 322–328 (1971).

Madrid, J.L.: Chemical hypophysectomy. Adv. Pain Res. Ther. *2:* 381–391 (1979).

Madrid, J.L.; Gozalo, A.; Fatela, L.V.; Lobato, R.D.: Low-dose cisternal morphine as a test for chronic intraventricular or intrathecal opiate therapy. Pain, suppl. 2, p. S342 (1984).

Magendie, F.: Expériences sur les fonctions des racines des nerfs rachidiens. J. Physiol., Paris *2:* 246–279 (1822).

Magora, F.; Olshwang, D.; Eimerl, D.; Shorr, J.; Katzenelson, R.; Cotev, S.; Davidson, J.T.: Observations on extradural morphine analgesia in various pain conditions. Br. J. Anaesth. *52:* 247–252 (1980).

Maiman, D.J.; Larson, S.J.; Sances, A.: Spinal cord stimulation for pain; in Myklebust, Cusick, Sances, Larson, Neural stimulation, vol. 1, pp. 147–154 (CRC Press, Boca Raton 1985).

Malone, P.S.; Duignan, J.P.; Hederman, W.P.: Transthoracic electrocoagulation (T.T.E.C.) — a new and simple approach to upper limb sympathectomy. Ir. med. J. *75:* 20–21 (1982).

Manart, F.D.; Sadler, T.R.; Schmitt, E.A.; Rainer, W.G.: Upper dorsal sympathectomy. Am. J. Surg. *150:* 762–766 (1985).

Mansuy, L.; Lecuire, J.; Acassat, L.: Technique de la myélotomie commissurale postérieure. J. Chir. *60:* 206–213 (1944).

Mansuy, L.; Sindou, M.; Fischer, G.; Brunon, J.: La cordotomie spino-thalamique dans les douleurs cancéreuses. Résultats d'une série de 124 malades opérés par abord direct postérieur. Neuro-chirurgie *22:* 437–444 (1976).

Mark, V.H.; Ervin, F.R.: Role of thalamotomy in treatment of chronic severe pain. Postgrad. Med. *37:* 563–571 (1965).

Mark, V.H.; Ervin, F.R.; Hackett, T.P.: Clinical aspects of stereotactic thalamotomy in the human. I. The treatment of chronic severe pain. Archs Neurol. *3:* 351–367 (1960).

Mark, V.H.; Ervin, F.R.; Yakovlev, P.I.: Correlation of pain relief, sensory loss and anatomical lesion sites in pain patients treated by stereotactic thalamotomy. Trans. Am. neurol. Ass. *86:* 86–90 (1961).

Mark, V.H.; Hackett, T.P.: Surgical aspects of thalamotomy in the human. Trans. Am. neurol. Ass. *84:* 92–94 (1959).

Martin, G.F.; Cabana, T.; Humbertson, A.U.; Laxson, L.C.; Panneton, W.M.: Spinal projections from the medullary reticular formation on the North American opossum: evidence for connectional heterogeneity. J. comp. Neurol. *196:* 663–682 (1981).

Martin, R.: In Lehrbuch der Anthropologie, pp. 579—1182 (Fischer, Jena 1928).

Martin, W.R.; Eades, C.G.; Fraser, H.F.; Wikler, A.: Use of hindlimb reflexes of the chronic spinal dog for comparing analgesics. J. Pharmac. exp. Ther. *144:* 8–11 (1964).

Martinez, S.N.; Bertrand, C.; Molina Negro, P.M.; Perez-Calvo, J.M.: Alteration of pain perception by stereotactic lesions of fronto-thalamic pathways. Confinia neurol. *37:* 113–118 (1975).

Maruta, T.; Swanson, D.W.; Finlayson, R.E.: Drug abuse and dependency in patients with chronic pain. Mayo Clin. Proc. *54:* 241–244 (1979).

Mattassi, R.; Miele, F.; D'Angelo, F.: Thoracic sympathectomy. Review of indications, results and surgical techniques. J. cardiovasc. Surg. *22:* 336–339 (1981).

Maxwell, R.E.: Surgical control of chronic migrainous neuralgia by trigeminal gangliorhizolysis. J. Neurosurg. *57:* 459–466 (1982).

Maxwell, R.E. Personal communication (1985).

Mayanagi, Y.; Hori, T.; Sano, K.: The posteromedial hypothalamus and pain, behavior, with special reference to endocrinological findings. Appl. Neurophysiol. *41:* 223–231 (1978).

Mayberg, M.R.; Zervas, N.T.; Moskowitz, M.A.: Trigeminal projections to supratentorial pial and dural blood vessels in cats demonstrated by horseradish peroxidase histochemistry. J. comp. Neurol. *223:* 46–56 (1984).

Mayer, D.J.; Price, D.D.: Central nervous system mechanism of analgesia. Pain *2:* 379–404 (1976).

Mayer, D.J.; Price, D.D.; Becker, D.P.: Neurophysiological characterization of the anterolateral spinal cord neurons contributing to pain perception in man. Pain *1:* 51–58 (1975a).

Mayer, D.J.; Price, D.D.; Becker, D.P.; Young, H.F.: Threshold for pain from anterolateral quadrant stimulation as a predictor to success of percutaneous cordotomy for relief of pain. J. Neurosurg. *43:* 445–447 (1975b).

Mayer, D.J.; Watkins, L.R.: Multiple endogenous opiate and non-opiate analgesia systems. Adv. Pain Res. Ther. *6:* 253–276 (1984).

Mayfield, F.H.: Causalgia (Thomas, Springfield 1951).

Mazars, G.: Etat actuel de la chirurgie de la douleur. Neuro-chirurgie *22:* suppl. 1 (1976).

Mazars, G.; Mérienne, L.; Ciolocca, C.: Stimulations thalamiques intermittentes antalgiques. Note préliminaire. Revue neurol. *128:* 273–279 (1973).

Mazars, G.; Mérienne, L.; Ciolocca, C.: Comparative study of electrical stimulation of posterior thalamic nuclei, periaqueductal gray, and other midline mesencephalic structures in man. Adv. Pain Res. Ther. *3:* 541–546 (1979).

Mazars, G.; Roge, R.; Pansini, A.: Stereotactic coagulation of the spinothalamic tract of intractable trigeminal pain. J. Neurol. Neurosurg. Psychiat. *23:* 352 (1960).

McCabe, J.S.; Low, F.N.: The subarachnoid angle: an area of transition in peripheral nerve. Anat. Rec. *164:* 15–34 (1969).

McCulloch, J.A.: Percutaneous radiofrequency lumbar rhizolysis (rhizotomy). Appl. Neurophysiol. *39:* 87–96 (1976/77).

Meglio, M.: Percutaneously implantable chronic electrode for radiofrequency stimulation of the Gasserian ganglion. A new perspective in the management of trigeminal pain. Acta neurochir., suppl. 33, pp. 521–525 (1984).

Meglio, M.; Cioni, B.; Dal Lago, A.; De Santis, M.; Pola, P.; Serricchio, M.: Pain control and improvement of peripheral blood flow following epidural spinal cord stimulation. Case report. J. Neurosurg. *54:* 821–823 (1981).

Meglio, M.; Cioni, B.; D'Annunzio, V.; Rossi, G.F.: A comparison of the results of treatment of trigeminal neuralgia using Gasserian ganglion percutaneous microcompression and selective thermocoagulation. J. Neurosurg. Sci. *29:* 166–167 (1985).

Mehler, W.R.: The anatomy of the so-called 'pain tract' in man: an analysis of the course and distribution of the ascending fibers of the fasciculus anterolateralis; in French, Porter, Basic research in paraplegia, pp. 26–55 (Thomas, Springfield 1962).

Mehler, W.R.: Some neurological species differences. Ann. N.Y. Acad. Sci. *167:* 424–468 (1969).

Mehler, W.R.; Feferman, M.E.; Nauta, W.J.H.: Ascending axon degeneration following anterolateral cordotomy. An experimental study in the monkey. Brain *83:* 718–751 (1960).

Mehta, L.; Fatani, J.; Rao, G.: Superior cerebellar artery in the pontine zone. Saudi med. J. *2:* 213–216 (1981).

Mehta, M.; Sluijter, M.E.: The treatment of chronic back pain. Anesthesia *34:* 768–775 (1979).

Melzack, R.; Loeser, J.D.: Phantom body pain in paraplegics: evidence for a central 'pattern generating mechanism' for pain. Pain *4:* 195–210 (1978).

Melzack, R.; Wall, P.D.: Pain mechanisms: a new theory. Science *150:* 971–978 (1965).

Menétry, D.; Roudier, F.; Besson, J.M.: Spinal neurons reaching the lateral reticular nucleus as studied in the rat by retrograde transport of horseradish peroxidase. J. comp. Neurol. *220:* 439–452 (1983).

Menzel, J.: Operative Behandlung der Trigeminusneuralgie. Dt. med. Wschr. *111:* 1247–1250 (1986).

Menzel, J.; Piotrowski, W.; Penzholz, H.: Long-term results of Gasserian ganglion electrocoagulation. J. Neurosurg. *42:* 140–143 (1975).

Merskey, H.: Pain terms. Pain *6:* 249–252 (1979).

Merskey, H.: Pain terms: a supplementary note. Pain *14:* 205–206 (1982).

Meyer, G.A.: Cingulotomy for pain. Presented to the Am. College of Surgeons, Miami 1973.

Meyer, G.A.; Fields, H.L.: Causalgia treated by selective large fibre stimulation of peripheral nerve. Brain *95:* 163–168 (1972).

Meyerson, B.A.: Electrostimulation procedures: effects, presumed rationale, and possible mechanisms. Adv. Pain Res. Ther. *5:* 495–534 (1983).

Meyerson, B.A.: Aspects on the present state of intracerebral stimulation for pain; in Tsubokawa, Brain stimulation and neuronal plasticity, pp. 34–54 (Tokyo 1985).

Meyerson, B.A.; Arnér, S.; Linderoth, B.: I. Pelvic cancer pain (somatogenic pain). Pros and cons of different approaches to the management of pelvic cancer pain. Acta neurochir., suppl. 33, pp. 407–419 (1984).

Meyerson, B.A.; Boethius, J.; Carlsson, A.M.: Alleviation of malignant pain by electrical stimulation in the periventricular-periaqueductal region: pain relief as related to stimulation sites. Adv. Pain Res. Ther. *3:* 525–533 (1979).

Meyerson, B.A.; Brodin, E.; Linderoth, B.: Possible neurohymoral mechanisms in CNS stimulation for pain suppression. Appl. Neurophysiol. *48:* 175–180 (1985).

Meyerson, B.A.; Håkanson, S.: Alleviation of atypical trigeminal pain by stimulation of the Gasserian ganglion via an implanted electrode. Acta neurochir., suppl. 30, pp. 303–309 (1980).

Meyerson, B.A.; Håkanson, S.: Suppression of pain in trigeminal neuropathy by electrical stimulation of the Gasserian ganglion. Neurosurgery *18:* 59–66 (1986).

Meynadier, J.; Dubar, M.; Blond, S.; Combelles-Pruvot, M.: Intrathecal morphine in treatment of intractable pain in cancer patients. Pain Clinic *I:* 87–91 (1985).

Michotey, G.; Sastre, B.; Argeme, M.; Mannara, P.; Crespy, B.: La splanchnicectomie par voie transhiatale de Dubois. A propos de 25 sections. J. Chir., Paris *120:* 487–491 (1983).

Miles, J.: Chemical hypophysectomy. Adv. Pain Res. Ther. *2:* 373–380 (1979).

Miles, J.: Pituitary destruction; in Wall, Melzack, Textbook of pain, pp. 656–665 (Churchill-Livingstone, Edinburgh 1984).

Miles, J.; Lipton, S.: Mode of action by which pituitary alcohol injection relieves pain. Adv. Pain Res. Ther. *1:* 867–869 (1976).

Miller, N.E.; Jensen, D.D.; Myers, A.: Injury and excitation by electric currents. B. A comparison of the Lilly waveform and the sixty-cycle sine wave; in Sheer, Electrical stimulation of the brain, pp. 64 (University of Texas Press, Austin 1961).

Mitchell, S.W.: Injuries of nerves and their consequences (Lippincott, Philadelphia 1872).

Mittal, B.; Thomas, D.G.T.: Controlled thermocoagulation in trigeminal neuralgia. J. Neurol. Neurosurg. Psychiat. *49:* 932–936 (1986).

Modesti, L.M.; Waszak, M.: Firing pattern of cells in human thalamus during dorsal column stimulation. Appl. Neurophysiol. *38:* 251–258 (1975).

Mokhtar, A.; Farouk, Y.; Martin, J.: The spinal nerve root 'innervation', and a new concept of the clinicopathological interrelations in back pain and sciatica. Neurochirurgie *24:* 137–141 (1981).

Moniz, E.: Tentatives opératoires dans le traitement de certaines psychoses (Masson, Paris 1936).

Monnier, M.: Les résultats de la coagulation du thalamus chez l'homme (noyau ventropostérieur). Acta neurochir., suppl. 3, pp. 291–307 (1955).

Monnier, M.; Fischer, R.: Localisation, stimulation et coagulation du thalamus chez l'homme. J. Physiol., Paris *43:* 818 (1951).

Morales, F.; Albert, P.; Alberca, R.; De Valle, B.; Narros, A.: Glossopharyngeal and vagal neuralgia secondary to vascular compression of the nerves. Surg. Neurol. *8:* 431–433 (1977).

Morley, T.P.: Case against microvascular decompression in the treatment of trigeminal neuralgia. Archs Neurol. *42:* 801–802 (1985).

Mortimer, J.T.; Shealy, N.; Wheeler, C.: Experimental nondestructive electrical stimulation of the brain and spinal cord. J. Neurosurg. *32:* 553–559 (1970).

Moulin, D.E.; Inturrisi, C.E.; Foley, K.M.: Cerebrospinal fluid pharmacokinetics of intrathecal morphine sulfate and D-Ala^2-D-Leu^5-enkephalin in cancer patients with chronic pain. Ann. Neurol. *20:* 218–222 (1986).

Moulin, D.E.; Max, M.; Kaiko, R.; Inturrisi, C.; Maggard, J.; Foley, K.: The analgesic efficacy of intrathecal (IT) D-Ala^2-D-Leu^5-enkephalin (DADL) in cancer patients with chronic pain. Pain, suppl. 2, p. S343 (1984).

Mullan, S.: Personal communication (1987).

Mullan, S.: Percutaneous cordotomy. J. Neurosurg. *35:* 360–366 (1971).

Mullan, S.; Harper, P.V.; Hekmatpanah, J.; Torres, H.; Dobben, G.: Percutaneous interruption of spinal-pain tracts by means of a strontium needle. J. Neurosurg. *20:* 931–939 (1963).

Mullan, S.; Hekmatpanah, J.; Dobben, G.; Beckman, F.: Percutaneous, intramedullary cordotomy utilizing the unipolar anodal electrolytic lesion. J. Neurosurg. *22:* 548–553 (1965).

Mullan, S.; Lichtor, T.: Percutaneous microcompression of the trigeminal ganglion for trigeminal neuralgia. J. Neurosurg. *59:* 1007–1012 (1983).

Müller, H.; Stoyanov, M.; Borner, U.; Hempelmann, G.: Epidural opiates for relief of cancer pain; in Yaksh et al., Anaesthesia and intensive care medicine, pp. 125–137 (Springer, Heidelberg 1981).

Müller, J.: Praktische Bemerkungen über die Kur des halbseitigen Kopfwehes oder der sogenannten Migraine mit beigefügten diatetischen Vorschriften für Nervenkranke und Hypochondristen (Bronner, Frankfurt am Main 1813).

Mundinger, F.; Salomao, J.F.: Deep brain stimulation in mesencephalic lemniscus medialis for chronic pain. Acta neurochir., suppl. 30, pp. 245–258 (1980).

Myklebust, J.B.; Cusick, J.F.; Sances, A.; Larson, S.J.: Neural stimulation, vol. 1 (CRC Press, Boca Raton 1985).

Myklebust, J.B.; Maiman, D.J.; Larson, S.J.; Sances, A.: Electrophysiological effects of lumbar dorsal root stimulation. Neurosurgery *14:* 682–687 (1984).

Nagaro, T.; Kimura, S.; Arai, T.: A mechanism of new pain following cordotomy; reference of sensation. Pain *30:* 89–91 (1987).

Nagashima, C.; Sakaguchi, A.; Kamisasa, A.; Kawanuma, S.: Cardiovascular complications on upper vagal rootlet section for glossopharyngeal neuralgia. Case report. J. Neurosurg. *44:* 248–253 (1976).

Nahin, R.L.; Madsen, A.M.; Giesler, G.J.: Anatomical and physiological studies of the gray matter surrounding the spinal cord central canal. J. comp. Neurol. *220:* 321–335 (1983).

Nahin, R.L.; Madsen, A.M.; Micevych, P.E.; Terman, G.W.; Haist, F.; Giesler, G.J.: Studies of the area around the central canal: efferents and afferents. Neurosci. Abstr. *10:* 487 (1984).

Nakamura, S.; Tsubokawa, T.: Evaluation of spinal cord stimulation for postapoplectic spastic hemiplegia. Neurosurgery *17:* 253–259 (1985).

Nakata, Y.; Kusakan, Y.; Segawa, T.: Supersensitivity to substance P after dorsal root section. Life Sci. *24:* 1651–1654 (1979).

Nally, F.F.: A 22-year study of paroxysmal trigeminal neuralgia in 211 patients with a 3-year appraisal of the role of cryotherapy. Oral Surg. Oral Med. Oral Pathol. *58:* 17–23 (1984).

Nashold, B.S.: Extensive cephalic and oral pain relieved by midbrain tractotomy. Confinia neurol. *34:* 382–388 (1972).

Nashold, B.S.: Modification of DREZ lesion technique. J. Neurosurg. *55:* 1012 (1981).

Nashold, B.S.: Brainstem stereotaxic procedures; in Schaltenbrand, Walker, Stereotaxy of the human brain; 2nd ed., pp. 475–494 (Thieme, Stuttgart 1982).

Nashold, B.S.; Bullitt, E.: Dorsal root entry zone lesions to control central pain in paraplegics. J. Neurosurg. *55:* 414–419 (1981).

Nashold, B.S.; Friedman, A.H.: Dorsal column stimulation for control of pain. Preliminary report on 30 patients. J. Neurosurg. *36:* 590–596 (1972).

Nashold, B.S.; Goldner, J.L.: Electrical stimulation of peripheral nerves for relief of intractable chronic pain. Med. Instrum. *9:* 224–225 (1975).

Nashold, B.S.; Goldner, J.L.; Bright, D.S.: Electrical stimulation of peripheral nerves with micro-electrical implants for pain relief; in Omer, Spinner, Management of peripheral nerve problems, pp. 254–271 (Saunders, Philadelphia 1980).

Nashold, B.S.; Goldner, J.L.; Mullen, J.B.; Bright, D.S.: Long-term pain control by direct peripheral nerve stimulation. J. Bone Jt Surg. *64-A:* 1–10 (1982).

Nashold, B.S.; Lopes, H.; Choda-Kiewitz, J.; Bronec, P.: Trigeminal DREZ for craniofacial pain; in Samii, Surgery in and around the brain stem, pp. 53–58 (Springer, Heidelberg 1986).

Nashold, B.S.; Moossy, J.; Higgins, A.C.; Blumenkopf, M.B.; Friedman, A.H.: The DREZ operation; in Modern technics in surgery, neurosurgery, vol. 35, pp. 1–17 (Futura, New York 1984).

Nashold, B.S.; Mullen, J.B.; Avery, R.: Peripheral nerve stimulation for pain relief using a multicontact electrode system. J. Neurosurg. *51:* 872–873 (1979).

Nashold, B.S.; Ostdahl, R.H.: Dorsal root entry zone lesions for pain relief. J. Neurosurg. *51:* 59–69 (1979).

Nashold, B.S.; Ovelmen-Levitt, J.; Sharpe, R.; Higgins, A.C.: Intraoperative evoked potentials recorded in man directly from dorsal roots and spinal cord. J. Neurosurg. *62:* 680–693 (1985).

Nashold, B.S.; Slaughter, D.G.; Wilson, W.P.; Zorub, D.: Stereotactic mesencephalotomy. Prog. neurol. Surg., vol. 8, pp. 35–49 (Karger, Basel 1977).

Nashold, B.S.; Somjen, G.G.; Friedman, A.H.: Paresthesias and EEG potentials evoked by stimulation of the dorsal funiculi in man. Expl Neurol. *36:* 273–287 (1972).

Nashold, B.S.; Urban, B.; Zorub, D.S.: Phantom pain relief by focal destruction of the substantia gelatinosa of Rolando. Adv. Pain Res. Ther. *1:* 959–963 (1976).

Nashold, B.S.; Walker, J.S.: Laser effect on spinal cord. J. Neurosurg. *60:* 870 (1984).

Nashold, B.S.; Wilson, W.P.: Central pain. Observations in man with chronic implanted electrodes in the midbrain tegmentum. Confinia neurol. *27:* 30–44 (1966).

Nashold, B.S.; Wilson, W.P.; Slaughter, D.G.: Sensations evoked by stimulation in the midbrain of man. J. Neurosurg. *30:* 14–24 (1969a).

Nashold, B.S.; Wilson, W.P.; Slaughter, D.G.: Stereotaxic midbrain lesions for central dysesthesia and phantom pain. J. Neurosurg. *30:* 116–126 (1969b).

Nashold, B.S.; Wilson, W.P.; Slaughter, D.G.: The midbrain and pain. Adv. Neurol. *4:* 191–196 (1974).

Nathan, P.W.: Micturition reflexes in man. J. Neurol. Neurosurg. Psychiat. *15:* 148–149 (1952).

Nathan, P.W.: Reference of sensation at the spinal level. J. Neurol. Neurosurg. Psychiat. *19:* 88–100 (1956).

Nathan, P.W.: Results of antero-lateral cordotomy for pain in cancer. J. Neurol. Neurosurg. Psychiat. *26:* 353–362 (1963a).

Nathan, P.W.: The descending respiratory pathway in man. J. Neurol. Neurosurg. Psychiat. *26:* 487–499 (1963b).

Nathan, P.W.; Rudge, P.: Testing the gate-control theory of pain in man. J. Neurol. Neurosurg. Psychiat. *37:* 1366–1372 (1974).

Nathan, P.W.; Smith, M.C.: The centripetal pathway from the bladder and urethra within the spinal cord. J. Neurol. Neurosurg. Psychiat. *14:* 262–280 (1951).

Nathan, P.W.; Smith, M.C.: Spinal pathways subserving defaecation and sensation from the lower bowel. J. Neurol. Neurosurg. Psychiat. *16:* 245–256 (1953).

Nathan, P.W.; Smith, M.C.: The centrifugal pathway for micturition within the spinal cord. J. Neurol. Neurosurg. Psychiat. *21:* 177–189 (1958).

Nathan, P.W.; Smith, M.C.: Fasciculi proprii of the spinal cord in man; review of present knowledge. Brain *82:* 610–668 (1959).

Nathan, P.W.; Smith, M.C.: Some tracts of the anterior and lateral columns of the spinal cord; in Knighton, Dumke, Pain, pp. 47–57 (Little, Brown, Boston 1966).

Nathan, P.W.; Smith, M.C.: Effects of two unilateral cordotomies on the modality of the lower limbs. Brain *96:* 471–494 (1973).

Nathan, P.W.; Smith, M.C.: Clinico-anatomical correlation in anterolateral cordotomy. Adv. Pain Res. Ther. *3:* 921–926 (1979).

Nathan, P.W.; Smith, M.C.: Dysesthésie après cordotomie. Méd. Hyg. *42:* 1788–1790 (1984).

Nathan, P.W.; Smith, M.C.: The location of descending fibres to sympathetic neurons supplying the eye and sudomotor neurons supplying the head and neck. J. Neurol. Neurosurg. Psychiat. *49:* 187–194 (1986).

Nathan, P.W.; Smith, M.C.: The location of descending fibres to sympathetic preganglionic vasomotor and sudomotor neurons in man. J. Neurol. Neurosurg. Psychiat. *50:*1253–1262 (1987).

Nielson, K.D.; Adams, J.E.; Hosobuchi, Y.: Phantom limb pain, treatment with dorsal column stimulation. J. Neurosurg. *42:* 301–307 (1975a).

Nielson, K.D.; Adams, J.E.; Hosobuchi, Y.: Experience with dorsal column stimulation for relief of chronic intractable pain: 1968–1973. Surg. Neurol. *4:* 148–152 (1975b).

Niizuma, H.; Kwak, R.; Saso, S.; Sakamoto, T.; Ohi, T.; Ohyama, H.; Suzuki, J.: Follow-up results of center median thalamotomy for central pain. Appl. Neurophysiol. *43:* 336 (1980).

Nobili, C.; Ambrosino, A.; Formenti, S.; Izzo, V.; Piva, L.; Severgnini, A.; Tiengo, M.: Home treatment of terminal cancer pain by epidural morphine. Pain, suppl. 2, p. S335 (1984).

Noordenbos, W.: Pain (Elsevier, Amsterdam 1959).

North, R.B.; Fischell, T.A.; Long, D.M.: Chronic stimulation via percutaneously inserted epidural electrodes. Neurosurgery *1:* 215 (1977).

North, R.B.; Fischell, T.A.; Long, D.M.: Chronic dorsal column stimulation via percutaneously inserted epidural electrodes. Appl. Neurophysiol. *40:* 184–191 (1977/78).

Nugent, G.R.: Trigeminal neuralgia: treatment by percutaneous electrocoagulation; in Wilkins, Rengachary, Neurosurgery, vol. 3, pp. 2345–2350 (McGraw-Hill, New York 1985).

Nugent, G.R.; Berry, B.: Trigeminal neuralgia treated by percutaneous radiofrequency coagulation of the Gasserian ganglion. J. Neurosurg. *40:* 517–523 (1974).

Nurchi, G.: Use of intraventricular and intrathecal morphine in intractable pain associated with cancer. Neurosurgery *15:* 801–803 (1984).

Nyquist, J.K.; Greenhoot, J.H.: Responses evoked from the thalamic centrum medianum painful input: suppression by dorsal funiculus conditioning. Expl Neurol. *39:* 215–222 (1973).

Obbens, E.A.M.T.; Hill, C.S.; Leavens, M.E.; Ruthenbeck, S.S.; Otis, F.: Intraventricular morphine administration for control of chronic cancer pain. Pain *28:* 61–68 (1987).

Obrador, S.: Actions of certain drugs injected into the ventricular system of man (Intraventricular encephalo-pharmaco-therapy). J. Neurosurg. *22:* 441–448 (1965).

O'Brien, M.D.; MacCabe, J.J.: Trigeminal nerve section for unremitting migrainous neuralgia. 3rd Int. Symp. Migraine Trust, London 1980 (cited by Campbell, 1984).

Ochoa, J.; Cline, M.; Comstock, W.; Culp, W.J.; Dotson, R.; Marchettini, P.; Torebjörk, H.E.: Painful syndrome disentangled: polymodal hyperalgesia with cross modality threshold modulation and rubor. Its basis: sensitized nociceptors plus antidromic vasodilatation. Pain, suppl. 4, p. S344 (1987).

Ojemann, G.A.; Fedio, D.; Van Buren, J.M.: Anomia from pulvinar and subcortical parietal stimulation. Brain *91:* 99–117 (1968).

Olafson, R.A.; Rushton, J.G.; Sayre, G.P.: Trigeminal neuralgia in a patient with multiple sclerosis. An autopsy report. J. Neurosurg. *24:* 755–759 (1966).

Olds, J.; Milner, B.: Positive reinforcement produced by electrical stimulation of the septal area and other regions of the rat brain. J. comp. physiol. Psychol. *47:* 419 (1954).

Oliveras, J.L.; Bougoin, S.; Hery, F.; Besson, J.M.; Hamon, M.: The topographical distribution of serotonergic terminals in the spinal cord of the cat: biochemical mapping by the combined use of microdissection and microassay procedures. Brain Res. *138:* 393–406 (1977).

Olszewski, J.: On the anatomical and functional organization of the spinal trigeminal nucleus. J. comp. Neurol. *92:* 401–413 (1950).

Omer, G.; Thomas, S.: Treatment of causalgia. Review of cases at Brooke General Hospital. Tex. Med. *67:* 93–96 (1971).

Onofrio, B.M.: Rhizotomy: what is its place in the treatment of pain? Adv. Neurol. *4:* 621–627 (1974).

Onofrio, B.M.: Radiofrequency percutaneous Gasserian ganglion lesions. Results in 140 patients with trigeminal pain. J. Neurosurg. *42:* 132–139 (1975).

Onofrio, B.M.; Campa, H.K.: Evaluation of rhizotomy. Review of 12 years' experience. J. Neurosurg. *36:* 751–755 (1972).

Onofrio, B.M.; Campbell, J.K.: Surgical treatment of chronic cluster headache. Mayo Clin. Proc. *61:* 537–544 (1986).

Onofrio, B.M.; Yaksh, T.L.: Intrathecal delta-receptor ligand produces analgesia in man. Lancet *i:* 1386–1387 (1983).

Onofrio, B.M.; Yaksh, T.L.; Arnold, P.G.: Continuous low-dose intrathecal morphine administration in the treatment of chronic pain of malignant origin. Mayo Clin. Proc. *56:* 516–520 (1981).

Opperman, J.: Dissertatio medica qua inauguralis de hemicrania horologica (Hilliger, Halle 1747).

Organ, L.W.: Electrophysiologic principles of radiofrequency lesion making. Appl. Neurophysiol. *39:* 69–76 (1976/77).

Ori, C.; Salar, G.; Giron, G.P.: Cardiovascular and cerebral complications during glossopharyngeal nerve thermocoagulation. Anaesthesia *40:* 433–437 (1985).

Orthner, H.; Roeder, F.: Further clinical and anatomical experience with stereotactic operations for relief of pain. Confinia neurol. *27:* 418–430 (1966).

Osgood, C.P.: Personal communication (1982).

Osgood, C.P.; Dujovny, M.; Faille, R.; Abassy, M.: Microsurgical lumbosacral ganglionectomy, anatomic rationale, and surgical results. Acta neurochir. *35:* 197–204 (1976).

Ouaknine, G.; Nathan, H.: Anastomotic connections between the eleventh nerve and the posterior root of the first cervical nerve in humans. J. Neurosurg. *38:* 189–197 (1973).

Ouaknine, G.E.; Robert, F.; Molina-Negro, P.; Hardy, J.: Geniculate neuralgia and audiovestibular disturbances due to compression of the intermediate and eighth nerves by the postero-inferior cerebellar artery. Surg. Neurol. *13:* 147–150 (1979).

Oudenhoven, R.C.: Paraspinal electromyography following facet rhizotomy. Spine *2:* 299–304 (1977).

Ovelmen-Levitt, J.; Johnson, B.; Bedenbaugh, P.; Nashold, B.S.: Dorsal root rhizotomy and avulsion in the cat: a comparison of long-term effects on dorsal horn neuronal activity. Neurosurgery *15:* 921–927 (1984).

Oyama, T.; Jin, T.; Yamaya, R.; Ling, N.; Guillemin, R.: Profound analgesic effects of beta-endorphin in man. Lancet *i:* 122–124 (1980).

Pagni, C.A.: Central pain and painful anesthesia: pathophysiology and treatment of sensory deprivation syndromes due to central and peripheral nervous system lesions; in Krayenbühl, Maspes, Sweet, Prog. neurol. surg., vol. 8, pp. 132–257 (Karger, Basel 1976).

Paillas, J.W.; Pellet, W.: Dorsal nerve root section in the treatment of refractory peripheral pain; in Janzen, Keidel, Herz, Steichele, Pain, pp. 209–213 (Thieme, Stuttgart 1972).

Panagopoulos, K.; Chakraborty, M.; Deopujari, C.E.; Sengupta, R.P.: Neurovascular decompression for cranial rhizopathies. Br. J. Neurosurg. *1:* 235–241 (1987).

Pàpez, J.W.: A proposed mechanism of emotion. Archs Neurol. Psychiat. *38:* 725–743 (1937).

Papo, I.; Luongo, A.: High cervical commissural myelotomy in the treatment of pain. J. Neurol. Neurosurg. Psychiat. *39:* 705–710 (1976).

Parker, H.L.: Trigeminal neuralgic pain associated with multiple sclerosis. Brain *51:* 46–62 (1928).

Pasqualucci, V.; Tantucci, C.; Paoletti, F.; Dottorini, M.L.; Bifarini, G.; Belfiori, R.; Berioli, M.B.; Grassi, V.; Sorbini, C.A.: Buprenorphine vs. morphine via the epidural route: a controlled comparative clinical study of respiratory effects and analgesic activity. Pain *29:* 273–286 (1987).

Patrick, B.S.: Personal communication (1985).

Paturet, G.: Traité d'anatomie humaine, tome 1 (Masson, Paris 1957).

Pawl, R.P.: Microsurgical ganglionectomy for treatment of arachnoiditis-related unilateral sciatica. Presented to the Am. Pain Society, 3rd Gen. Meet., Miami 1982.

Pedersen, H.E.; Blunck, C.F.J.; Gardner, E.: The anatomy of lumbosacral posterior rami and meningeal branches of spinal nerves (sinu-vertebral nerves). J. Bone Jt Surg. *38A:* 377–391 (1956).

Peet, M.M.; Schneider, R.C.: Trigeminal neuralgia. A series of 689 cases with a follow-up study in 65% of the group. J. Neurosurg. *9:* 367–377 (1952).

Pelletier, V.A.; Poulos, D.A.; Lende, R.A.: Functional localization in the trigeminal root. J. Neurosurg. *40:* 504–513 (1974).

Penfield, W.; Jasper, H.: Epilepsy and functional anatomy of the human brain (Little, Brown, Boston 1954).

Penn, R.D.; Paice, J.A.: Chronic intrathecal morphine for intractable pain. J. Neurosurg. *67:* 182–186 (1987).

Penn, R.D.; Paice, J.A.; Gottschalk, W.; Ivankovich, A.D.: Cancer pain relief using chronic morphine infusion. J. Neurosurg. *61:* 302–306 (1984).

Penzholz, H.: Die Neuralgien im Kopf-Halsbereich aus neurochirurgischer Sicht. HNO *34:* 56–60 (1986).

Penzholz, H.; Menzel, J.; Hagenlocher, H.-U.: Results of surgical treatment of idiopathic trigeminal neuralgia using different operative techniques (a co-operative study). Adv. Neurosurg. *3:* 320–327 (1975).

Perez-Calvo, J.M.; Gonzalez Martinez, E.; Peraita, P.: Tratamiento de la neuralgia del trigémino con coagulacion percutanea del ganglio de Gasser. Rev. Clin. Esp. *171:* 337–339 (1983).

Perl, E.R.: Pain and nociception; in Darian-Smith, Handbook of physiology, section 1, vol. III, part 2, pp. 915–975 (Am. Physiological Society, Bethesda 1984).

Perneczky, A.; Sunder-Plassmann, M.: Anterolateral cordotomy in cases of phantom limb pain. Adv. Neurosurg. *3:* 170–173 (1975).

Persson, A.V.; Anderson, L.A.; Padberg, F.T.: Selection of patients for lumbar sympathectomy. Surg. Clins N. Am. *65:* 393–403 (1985).

Pert, C.B.; Kuhar, M.J.; Snyder, S.H.: Autoradiographic localization of the opiate receptor in rat brain. Life Sci. *16:* 1849–1854 (1975).

Pertuiset, B.; Philippon, J.; Nachanakian, A.; Van Effenterre, R.: Névralgie faciale: traitement par électrothermie différentielle rétrogassérienne. 100 observations. Nouv. Presse méd. *6:* 3717–3720 (1977).

Peschanski, M.; Besson, J.M.: Diencephalic connections of the raphe nuclei of the rat brainstem: an anatomical study with reference to the somatosensory system. J. comp. Neurol. *224:* 509–534 (1984).

Piatt, J.H.; Wilkins, R.H.: Treatment of tic douloureux and hemifacial spasm by posterior fossa exploration: therapeutic implications of various neurovascular relationships. Neurosurgery *14:* 462–471 (1984).

Picaza, J.A.; Cannon, B.W.; Hunter, S.E.; Boyd, A.S.; Cuma, J.; Maurer, D.: Pain suppression by peripheral nerve stimulation. II. Observations with implanted devices. Surg. Neurol. *4:* 115–126 (1975).

Picaza, J.A.; Hunter, S.E.; Cannon, B.W.: Pain suppression by peripheral nerve stimulation. Appl. Neurophysiol. *40:* 223–234 (1977/78).

Pieri, G.: Contributi clinici alla chirurgia del sistema nervoso vegetativo; la cura della nevrite ascendente. Arch. Ital. Chir. *27:* 288–298 (1930).

Pilon, R.N.; Baker, A.R.: Chronic pain control by means of an epidural catheter. Cancer *37:* 903–905 (1976).

Pineda, A.: Dorsal column stimulation and its prospects. Surg. Neurol. *4:* 157–163 (1975).

Piscol, K.: Open spinal surgery for (intractable) pain. Adv. Neurosurg. *3:* 157–169 (1975).

Plotkin, R.: Results in 60 cases of deep brain stimulation for chronic intractable pain. Appl. Neurophysiol. *45:* 173–178 (1982).

Poletti, C.E.: Open cordotomy — new techniques; in Schmidek, Sweet, Operative neurosurgical techniques: indications, methods and results, vol. 2, pp. 1119–1136 (Grune & Stratton, New York 1982).

Ponti, L.; Valerio, M.: Results of resection of the greater superficial nerve in several cases of post-otitis headache and of cranio-facial neuralgia. Clin. Otorhinolaryng. *12:* 409–418 (1960).

Portenoy, R.K.; Foley, K.M.: Chronic use of opioid analgesics in non-malignant pain: report of 38 cases. Pain *25:* 171–186 (1986).

Portenoy, R.K.; Jarden, J.O.: Sidtis, J.J.; Lipton, R.B.; Foley, K.M.; Rottenberg, D.A.: Compulsive thalamic self-stimulation: a case with metabolic, electrophysiologic and behavioral correlates. Pain *27:* 277–290 (1986).

Porter, R.W.; Hohmann, G.W.; Bors, E.; French, J.D.: Cordotomy for pain following cauda equina injury. Archs Surg. *92:* 765–770 (1966).

Powers, S.K.: Laser-induced DREZ lesions. J. Neurosurg. *60:* 871 (1984).

Powers, S.K.: Presented at the DREZ Symp., Durham 1987.

Powers, S.K.; Adams, J.E.; Edwards, M.S.B.; Bogga, J.E.; Hosobuchi, Y.: Pain relief from dorsal root entry zone lesions made with argon and carbon dioxide microsurgical lasers. J. Neurosurg. *61:* 841–847 (1984).

Price, D.D.: Presented at the 8th Int. Congr. of Neurological Surgery, Toronto 1985.

Prince, D.A.: Neurophysiology of epilepsy. Annu. Rev. Neurosci. *1:* 395–415 (1978).

Pudenz, R.H.; Bullara, L.A.; Dru, D.; Talalla, A.: Electrical stimulation of the brain. II. Effects on the blood-brain barrier. Surg. Neurol. *4:* 265 (1975).

Pudenz, R.H.; Shelden, C.H.: Experiences with foraminal decompression in the surgical treatment of tic douloureux. Presented at the 14th Annu. Meet. American Academy of Neurological Surgery, New York 1952.

Pulec, J.L.: Geniculate neuralgia: diagnosis and surgical management. Laryngoscope *86:* 955–964 (1976).

Putnam, T.J.: Myelotomy of the commissure, a new method of treatment for pain in the upper extremities. Archs Neurol. Psychiat. *32:* 1189–1193 (1934).

Putti, V.: New conceptions in the pathogenesis of sciatic pain. Lancet *ii:* 53–60 (1927).

Rachlin, J.R.; Fessler, R.G.; Duda, E.E.; Brown, F.D.; Fang, V.; Mullan, S.: Beta-endorphin-like immunoreactivity increases in human lumbar cerebrospinal fluid following routine metrizamide myelography. J. Neurosurg. *60:* 800–802 (1984).

Ramirez, L.F.; Levin, A.B.: Pain relief after hypophysectomy. Neurosurgery *14:* 499–504 (1984).

Ranck, J.B.: Which elements are excited in electrical stimulation of mammalian central nervous system: a review. Brain Res. *98:* 417–440 (1975).

Rand, R.W.: Stereotactic transsphenoidal cryohypophysectomy. Bull. Los Angeles neurol. Soc. *29:* 40–48 (1964).

Rand, R.W.: Functional and anatomical localization in the trigeminal root: in support of Dandy; in Morley, Current controversies in neurosurgery, pp. 533–538 (Saunders, Philadelphia 1976).

Ranson, S.W.: The course within the spinal cord of the non-medullated fibers of the spinal dorsal roots: a study of Lissauer's tract in the cat. J. comp. Neurol. *23:* 259–274 (1913).

Ranson, S.W.; Billingsley, P.R.: The conduction of painful afferent impulses in the spinal nerves. Studies in vasomotor reflex arc II. Am. J. Physiol. *40:* 571–584 (1916).

Rappaport, Z.H.: Percutaneous retrogasserian glycerol injection for trigeminal neuralgia: one year follow-up. Pain Clinic *1:* 57–61 (1986).

Rasmussen, T.B.; Freedman, H.: Treatment of causalgia. An analysis of 100 cases. J. Neurosurg. *3:* 165–173 (1946).

Ray, B.S.; Console, A.D.: The relief of pain in chronic (calcareous) pancreatitis by sympathectomy. Surgery Gynec. Obstet. *89:* 1–8 (1949).

Ray, C.D.: Percutaneous spinal cord stimulation: technique; in Hosobuchi, Corbin, Indications for spinal cord stimulation, pp. 17–30 (Excerpta Medica, Amsterdam 1981).

Ray, C.D.; Burton, C.V.; Lifson, A.: Neurostimulation as used in a large clinical practice. Appl. Neurophysiol. *45:* 160–166 (1982).

Redman, D.R.O.; Robinson, P.N.; Al-Kutoubi, M.A.: Computerised tomography guided lumbar sympathectomy. Anaesthesia *41:* 39–41 (1986).

Rees, S.: Disconnective neurosurgery; in Rees, The treatment of pain as the major disability; 2nd ed. (Visual Abstracts, Australia 1975).

Reid, W.; Watt, J.K.; Gray, T.G.: Phenol injection of the sympathetic chain. Br. J. Surg. *57:* 45–50 (1970).

Reiz, S.; Westberg, M.: Side-effects of epidural morphine. Lancet *i:* 203–204 (1980).

Rengachary, S.S.; Watanabe, I.S.; Singer, P.; Bopp, W.J.: Effect of glycerol on peripheral nerve: an experimental study. Neurosurgery *13:* 681–688 (1983).

Reynolds, D.V.: Surgery in the rat during electrical analgesia induced by focal brain stimulation. Science *164:* 444–445 (1969).

Rhoton, A.: Personal communication (1985).

Richards, D.E.; Tyner, C.F.; Shealy, C.N.: Focussed ultrasonic spinal commissurotomy. Experimental evaluation. J. Neurosurg. *24:* 701–707 (1966).

Richardson, D.E.: Thalamotomy for intractable pain. Confinia neurol. *29:* 139–145 (1967).

Richardson, D.E.: Thalamotomy for control of chronic pain. Acta neurochir., suppl. 21, pp. 77–88 (1974).

Richardson, D.E.; Akil, H.: Long-term results of periventricular gray self-stimulation. Neurosurgery *1:* 199–202 (1977a).

Richardson, D.E.; Akil, H.: Pain reduction by electrical brain stimulation in man. I. Acute administration in periaqueductal and periventricular sites. J. Neurosurg. *47:* 178–183 (1977b).

Richardson, D.E.; Akil, H.: Pain reduction by electrical brain stimulation in man. II. Chronic self-administration in the periventricular gray matter. J. Neurosurg. *47:* 184–194 (1977c).

Richardson, D.E.; Zorub, D.S.: Sensory function of the pulvinar. Confinia neurol. *32:* 165–173 (1970).

Richardson, R.R.; Meyer, P.R.; Cerullo, L.J.: Neurostimulation in the modulation of intractable paraplegic and traumatic neuroma pains. Pain *8:* 75–84 (1980).

Richardson, R.R.; Sequeira, E.B.; Cerullo, L.J.: Spinal epidural neurostimulation for treatment of acute and chronic intractable pain — initial and long-term results. Neurosurgery *5:* 344–348 (1979).

Richter, H.-P.; Schachenmayr, W.: Is the substantia gelatinosa the target in dorsal root entry zone lesions? An autopsy report. Neurosurgery *15:* 913–916 (1984).

Richter, H.-P.; Seitz, K.: Dorsal root entry zone lesions for the control of deafferentation pain: experiences in ten patients. Neurosurgery *15:* 956–959 (1984).

Rifkinson, N.: Personal communication (1987).

Riley, H.A.; German, W.J.; Wortis, H.; Herbert, C.; Zahn, D.; Eichna, L.: Glossopharyngeal neuralgia initiating or associated with cardiac arrest. Trans. Am. neurol. Ass. *68:* 28–29 (1942).

Rippe, E.S.; Kresel, J.J.; Coombs, D.W.; Mroza, W.T.; Smith, C.R.: Effect of morphine sulfate concentration on flow rate in an implantable reservoir pump. Am. J. Hosp. Pharm. *41:* 496–500 (1984).

Rish, B.L.: Cerebrovascular accident after percutaneous RF thermocoagulation of the trigeminal ganglion. J. Neurosurg. *44:* 376–377 (1976).

Rodan, B.A.; Cohen, F.L.; Bean, W.J.; Martyak, S.N.: Fibrous mass complicating epidural morphine infusion. Neurosurgery *16:* 68–70 (1985).

Roeder, F.; Orthner, H.: Erfahrungen mit stereotaktischen Eingriffen. Confinia neurol. *21:* 51–97 (1961).

Roquefeuil, B.; Benezech, J.; Batier, C.: Intérêt de l'analgésie morphinique par voie ventriculaire dans les algies rebelles néoplasiques; in Simon, Roquefeuil, Pelissier, La douleur chronique, pp. 212 (Masson, Paris 1985).

Roquefeuil, B.; Benezech, J.; Batier, C.; Blanchet, P.; Gros, C.; Mathieu-Daude, J.-C.: Intérêt de l'analgésie morphinique par voie ventriculaire dans les algies rebelles néoplasiques. Neuro-chirurgie *29:* 135–141 (1983).

Roquefeuil, B.; Benezech, J.; Blanchet, P.; Batier, C.; Frerebeau, P.; Gros, C.: Intraventricular administration of morphine in patients with neoplastic intractable pain. Surg. Neurol. *21:* 155–158 (1984).

Rose, W.: Surgical treatment of trigeminal neuralgia (Abstract of the Lettsomian Lectures). Lancet *Jan. 9* (1892).

Rösner, K.; Goldberg, S.: Der Stellenwert der thorakoskopischen Sympathikotomie bei der Behandlung des Raynaud-Syndrom. Z. ges. inn. Med. *34:* 127–128 (1979).

Rosomoff, H.L.: Cordotomy: 1967. Lancet *ii:* 23–27 (1968).

Rosomoff, H.L.; Carroll, F.; Brown, J.; Sheptak, P.: Percutaneous radiofrequency cervical cordotomy technique. J. Neurosurg. *23:* 639–644 (1965).

Rosomoff, H.L.; Kreiger, A.J.; Kuperman, A.S.: Effects of percutaneous cervical cordotomy on pulmonary function. J. Neurosurg. *31:* 620–627 (1969).

Rovit, R.: Personal communication (1985).

Rowe, S.N.: Discussion of Jaeger, R.: The results of injecting hot water into the gasserian ganglion for the relief of tic douloureux. J. Neurosurg. *16:* 662 (1959).

Rowland, V.; MacIntyre, W.J.; Bidder, T.G.: The production of brain lesions with electrical currents. II. Bidirectional currents. J. Neurosurg. *17:* 55 (1960).

Rushton, J.G.; Stevens, J.C.; Miller, R.H.: Glossopharyngeal (vagoglossopharyngeal) neuralgia. Archs Neurol. *38:* 201–205 (1981).

Saadé, N.E.; Atweh, S.F.; Tabet, M.S.; Jabbur, S.J.: Inhibition of nociceptive withdrawal flexion reflexes through a dorsal column-brainstem-spinal loop. Brain Res. *335:* 306–308 (1985).

Saadé, N.E.; Tabet, M.S.; Soueidan, S.A.; Bitar, M.; Atweh, S.F.; Jabbur, S.J.: Supraspinal modulation of nociception in awake rats by stimulation of the dorsal column nuclei. Brain Res. *369:* 307–310 (1986).

Sachs, E., Jr.: The role of the nervus intermedius in facial neuralgia. Report of four cases with observations on the pathways for taste, lacrimation, and pain in the face. J. Neurosurg. *28:* 54–60 (1968).

Sachs, E., Jr.: Further observations on surgery of the nervus intermedius. Headache *9:* 159–161 (1969).

Sachs, E., Jr.: Personal communication (1976).

Sadar, E.S.; Hardy, R.W.: Thoracic splanchnicectomy and sympathectomy for relief of pancreatic pain; in Copperman, Hoerr, Surgery of the pancreas, pp. 141–152 (Mosby, St. Louis 1978).

Saini, S.S.: Retrogasserian anhydrous glycerol injection therapy in trigeminal neuralgia: observations in 552 patients. J. Neurol. Neurosurg. Psychiat. *50:* 1536–1538 (1987).

Sakai, Y.; Nishijima, Y.; Mikuni, N.; Iwata, N.: An experimental model of hyperirritability in the trigeminal skin field of the rat. Pain *7:* 147–157 (1979).

Salar, G.; Iob, I.; Ori, C.: Combined thermocoagulation of the 5th and 9th cranial nerves for oral pain of neoplastic aetiology. J. max.-fac. Surg. *14:* 1–4 (1986).

Samii, M.; Moringlane, J.R.: Thermocoagulation of the dorsal root entry zone for the treatment of intractable pain. Neurosurgery *15:* 953–955 (1984).

Samuelsson, H.; Nordberg, G.; Hedner, T.: CSF and plasma morphine concentrations during chronic epidural therapy. Pain, suppl. 4, p. S70 (1987a).

Samuelsson, H.; Nordberg, G.; Hedner, T.; Lindqvist, J.: CSF and plasma morphine concentrations in cancer patients during chronic epidural morphine therapy and its relation to pain relief. Pain *30:* 303–310 (1987b).

Sances, A.; Myklebust, J.; Larson, S.; Darin, J.; Swiontek, T.; Prieto, T.; Chilbert, M.; Cusick, J.: Experimental electrical injury studies. J. Trauma *21:* 589 (1981).

Sano, K.: Intralaminar thalamotomy (thalamolaminotomy) and postero-medial hypothalamotomy in the treatment of intractable pain. Prog. neurol. Surg., vol. 8, pp. 50–103 (Karger, Basel 1977).

Sano, K.: Stereotaxic thalamolaminotomy and postero-medial hypothalamotomy for the relief of intractable pain. Adv. Pain Res. Ther. *2:* 475–485 (1979).

Sano, K.; Yoshioka, M.; Ogashiwa, M.; Ishijima, B.; Ohye, C.: Thalamolaminotomy. A new operation for relief of intractable pain. Confinia neurol. *27:* 63–66 (1966).

Sano, K.; Yoshioka, M.; Sekino, H.; Mayanagi, Y.; Yoshimasu, N.; Tsukamoto, Y.: Functional organization of the internal medullary lamina in man. Confinia neurol. *32:* 374–380 (1970).

Saris, S.C.; Iacono, R.P.; Nashold, B.S.: Dorsal root entry zone lesions for post-amputation pain. J. Neurosurg. *62:* 72–76 (1985).

Saunders, R.L.; Weider, D.: Tympanic membrane sensation. Brain *108:* 387–404 (1985).

Scadding, J.W.: Development of ongoing activity, mechanosensitivity, and adrenaline sensitivity in severed peripheral nerve axons. Expl Neurol. *73:* 345–364 (1981).

Schaltenbrand, G.; Bailey, P.: Introduction to stereotaxis with an atlas of the human brain (Thieme, Stuttgart 1959).

Schild, H.; Grönniger, J.; Günther, R.; Thelen, M.; Schwab, R.: Transabdominelle CT-gesteuerte Sympathektomie. Fortschr. Röntgenstr. *141:* 504–508 (1984).

Schloesser, K.: Erfahrungen in der Neuralgiebehandlung mit Alkoholeinspritzungen. Klin. Wschr. *44:* 533–534 (1907).

Schmauss, C.; Yaksh, T.L.: In vivo studies on spinal opiate receptor systems mediating antinociception. II. Pharmacological profils suggesting differential association of mu, delta and kappa receptors with visceral chemical and cutaneous thermal stimuli in the rat. J. Pharmac. exp. Ther. *228:* 1–11 (1984).

Schmidek, H.: Ganglion cells located in the root of the trigeminal nerve in man. Neurochirurgia *11:* 74–77 (1968).

Schmidt, B.; Richter-Rau, G.; Thoden, U.: Suchtähnliches Verhalten bei Selbstreizung des mediobasalen Thalamus mit intracerebralen Dauerelektroden. Arch. Psychiat. NervKrankh. *230:* 55–61 (1981).

Schoenen, J.: Organisation neuronale de la moelle épinière de l'homme; thèse, Liège (1980).

Schoenen, J.; Lotstra, F.; Vierendeels, G.; Reznik, M.; Vanderhaeghen, J.J.: Substance P, enkephalins, somatostatin, cholecystokinin, oxytocin, and vasopressin in human spinal cord. Neurology *35:* 881–890 (1985).

Schürmann, K.; Butz, M.; Brock, M.: Temporal retrogasserian resection of trigeminal root versus controlled selective percutaneous electrocoagulation of the ganglion of Gasser in the treatment of trigeminal neuralgia. Report on a series of 531 cases. Acta neurochir. *26:* 33–53 (1972).

Schürmann, E.; Schürmann, K.: Controlled and partial percutaneous electrocoagulation of the Gasserian ganglion in facial pain. Adv. Neurosurg. *3:* 301–313 (1975).

Schvarcz, J.R.: Stereotactic trigeminal tractotomy. Confinia neurol. *37:* 73–77 (1975).

Schvarcz, J.R.: Functional exploration of the spinomedullary junction. Acta neurochir., suppl. 24, pp. 179–185 (1977a).

Schvarcz, J.R.: Periaqueductal mesencephalotomy for facial central pain; in Sweet, Obrador, Martin-Rodriguez, Neurosurgical treatment in psychiatry, pain and epilepsy, pp. 661–667 (University Park Press, Baltimore 1977b).

Schvarcz, J.R.: Spinal cord stereotactic techniques re trigeminal nucleotomy and extralemniscal myelotomy. Appl. Neurophysiol. *41:* 99–112 (1978).

Schvarcz, J.R.: Stereotactic spinal trigeminal nucleotomy for dysesthetic facial pain. Adv. Pain Res. Ther. *3:* 331–336 (1979).

Schvarcz, J.R.: Chronic self-stimulation of the medial posterior inferior thalamus for the alleviation of deafferentation pain. Acta neurochir., suppl. 30, pp. 295–301 (1980).

Schvarcz, J.R.: Trigeminal, glosso-vagal and high cervical post-herpetic neuralgia treated by stereotactic spinal trigeminal nucleotomy. Presented at the 8th Int. Congr. of Neurological Surgery, Toronto 1985a.

Schvarcz, J.R.: Chronic stimulation of the septal area for the relief of intractable pain. Appl. Neurophysiol. *48:* 191–194 (1985b).

Schwartz, H.G.: Gasserian gangliolysis for trigeminal neuralgia. Sth. med. J. *48:* 189–192 (1955).

Schwartz, H.G.: High cervical cordotomy — technique and results. Clin. Neurosurg. *8:* 282–293 (1960).
Schwartz, H.G.; O'Leary, J.L.: Section of the spinothalamic tract in the medulla with observations on the pathway for pain. Surgery *9:* 183–193 (1941).
Schwartzman, R.J.; McLellan, T.L.: Reflex sympathetic dystrophy. Archs Neurol. *44:* 555–561 (1987).
Schwarz, M.; Tindall, G.T.; Nixon, D.W.: Transsphenoidal hypophysectomy in disseminated breast cancer. Sth. med. J. *73:* 315–317 (1981).
Scott, D.B.; Littlewood, D.G.: Chemical lumbar sympathectomy with radiological assessment. Ann. R. Coll. Surg. *64:* 135 (1982).
Scott, P.V.; Bowen, F.E.; Cartwright, P.; Mohan Rao, B.C.; Deeley, D.; Wotherspoon, H.G.; Sumrein, I.M.A.: Intrathecal morphine as sole analgesic during labour. Br. med. J. *281:* 351–353 (1980).
Scott, W.W.; Schirmer, H.K.A.: Hypophysectomy for disseminated prostatic cancer; in Haddow et al., On cancer and hormones: Essays in experimental biology, pp. 175–204 (University of Chicago Press, Chicago 1962).
Scoville, W.B.: Extradural spinal sensory rhizotomy. J. Neurosurg. *25:* 94–95 (1966).
Sedan, R.; Lazorthes, Y.: La neurostimulation électrique thérapeutique. Neuro-chirurgie *24:* suppl. 1, pp. 1–138 (1978).
Sekhar, L.; Heros, R.C.; Kerber, C.W.: Carotid-cavernous fistula following percutaneous retrogasserian procedures. Report of two cases. J. Neurosurg. *51:* 700–706 (1979).
Seltzer, Z.; Devor, M.: Ephaptic transmission in chronically damaged peripheral nerves. Neurology *29:* 1061–1064 (1979).
Sessle, B.J.; Greenwood, L.F.: Inputs to trigeminal brain stem neurones from facial, oral, tooth pulp and pharyngolaryngeal tissues. I. Responses to innocuous and noxious stimuli. Brain Res. *117:* 211–226 (1976).
Shaw, R.S.: Pathologic malingering. The painful disabled extremity. New Engl. J. Med. *271:* 22–26 (1964).
Shealy, C.N.: Percutaneous radiofrequency denervation of spinal facets. Treatment for chronic back pain and sciatica. J. Neurosurg. *43:* 448–451 (1975).
Shealy, C.N.; Mortimer, J.T.; Hagfors, N.R.: Dorsal column electroanalgesia. J. Neurosurg. *32:* 560–564 (1970).
Shealy, C.N.; Mortimer, J.T.; Reswick, J.: Electrical inhibition of pain by stimulation of the dorsal column: preliminary clinical reports. Anesth. Analg. *46:* 489–491 (1967).
Sheer, D.E.: Electrical stimulation of the brain (University of Texas Press, Austin 1961).
Shelden, C.H.: Compression procedure for trigeminal neuralgia: Review and clinical appraisal of ten years' experience. Presented at the 26th Annu. Meet. American Academy of Neurological Surgery, Key Biscayne 1964.
Shelden, C.H.: Depolarization in the treatment of trigeminal neuralgia; in Knighton, Dumke, Pain, pp. 373–386 (Little, Brown, Boston 1966).
Shelden, C.H.; Paul, F.; Jacques, B.; Pudenz, R.H.: Electrical stimulation of the nervous system. Surg. Neurol. *4:* 127–132 (1975).
Shelden, C.H.; Pudenz, R.H.; Freshwater, D.B.; Crue, B.L.: Compression rather than decompression for trigeminal neuralgia. J. Neurosurg. *12:* 123–126 (1955).
Sherwood, A.M.: Biomedical engineering aspects of spinal cord stimulation. Appl. Neurophysiol. *44:* 126–132 (1981).
Shetter, A.G.; Hadley, M.N.: Glycerol gangliolysis for trigeminal neuralgia. Presented at the Am. Pain Society, 6th Gen. Meet., Washington 1986.

Shetter, A.G.; Hadley, M.N.; Wilkinson, E.: Administration of intraspinal morphine sulfate for treatment of intractable cancer pain. Neurosurgery *18:* 740–747 (1986).

Shieff. C.; Nashold, B.S.: Stereotactic mesencephalic tractotomy for thalamic pain. Neurol. Res. *9:* 101–104 (1987).

Shulman, R.; Turnbull, I.M.; Diewold, P.: Psychiatric aspects of thalamic stimulation for neuropathic pain. Pain *13:* 127–135 (1982).

Sicard, R.; Robineau: Algie vélo-pharyngée essentielle. Traitement chirurgical. Revue neurol. *36:* 256–257 (1920).

Siebert, H.: Über Erkrankungen peripherischer Nerven. Mschr. Psychiat. Neurol. *49:* 364–370 (1921).

Siegfried, J.: Stereotactic pulvinarotomy in the treatment of intractable pain. Prog. neurol. Surg., vol. 8, pp. 104–113 (Karger, Basel 1977a).

Siegfried, J.: 500 percutaneous thermocoagulations of the Gasserian ganglion for trigeminal pain. Surg. Neurol. *8:* 126–131 (1977b).

Siegfried, J.: Percutaneous controlled thermocoagulation of Gasserian ganglion in trigeminal neuralgia. Experiences with 1000 cases; in Samii, Jannetta, The cranial nerves, pp. 322–330 (Springer, Berlin 1981).

Siegfried, J.: Long-term results of percutaneous controlled thermocoagulation of Gasserian ganglion in trigeminal neuralgia; in Rizzi, Visentin, Pain therapy, pp. 309–320 (Elsevier, Amsterdam 1983a).

Siegfried, J.: Long-term results of electrical stimulation in the treatment of pain by means of implanted electrodes (epidural spinal cord and deep brain stimulation); in Rizzi, Visentin, Pain therapy, pp. 463–475 (Elsevier, Amsterdam 1983b).

Siegfried, J.: Personal communication (1985).

Siegfried, J.; Comte, P.; Meier, R.: Intracerebral electrode implantation system. J. Neurosurg. *59:* 356 (1983).

Siegfried, J.; Hood, T.: Current status of functional neurosurgery. Adv. Tech. Stand. Neurosurg. *10:* 19–79 (1983).

Siegfried, J.; Krayenbühl, H.: Einige Erfahrungen über die chirurgische Behandlung medikamentös nicht beinflussbarer Schmerzzustände; in Janzen, Keidel, Herz, Steichele, Schmerz: Grundlagen — Pharmakologie — Therapie, pp. 216–218 (Thieme, Stuttgart 1972).

Siegfried, J.; Lazorthes, Y.: Long-term follow-up of dorsal cord stimulation for chronic pain syndrome after multiple lumbar operations. Appl. Neurophysiol. *45:* 201–204 (1982).

Siegfried, J.; Vosmansky, M.: Technique of the controlled thermocoagulation of trigeminal ganglion and spinal roots. Adv. Tech. Stand. Neurosurg. *2:* 199–209 (1975).

Silverberg, G.D.: Hypophysectomy in the treatment of disseminated prostate carcinoma. Cancer *39:* 1727–1731 (1977).

Silverberg, G.D.; Britt, R.H.: Percutaneous radiofrequency rhizotomy in the treatment of trigeminal neuralgia. West. J. Med. *129:* 97–100 (1978).

Simeone, F.A.: The anatomy of the lumbar sympathetic trunks in man (with special reference to the question of regeneration after sympathectomy). J. cardiovasc. Surg. *20:* 283–285 (1979).

Sindou, M.: Etude de la jonction radiculo-médullaire postérieure. La radicellotomie postérieure sélective dans la chirurgie de la douleur; thèse, Lyon (1972).

Sindou, M.; Daher, A.: Spinal cord ablation procedures for pain; in Dubnèr, Gebhart, Bond, Pain research and clinical management, vol. 3, pp. 477–495 (Elsevier, Amsterdam, 1988).

Sindou, M.; Fischer, G.; Goutelle, A.; Mansuy, L.: La radicellotomie postérieure selective. Premiers résultats dans la chirurgie de la douleur. Neuro-chirurgie *20:* 397–408 (1974a).
Sindou, M.; Fischer, G.; Goutelle, A.; Schott, B.; Mansuy, L.: La radicellotomie postérieure sélective dans le traitement des spasticités. Revue neurol. *130:* 201–215 (1974b).
Sindou, M.; Fischer, G.; Mansuy, L.: Posterior spinal rhizotomy and selective posterior rhizidiotomy. Prog. neurol. Surg., vol. 7, pp. 201–250 (Karger, Basel 1976).
Sindou, M.; Goutelle, A.: Surgical posterior rhizotomies for the treatment of pain. Adv. Tech. Stand. Neurosurg. *10:* 147–185 (1983).
Sindou, M.; Keravel, Y.: Thermocoagulation percutanée du trijumeau dans le traitement de la névralgie faciale essentielle. Neuro-chirurgie *25:* 166–172 (1979).
Sindou, M.; Keravel, Y.: Analgésie par la méthode d'électrostimulation transcutanée. Résultats dans les douleurs d'origine neurologique. A propos de 180 cas. Neuro-chirurgie *26:* 153–157 (1980).
Sindou, M.; Keravel, Y.; Abdennebi, B.; Szapiro, J.: Traitement neuro-chirurgical de la névralgie trigéminale. Abord direct ou méthode percutanée? Neuro-chirurgie *33:* 89–111 (1987).
Sindou, M.; Lapras, C.: Neurosurgical treatment of pain in the Pancoast-Tobias syndrome: selective posterior rhizotomy and open anterolateral C2-cordotomy. Adv. Pain Res. Ther. *4:* 199–206 (1982).
Sindou, M.; Mifsud, J.J.; Boisson, D.; Goutelle, A.: Selective posterior rhizotomy in the dorsal root entry zone for treatment of hyperspasticity and pain in the hemiplegic upper limb. Neurosurgery *18:* 587–595 (1986).
Sindou, M.; Quoex, C.; Baleydier, C.: Fiber organization at the posterior spinal cord-rootlet junction in man. J. comp. Neurol. *153:* 15–26 (1974c).
Sjaastad, O.; Dale, I.: A new clinical headache entity 'chronic paroxysmal hemicrania'. Acta neurol. scand. *54:* 140–159 (1976).
Sjöqvist, O.: Studies on pain conduction in the trigeminal nerve. Acta psychiat. neurol., suppl. 17, pp. 1–139 (1938).
Slettebo, H.; Lindegaard, K.F.; Hirschberg, H.: Trigeminal neuralgia treated by glycerol injection. Acta neurochir. *84:* 150 (1987).
Sluijter, M.E.; Mehta, M.: Treatment of chronic back and neck pain by percutaneous thermal lesions; in Lipton, Miles, Persistent pain: modern methods of treatment vol. 3, pp. 141–179 (Academic Press, London/Grune & Stratton, New York 1981).
Smith, F.P.: Trans-spinal ganglionectomy for relief of intercostal pain. J. Neurosurg. *32:* 574–577 (1970).
Smith, G.W.; Miller, J.M.: The treatment of tic douloureux with stilbamidine. Bull. Johns Hopkins Hosp. *96:* 146–149 (1955).
Smith, H.P.; McWhorter, J.M.; Challa, V.R.: Radiofrequency neurolysis in a clinical model. Neuropathological correlation. J. Neurosurg. *55:* 246–253 (1981).
Smolik, E.A.; Nash, F.P.; Machek, O.: Spinal cordectomy in the management of spastic paraplegia. Am. Surg. *26:* 639–645 (1960).
Snyder, R.: The organization of the dorsal root entry zone in cats and monkeys. J. comp. Neurol. *174:* 47–70 (1977).
Sourek, K.: Commissural myelotomy. J. Neurosurg. *31:* 524–527 (1969).
Sourek, K.: Mediolongitudinal myelotomy. Prog. neurol. Surg., vol. 8, pp. 15–34 (Karger, Basel 1977).

Sourek, K.: Central thermomyelo-coagulation for intractable chronic pain and opioid peptides. Presented at the 8th Int. Congr. Neurological Surgery, Toronto 1985, Abstr. 221.

Sourek, K.: Personal communication (1987).

Spalteholz, W.: Handatlas der Anatomie des Menschen, vol. III (Hirzel, Leipzig 1940).

Spiller, W.G.; Frazier, C.H.: The division of the sensory root of the trigeminus for the relief of tic douloureux; an experimental, pathological and clinical study, with a preliminary report of one surgically successful case. Philad. med. J. *8:* 1039–1049 (1901).

Spiller, W.G.; Martin, E.: The treatment of persistent pain of organic origin in the lower part of the body by division of the anterolateral column of the spinal cord. J. Am. med. Ass. *58:* 1489–1490 (1912).

Spurling, R.G.: Causalgia of the upper extremity. Treatment by dorsal sympathetic ganglionectomy. Archs Neurol. Psychiat. *23:* 784–788 (1930).

Steinbusch, H.W.M.: Distribution of serotonin-immunoreactivity in the central nervous system of the rat — cell bodies and terminals. Neuroscience *6:* 557–618 (1981).

Sternbach, R.A.: Letters to the editor. Pain *29:* 257–258 (1987).

Steude, U.: Radiofrequency electrical stimulation of the Gasserian ganglion in patients with atypical trigeminal pain: methods of percutaneous temporary test-stimulation and permanent implantation of stimulation devices. Acta neurochir., suppl. 33, pp. 481–486 (1984).

Stewart, W.A.; King, R.B.: Fiber projections from the nucleus caudalis of the spinal trigeminal nucleus. J. comp. Neurol. *121:* 271–286 (1963).

Stewart, W.A.; Stoops, W.L.; Pillone, P.R.; King, R.B.: An electrophysiologic study of ascending pathways from nucleus caudalis of the spinal trigeminal nuclear complex. J. Neurosurg. *21:* 35–48 (1964).

Stibbe, E.P.: Surgical anatomy of subtentorial angle, with special reference to the acoustic and trigeminal nerves (Hunterian Lecture, abr.). Lancet *i:* 859–862, 918–921 (1939).

Stookey, B.: Further light on the transmission of pain and temperature within the spinal cord: human cordotomy to abolish pain sense without destroying temperature sense. J. nerv. ment. Dis. *69:* 552–557 (1929).

Stookey, B.; Ransohoff, J.: Trigeminal neuralgia. Its history and treatment (Thomas, Springfield 1959).

Storrs, D.G.; King, R.B.: A pharmacologic study of primary afferent preterminal excitability in trigeminal relay nuclei; in Dubner, Kawamura, Orofacial sensory and motor mechanisms, pp. 263–278 (Appleton Century Crofts, New York 1971).

Stowell, A.: The physiological mechanisms and treatment of headache. Trans. Am. neurol. Ass. *88:* 297 (1963).

Strait, T.A.; Hunter, S.E.: Intraspinal extradural sensory rhizotomy in patients with failure of lumbar disc surgery. J. Neurosurg. *54:* 193–196 (1981).

Ström-Olsen, R.; Carlisle, S.: Bifrontal stereotactic tractotomy: a follow-up study of its effects on 210 patients. Br. J. Psychiat. *118:* 141–154 (1971).

Sudeck, P.: Über die acute entzündliche Knochenatrophie. Arch. klin. Chir. *62:* 147–156 (1900).

Sudeck, P.: Die sogenannte akute Knochenatrophie als Entzündungsvorgang. Chirurgie *14:* 449–458 (1942).

Sugita, K.; Mutsuga, N.; Takaoka, Y.; Doi, T.: Results of stereotaxic thalamotomy for pain. Confinia neurol. *34:* 265–274 (1972).

Sugiura, Y.; Lee, C.L.; Perl, E.R.: Central projections of identified, unmyelinated (C) afferent fibers innervating mammalian skin. Science *234:* 358–361 (1986).

Sunderland, S.: Pain mechanisms in causalgia. J. Neurol. Neurosurg. Psychiat. *39:* 471–480 (1976).

Svien, H.J.; Love, J.G.: Results of decompression operation for trigeminal neuralgia four years plus after operation. J. Neurosurg. *16:* 653–655 (1959).

Swanson, S.E.; Farhat, S.M.: Neurovascular decompression with selective partial rhizotomy of the trigeminal nerve for tic douloureux. Surg. Neurol. *18:* 3–6 (1982).

Sweet, W.H.: Trigeminal neuralgias; in Alling, Facial pain, pp. 89–106 (Lea & Febiger, Philadelphia 1968).

Sweet, W.H.: Treatment of medically intractable mental disease by limited frontal leucotomy — justifiable? New Engl. J. Med. *289:* 1117–1125 (1973).

Sweet, W.H.: Recent observations pertinent to improving anterolateral cordotomy. Clin. Neurosurg. *23:* 89–95 (1976a).

Sweet, W.H.: Treatment of facial pain by percutaneous differential thermal trigeminal rhizotomy. Prog. neurol. Surg., vol. 7, pp. 153–179 (Karger, Basel 1976b).

Sweet, W.H.: Control of pain by direct electrical stimulation of peripheral nerves. Clin. Neurosurg. *23:* 103–111 (1976c).

Sweet, W.H.: Animal models of chronic pain: their possible validation from human experience with posterior rhizotomy and congenital analgesia. Pain *10:* 275–295 (1981).

Sweet, W.H.: Cerebral localization of pain; in Thompson, Green, New perspectives in cerebral localization, pp. 205–242 (Raven Press, New York 1982a).

Sweet, W.H.: Commentary: percutaneous rhizotomy; in Schmidek, Sweet, Operative neurosurgical techniques: indications, methods and results, vol. 2, pp. 1101–1106 (Grune & Stratton, New York 1982b).

Sweet, W.H.: Deafferentation pain after posterior rhizotomy, trauma to a limb and herpes zoster. Neurosurgery *15:* 928–932 (1984).

Sweet, W.H.: The history of the development of treatment for trigeminal neuralgia. Clin. Neurosurg. *32:* 294–318 (1985).

Sweet, W.H.: Treatment of trigeminal neuralgia by percutaneous rhizotomy; in Youmans, Neurological surgery; 3rd ed. (Saunders, Philadelphia 1988a).

Sweet, W.H.: Sympathectomy for pain; in Youmans, Neurological surgery; 3rd ed. (Saunders, Philadelphia 1988b).

Sweet, W.H.: Retrogasserian glycerol injection as treatment for trigeminal neuralgia; in Schmidek, Sweet, Operative neurosurgical techniques; 3rd ed., vol. 2, pp. 1129–1137 (Grune & Stratton, New York 1988c).

Sweet, W.H.: Vagoglossopharyngeal neuralgia; in Long, Current therapy in neurological surgery (Decker, Philadelphia 1988d).

Sweet, W.H.; Graham, J.R.; Poletti, C.E.: Surgical treatment of chronic migrainous neuralgia (chronic cluster headache). To be published 1989.

Sweet, W.H.; Mark, V.H.; Hamlin, H.: Radiofrequency lesions in the central nervous system of man and cat: including case reports of eight bulbar pain-tract interruptions. J. Neurosurg. *17:* 213–225 (1960).

Sweet, W.H.; Poletti, C.E.: Retrogasserian glycerol injection as treatment for trigeminal neuralgia; in Schmidek, Sweet, Operative neurosurgical techniques: indications, methods and results, vol. 2, pp. 1107–1117 (Grune & Stratton, New York 1982).

Sweet, W.H.; Poletti, C.E.: Operations in the brain stem and spinal canal with an appendix on open cordotomy; in Wall, Melzack, Textbook of pain, pp. 615–631 (Churchill-Livingstone, Edinburgh 1984a).

Sweet, W.H.; Poletti, C.E.: Appendix: open cervical and thoracic cordotomy; in Wall, Melzack, Textbook of pain, pp. 624–631 (Churchill-Livingstone, Edinburgh 1984b).

Sweet, W.H.; Poletti, C.E.: Problems with retrogasserian glycerol in the treatment of trigeminal neuralgia. Appl. Neurophysiol. *48:* 252–257 (1985).

Sweet, W.H.; Poletti, C.E.: Complications of percutaneous rhizotomy and microvascular decompression operations for facial pain. Section I; in Youmans, Neurological surgery; 3rd ed. (Saunders, Philadelphia 1988).

Sweet, W.H.; Poletti, C.E.; Macon, J.B.: Treatment of trigeminal neuralgia and other facial pains by retrogasserian injection of glycerol. Neurosurgery *9:* 647–653 (1981).

Sweet, W.H.; Poletti, C.E.; Roberts, J.T.: Dangerous rises in blood pressure upon heating of trigeminal rootlets; increased bleeding times in patients with trigeminal neuralgia. Neurosurgery *17:* 843–844 (1985).

Sweet, W.H.; Poletti, C.E.; Umansky, F.: Neurosurgical techniques to control the pain of superior pulmonary sulcus and other tumors in this region. Adv. Pain Res. Ther. *4:* 211–233 (1982).

Sweet, W.H.; Wepsic, J.G.: Treatment of chronic pain by stimulation of fibers of primary afferent neuron. Trans. Am. neurol. Ass. *93:* 103–105 (1968).

Sweet, W.H.; Wepsic, J.G.: Stimulation of the posterior columns of the spinal cord for pain control: indications, technique and results. Clin. Neurosurg. *21:* 278–310 (1974a).

Sweet, W.H.; Wepsic, J.G.: Controlled thermocoagulation of trigeminal ganglion and rootlets for differential destruction of pain fibers. 1. Trigeminal neuralgia. J. Neurosurg. *39:* 143–156 (1974b).

Sweet, W.H.; White, J.C.; Selverstone, B.; Nilges, R.: Sensory responses from anterior roots and from surface and interior of spinal cord in man. Trans. Am. neurol. Ass. *75:* 165–169 (1950).

Swiontek, T.; Maiman, D.; Sances, A.; Myklebust, J.; Larson, S.; Hemmy, D.: Effect of electrical current on temperature and pH in cerebellum and spinal cord. Surg. Neurol. *14:* 365 (1980).

Symonds, C.: A particular variety of headache. Brain *79:* 217–232 (1956).

Taarnhøj, P.: Decompression of the trigeminal root and the posterior part of the ganglion as treatment in trigeminal neuralgia. Preliminary communication. J. Neurosurg. *9:* 288–290 (1952).

Taarnhøj, P.: Decompression of the posterior trigeminal root in trigeminal neuralgia. A 30-year follow-up review. J. Neurosurg. *57:* 14–17 (1982).

Takagi, H.; Satoh, M.; Akaike, A.; Shibata, T.; Yajuma, H.; Ogawa, H.: Analgesia by enkephalins injected into the nucleus reticularis gigantocellularis of the rat medulla oblongata. Eur. J. Pharmacol. *49:* 113–116 (1978).

Takeda, F.; Fujii, T.; Tozawa, R.; Kitani, Y.; Fujita, T.: Endocrinological aspects of transsphenoidal adenohypophyseal neurolysis for cancer pain. 2nd World Congr. IASP, Montreal 1978, abstr., p. 145.

Takusagawa, Y.; Wakiya, K.; Fukushima, T.: Treatment of trigeminal neuralgia by percutaneous gasserian ganglion glycerol injection. Presented at the 8th Int. Congr. of Neurological Surgery, Toronto 1985, abstr., p. 143.

Talairach, J.; Aboulker, J.; Tournoux, P.; David, M.: Technique stéréotaxique de la chirurgie hypophysaire par voie nasale. Suites opératoires — indications thérapeutiques. Neuro-chirurgie *2:* 3–20 (1956).

Tallis, R.C.; Illis, L.S.; Sedgwick, E.M.; Hardwidge, C.; Garfield, J.S.: Spinal cord stimulation in peripheral vascular disease. J. Neurol. Neurosurg. Psychiat. *46:* 478–484 (1983).

Tamsen, A.; Gordh, T.: Epidural clonidine produces analgesia. Lancet *ii:* 231–232 (1984).

Taren, J.A.; Davis, R.; Crosby, E.C.: Target physiologic corroboration in stereotaxic cervical cordotomy. J. Neurosurg. *30:* 569–584 (1969).

Taren, J.A.; Kahn, E.A.: Thoracic anterolateral cordotomy; in Knighton, Dumke, Pain, pp. 299–310 (Little, Brown, Boston 1966).

Tarlov, E.: Posterior fossa surgery for typical trigeminal neuralgia. Presented to the New England Neurosurgical Society, Dedham 1985.

Tasker, R.R.: Thalamotomy for pain: lesion localization by detailed thalamic mapping. Can. J. Surg. *12:* 62–74 (1969).

Tasker, R.R.: Open cordotomy. Prog. neurol. Surg., vol. 8, pp. 1–14 (Karger, Basel 1977).

Tasker, R.R.: Percutaneous cervical cordotomy. Appl. Neurophysiol. *39:* 114–121 (1976/77).

Tasker, R.R.: Thalamic stereotaxic procedures; in Schaltenbrand, Walker, Stereotaxy of the human brain; 2nd ed., pp. 484–497 (Thieme-Stratton, Stuttgart 1982a).

Tasker, R.R.: Percutaneous cordotomy — the lateral high cervical technique; in Schmidek, Sweet, Operative neurosurgical techniques: indications, methods and results, vol. 2, pp. 1137–1153 (Grune & Stratton, New York 1982b).

Tasker, R.R.: Deafferentation; in Wall, Melzack, Textbook of pain, pp. 119–132 (Churchill-Livingstone, Edinburgh 1984).

Tasker, R.R.; Organ, L.W.: Mapping of the somatosensory and auditory pathways in the upper midbrain and thalamus in man; in Somjen, Neurophysiology studied in man, pp. 169–187 (Excerpta Medica, Amsterdam 1972).

Tasker, R.R.; Organ, L.W.; Hawrylyshyn, P.: The sensory organization of the human thalamus. Appl. Neurophysiol. *39:* 137–154 (1977).

Tasker, R.R.; Organ, L.W.; Hawrylyshyn, P.: Deafferentation and causalgia; in Bonica, Pain, pp. 305–329 (Raven Press, New York 1980).

Tasker, R.R.; Organ, L.W.; Hawrylyshyn, P.: The thalamus and midbrain in man. A physiological atlas using electrical stimulation (Thomas, Springfield 1982).

Tasker, R.R.; Richardson, P.; Newcastle, B.; Emmers, R.: Anatomical correlation of detailed sensory mapping of the human thalamus. Confinia neurol. *34:* 184–196 (1972).

Tasker, R.R.; Tsuda, T.; Hawrylyshyn, P.: Clinical neurophysiological investigation of deafferentation pain. Adv. Pain Res. Ther. *5:* 713–738 (1983).

Taub, A.: Opioid analgesics in the treatment of chronic intractable pain of non-neoplastic origin; in Kitahata, Narcotic analgesics in anesthesiology, pp. 199–207 (Williams & Wilkins, New York 1982a).

Taub, A.: Relief of chronic intractable sciatica by dorsal root ganglionectomy. Presented at the Am. Pain Society 3rd, Gen. Meet., Miami 1982b.

Taub, A.: Ganglionectomy lectures presented to the Massachusetts General Hospital 1985.

Taub, A.: Suppression of post-ganglionectomy dysesthesia by systemic lidocaine. Presented to the Am. Pain Society, Washington 1986.

Terman, G.W.; Shavit, Y.; Lewis, J.W.; Cannon, J.T.; Liebeskind, J.C.: Intrinsic mechanisms of pain inhibition: activation by stress. Science *226:* 1270–1277 (1984).

Testut, J.L.: Traité d'anatomie humaine; 3e éd. vol. 1, pp. 1188 (Doin, Paris 1896).

Teuber, H.L.; Corkin, S.; Twitchell, T.E.: A study of cingulotomy in man. Appendix to Psychosurgery. Reports prepared for the National Commission for the Protection of

Human Subjects of Biomedical and Behavioral Research, US Dept. of Health, Education and Welfare, DHEW. Publ. No. (OS) 77-0002, 3: 1-115 (1977).

Tew, J.M.: Percutaneous rhizotomy in the treatment of intractable facial pain (trigeminal, glossopharyngeal and vagal nerves); in Schmidek, Sweet, Current techniques in operative neurosurgery, pp. 409-426 (Grune & Stratton, New York 1977).

Tew, J.M.; Keller, J.T.; Williams, D.S.: Application of stereotactic principles to the treatment of trigeminal neuralgia. Appl. Neurophysiol. *41:* 146-156 (1978).

Tew, J.M.; Tobler, W.D.; Van Loveren, H.: Percutaneous rhizotomy in the treatment of intractable facial pain (trigeminal, glossopharyngeal and vagal nerves); in Schmidek, Sweet, Operative neurosurgical techniques: indications, methods and results, vol. 2, pp. 1083-1106 (Grune & Stratton, New York 1982).

Tew, J.M.; Van Loveren, H.: Percutaneous rhizotomy in the treatment of intractable facial pain (trigeminal, glossopharyngeal, and vagal nerves); in Schmidek, Sweet, Operative neurosurgical techniques; 2nd ed., vol. 2, pp. 111-123 (Grune & Stratton, New York 1988).

Thiébaut, J.-B.; Blond, S.; Farcot, J.-M.; Thurel, C.; Matge, G.; Schach, G.; Meynadier, J.; Buchhiet, F.: La morphine par voie intra-ventriculaire dans le traitement des douleurs néoplasiques. Méd. Hyg. *43:* 636-646 (1985).

Thiry, S.: Expérience personnelle basée sur 225 cas de névralgie essentielle du trijumeau traités par électrocoagulation du ganglion de Gasser entre 1950 et 1962. Neurochirurgie *9:* 86-92 (1962).

Thiry, S.; Hotermans, J.M.: Traitement de la névralgie essentielle du trijumeau par stéréotaxie et électrocoagulation partielle sélective du ganglion de Gasser. Expérience portant sur 365 cas traites entre 1950 et 1970. Neuro-chirurgie *20:* 55-60 (1974).

Thomas, D.G.T.; Jones, S.J.: Dorsal root entry zone lesions (Nashold's procedure) in brachial plexus avulsion. Neurosurgery *15:* 966-968 (1984).

Thompson, J.B.; Greenberg, E.; Pazionos, A.; Pearson, O.H.: Hypophysectomy in metastatic prostate cancer. N.Y. State J. Med. *74:* 1006-1008 (1974).

Thompson, J.E.: The diagnosis and management of posttraumatic pain syndromes (causalgia). Aust. N.Z. J. Surg. *49:* 299-304 (1979).

Thurel, C.: Personal communication (1987).

Tindall, G.T.; Ambrose, S.S.; Christy, J.H.; Patton, J.M.: Hypophysectomy in the treatment of disseminated carcinoma of the breast and prostate gland. Sth. med. J. *69:* 579-583 (1976).

Tindall, G.T.; Payne, N.S.; Nixon, D.W.: Transsphenoidal hypophysectomy for disseminated carcinoma of the prostate gland; Results in 53 patients. J. Neurosurg. *50:* 275-282 (1979).

Tobler, W.D.; Tew, J.M.; Cosman, E.; Keller, J.T.; Quallen, B.: Improved outcome in the treatment of trigeminal neuralgia by percutaneous stereotactic rhizotomy with a new, curved tip electrode. Neurosurgery *12:* 313-317 (1983).

Torebjörk, H.E.; Hallin, R.G.: Responses in human A and C fibers to repeated electrical intradermal stimulation. J. Neurol. Neurosurg. Psychiat. *37:* 653-664 (1974).

Torebjörk, H.E.; Hallin, R.G.: Microneurographic studies of peripheral pain mechanisms in man. Adv. Pain Res. Ther. *3:* 121-131 (1979).

Torvik, A.: Sensory, motor, and reflex changes in two cases of intractable pain after stereotactic mesencephalic tractotomy. J. Neurol. Neurosurg. Psychiat. *22:* 299-305 (1959).

Touati, Y.; Mathieu, J.-P.; Houel, F.; Imbert, P.: Indications actuelles de la sympathectomie dorsale supérieure. A propos de 84 cas. J. Malad. Vasc., Paris *7:* 187–192 (1982).

Tower, S.; Bodian, D.; Howe, H.: Isolation of intrinsic and motor mechanisms of monkey's spinal cord. J. Neurophysiol. *4:* 388–397 (1941).

Trachtenberg, M.C.; Siegfried, J.: Pulvinar contribution to oculomotor and cortical EEG activities; in Cooper, The pulvinar — LP complex, pp. 118–133 (Thomas, Springfield 1973).

Tracy, G.D.; Cockett, F.B.: Pain in the lower limb after sympathectomy. Lancet *i:* 12–14 (1957).

Trowbridge, W.V.; French, J.D.; Bayless, A.E.: Greater superficial petrosal neurectomy for orbito-facial pain: Preliminary report. Neurology *3:* 707–713 (1953).

Truex, R.C.; Taylor, M.J.; Smythe, M.Q.; Gildenberg, P.L.: The lateral cervical nucleus of cat, dog and man. J. comp. Neurol. *139:* 93–104 (1970).

Tsou, K.; Yang, C.S.: Studies on the site of analgesic action of morphine by intracerebral microinjection. Scientia sin. *13:* 1099–1109 (1964).

Tsuboi, M.; Suzuki, K.; Nagao, S.; Nishimoto, A.: Glossopharyngeal neuralgia with cardiac syncope. A case successfully treated by microvascular decompression. Surg. Neurol. *24:* 279–283 (1985).

Tsubokawa, T.; Katayama, Y.; Nishimoto, H.; Kotani, A.; Moriyasu, N.: Emotional slow negative potential shift (CNV) in the thalamus. Appl. Neurophysiol. *39:* 261–267 (1976/77).

Tsubokawa, T.; Katayama, Y.; Yamamoto, T.; Hirayama, T.: Deafferentation pain and stimulation of the thalamic sensory relay nucleus: clinical and experimental study. Appl. Neurophysiol. *48:* 166–171 (1985).

Tsubokawa, T.; Moriyasu, N.: Follow-up results of centre median thalamotomy for relief of intractable pain. Confinia neurol. *37:* 280–284 (1975).

Tsubokawa, T.; Yamamoto, T.; Katayama, Y.; Hirayama, T.; Sibuya, H.: Thalamic relay nucleus stimulation for relief of intractable pain. Clinical results and beta-endorphin immunoreactivity in the cerebrospinal fluid. Pain *18:* 115–126 (1984).

Tsubokawa, T.; Yamamoto, T.; Katayama, Y.; Moriyasu, N.: Clinical results and physiological basis of thalamic relay nucleus stimulation for relief of intractable pain with morphine tolerance. Appl. Neurophysiol. *45:* 143–155 (1982).

Tung, A.S.; Yaksh, T.L.: Evaluation of epidural opiates in the cat. 8th Int. Congr. of Pharmacology, Tokyo 1981, abstr., p. 283.

Tung, A.S.; Yaksh, T.L.; Wang, J.-Y.: Tolerance to intrathecal opiates in the rat. Anesthesiology *55:* A171 (1981).

Turnbull, I.M.; Black, R.G.; Scott, J.W.: Reflex efferent impulses in the trigeminal nerve. J. Neurosurg. *17:* 746–752 (1961).

Turnbull, I.M.; Shulman, R.; Woodhurst, W.B.: Thalamic stimulation for neuropathic pain. J. Neurosurg. *52:* 486–493 (1980).

Uematsu, S.: Percutaneous electrothermocoagulation of spinal nerve trunk, ganglion and rootlets; in Schmidek, Sweet, Operative neurosurgical techniques: indications, methods and results, vol. 2, pp. 1177–1198 (Grune & Stratton, New York 1982).

Uematsu, S.; Konigsmark, B.; Walker, A.E.: Thalamotomy for alleviation of intractable pain. Confinia neurol. *36:* 88–96 (1974a).

Uematsu, S.; Udvarhelyi, G.B.; Benson, D.W.; Siebens, A.A.: Percutaneous radiofrequency rhizotomy. Surg. Neurol. *2:* 319–325 (1974b).

Uhrenholdt, A.; Dam, W.H.; Larsen, O.A.; Lassen, N.A.: Parodoxical effect on peripheral blood flow after sympathetic blockades in patients with gangrene due to arteriosclerosis obliterans. Vasc. Surg. *5:* 154–163 (1971).

Urabe, M.; Tsubokawa, T.: Stereotaxic thalamotomy for the relief of intractable pain. CEM-thalamotomy. Tohoku J. exp. Med. *85:* 286–300 (1965).

Urban, B.J.; Nashold, B.S.: Percutaneous epidural stimulation of the spinal cord for relief of pain. Long-term results. J. Neurosurg. *48:* 323–328 (1978).

Van der Stricht, J.: Signification de la thermométrie cutanée; application à l'étude circulatoire des membres. Journées Angéiologiques de Langues Française, pp. 233–237 (Expansion Scientifique, Paris 1972).

Van Gehuchten, P.; Brucher, J.M.: Sclérose en plaques et névralgie du trijumeau. Revue neurol. *106:* 257–265 (1962).

Van Hees, J.: De C-nociceptor bij de mens en zijn rol in pijnsensatie; thesis, Leuven (1979).

Van Loveren, H.; Tew, J.M.; Keller, J.T.; Nurre, M.A.: A 10-year experience in the treatment of trigeminal neuralgia. Comparison of percutaneous stereotaxic rhizotomy and posterior fossa exploration. J. Neurosurg. *57:* 757–764 (1982).

Van Roost, D.: Die kommissurale Myelotomie in der Schmerzbehandlung: neue Erkentnisse; Doktorarbeit, Bonn (1988).

Varma, T.R.K.; Frazer, A.K.: Exploration of the trigeminal nerve in the posterior fossa for trigeminal neuralgia. J. Neurol. Neurosurg. Psychiat. *47:* 424 (1984).

Ventafridda, V.; Figliuzzi, M.; Tamburini, M.; Gori, E.; Parolaro, D.; Sala, M.: Clinical observation on analgsia elicited by intrathecal morphine in cancer patients. Adv. Pain Res. Ther. *3:* 559–565 (1979).

Verdie, J.C.; Lazorthes, Y.: Thermocoagulation percutanée analgésique des racines rachidiennes. 218 cas. Nouv. Presse méd. *11:* 2131–2134 (1982).

Vieira, J.F.S.; Shieff, C.; Nashold, B.S.; Bullard, D.E.; Cosman, E.: Impedance measurements of the spinal cord of man and animals. Appl. Neurophysiol. *51:* 154–163 (1988).

Vierck, C.J.; Greenspan, J.D.; Ritz, L.A.; Yeomans, D.C.: The spinal pathways contributing to the ascending conduction and the descending modulation of pain sensations and reactions; in Yaksh, Spinal afferent processing, p. 275–329 (Plenum, New York 1986).

Vilkki, J.: Effects of pulvinotomy and ventrolateral thalamotomy on some cognitive functions; in Sweet, Obrador, Martin-Rodriguez, Neurosurgical treatment in psychiatry, pain and epilepsy, pp. 673–677 (University Park Press, Baltimore 1977).

Villanueva, L.; Le Bars, D.: Indirect effects of intrathecal morphine upon diffuse noxious inhibitory controls (DNICs) in the rat. Pain *26:* 233–243 (1986).

Villiger, E.: Brain and spinal cord (Lippincott, Philadelphia 1931).

Vlahovitch, B.; Fuentes, J.-M.: Résultats de la radicellotomie sélective postérieure à l'étage lombaire et cervical. Neuro-chirurgie *21:* 29–42 (1975).

Vogel, H.P.; Heppner, B.; Humbs, N.; Schramm, J.; Wagner, C.: Long-term effects of spinal cord stimulation in chronic pain syndromes. J. Neurol. *233:* 16–18 (1986).

Von Euler, C.; Hayward, J.M.; Martkla, I.; Wyman, R.J.: Respiratory neurons of the ventrolateral nucleus of the solitary tract of cat: vagal input, spinal connections and morphological identification. Brain Res. *61:* 1–22 (1973).

Voris, H.C.: Ipsilateral sensory loss following chordotomy; report of a case. Archs Neurol. Psychiat. *65:* 95–96 (1951).

Voris, H.C.; Whisler, W.W.: Results of stereotaxic surgery for intractable pain. Confinia neurol. *37:* 86–96 (1975).

Vosschulte, K.; Wagner, E.: Splanchnicectomy in chronic pancreatitis. Minn. Med. *53:* 1053–1059 (1970).

Vyklický, L.; Keller, O.; Jastreboff, P.; Vyklický, L., Jr.; Butkhuzi, S.M.: Spinal trigeminal tractotomy and nociceptive reactions evoked by tooth pulp stimulation in the cat. J. Physiol. *73:* 379–386 (1977).

Waisbrod, H.; Gerbershagen, H.U.: Spinal cord stimulation in patients with a battered root syndrome. Arch. Orthop. Trauma Surg. *104:* 62–64 (1985).

Wake, M.; Hitchcock, E.: A review of treatment modalities for periodic migrainous neuralgia. Pain *31:* 345–352 (1987).

Walker, A.E.: The spinothalamic tract in man. Archs Neurol. Psychiat. *43:* 284–298 (1940).

Walker, A.E.: Relief of pain by mesencephalic tractotomy. Archs Neurol. Psychiat. *48:* 865–883 (1942a).

Walker, A.E.: Somatotopic localization of spinothalamic and secondary trigeminal tracts in mesencephalon. Archs Neurol. Psychiat. *48:* 884–889 (1942b).

Walker, A.E.; Nulsen, F.: Electrical stimulation of the upper thoracic portion of the sympathetic chain in man. Archs Neurol. Psychiat. *59:* 559–560 (1948).

Walker, P.M.; Johnston, K.W.: Predicting the success of a sympathectomy: a prospective study using discriminant function and multiple regression analysis. Surgery *87:* 216–221 (1980).

Wall, P.D.: The origin of a spinal cord slow potential. J. Physiol. *164:* 508–526 (1962).

Wall, P.D.: Mechanisms of acute and chronic pain. Adv. Pain Res. Ther. *6:* 95–104 (1984).

Wall, P.D.; Gutnick, M.: Ongoing activity in peripheral nerves: the physiology and pharmacology of impulses originating from a neuroma. Expl Neurol. *43:* 580–593 (1974a).

Wall, P.D.; Gutnick, M.: Properties of afferent nerve impulses originating from a neuroma. Nature, London *248:* 740–743 (1974b).

Wall, P.D.; Noordenbos, W.: Sensory functions which remain in man after complete transection of dorsal columns. Brain *100:* 641–653 (1977).

Wall, P.D.; Scadding, J.W.; Tomkiewicz, M.M.: The production and prevention of experimental anesthesia dolorosa. Pain *6:* 175–182 (1979).

Wall, P.D.; Sweet, W.H.: Temporary abolition of pain in man. Science *155:* 108–109 (1967).

Walsh, J.A.; Glynn, C.J.; Cousins, M.J.; Basedow, R.W.: Blood flow, sympathetic activity and pain relief following lumbar sympathetic blockade or surgical sympathectomy. Anaesth. intens. Care *13:* 18–24 (1984).

Walsh, K.W.: Neuropsychological aspects of modified leucotomy; in Sweet, Obrador, Martin-Rodriguez, Neurosurgical treatment in psychiatry, pain and epilepsy, pp. 163–174 (University Park Press, Baltimore 1977).

Waltz, J.M.: Computerized percutaneous multi-level spinal cord stimulation in motor disorders. Appl. Neurophysiol. *45:* 73–92 (1982).

Waltz, J.M.; Davis, J.A.: Cervical cord stimulation in the treatment of athetosis and dystonia. Adv. Neurol. *37:* 225–237 (1983).

Waltz, T.A.; Dalessio, D.J.; Copeland, B.; Abbott, G.: The treatment of trigeminal neuralgia by the percutaneous placement of glycerol into the trigeminal cistern. Presented to the Am. Ass. of Neurological Surgeons, Dallas 1987.

Waltz, T.A.; Dalessio, D.J.; Ott, K.H.; Copeland, B.; Abbott, G.: Trigeminal cistern glycerol injections for facial pain. Headache *25:* 354–357 (1985).
Wang, J.K.: Intrathecal morphine for intractable pain secondary to cancer of pelvic organs. Pain *21:* 99–102 (1985).
Wang, J.K.; Nauss, L.A.; Thomas, J.E.: Pain relief by intrathecally applied morphine in man. Anesthesiology *50:* 149–151 (1979).
Watkins, L.R.; Mayer, D.J.: Organization of endogenous opiate and non-opiate pain control systems. Science *216:* 1185–1192 (1982).
Watson, C.P.N.; Morley, T.P.; Richardson, J.C.; Schutz, H.; Tasker, R.R.: The surgical treatment of chronic cluster headache. Headache *23:* 289–295 (1983).
Weale, F.E.: Upper thoracic sympathectomy by transthoracic electrocoagulation. Br. J. Surg. *67:* 71–72 (1980).
Weddel, S.J.; Ritter, R.R.: Epidural morphine: serum levels and pain relief. Anesthesiology *53:* S419 (1980).
Weinman, J.: Biphasic stimulation and electrical properties of metal electrodes. J. appl. Physiol. *20:* 787 (1965).
Wepfer, J.: Observationes medico-tracticae de affectibus capitis (Ziegler, Schaffhausen 1727).
Wertheimer, P.; Lecuire, J.: La myélotomie commissurale postérieure. A propos de 107 observations. Acta chir. belg. *6:* 568–574 (1953).
West, C.R.; Avellanosa, A.M.; Bremer, A.M.; Yamada, K.: Hypophysectomy for relief of pain of disseminated carcinoma of the prostate. Adv. Pain Res. Ther. *2:* 393–400 (1979).
Whisler, W.W.; Hill, B.J.: A simplified technique for injection of the Gasserian ganglion, using the fluoroscope for localization. Neurochirurgia *5:* 167–172 (1972).
Whisler, W.W.; Voris, H.C.: Mesencephalotomy for intractable pain due to malignant disease. Appl. Neurophysiol. *41:* 52–56 (1978).
White, J.C.: Spinothalamic tractotomy in the medulla oblongata. Archs Surg. *43:* 113–127 (1941).
White, J.C.: Cordotomy: assessment of its effectiveness and suggestions for its improvement. Clin. Neurosurg. *13:* 1–19 (1966).
White, J.C.; Kjellberg, R.M.: Posterior spinal rhizotomy: a substitute for cordotomy in the relief of localized pain in patients with normal life expectancy. Neurochirurgia *16:* 141–170 (1973).
White, J.C.; Richardson, E.P.; Sweet, W.H.: Upper thoracic cordotomy for relief of pain: post-mortem correlation of spinal incision with analgesic levels in 18 cases. Ann. Surg. *144:* 407–420 (1956).
White, J.C.; Smithwick, R.H.; Simeone, F.A.: The autonomic nervous system (Macmillan, New York 1962).
White, J.C.; Sweet, W.H.: Pain, its mechanisms and neurosurgical control (Thomas, Springfield 1955).
White, J.C.; Sweet, W.H.: Pain and the neurosurgeon. A forty-year experience (Thomas, Springfield 1969).
White, J.C.; Sweet, W.H.: Anterolateral cordotomy: open versus closed comparison of end results. Adv. Pain Res. Ther. *3:* 911–919 (1979).
White, J.C.; Sweet, W.H.; Hawkins, R.; Nilges, R.G.: Anterolateral cordotomy: results, complications and causes of failure. Brain *73:* 346–367 (1950).
Whitehorn, D.; Burgess, P.R.: Changes in polarization of central branches of myelinated mechanoreceptor and nociceptor fibers during noxious and innocuous stimulation of the skin. J. Neurophysiol. *36:* 226–237 (1973).

Whitelaw, G.P.; Smithwick, R.H.: Some secondary effects of sympathectomy with particular reference to disturbance of sexual function. New Engl. J. Med. *245:* 121–130 (1951).

Wiegand, H.; Winkelmüller, W.: Behandlung des Deafferentierungsschmerzes durch Hochfrequenzläsion der Hinterwurzeleintrittszone. Dt. med. Wschr. *110:* 216–220 (1985).

Wiesenfeld, Z.; Lindblom, U.: Behavioral and electrophysiological effects of various types of peripheral nerve lesions in the rats: a comparison of possible models for chronic pain. Pain *8:* 285–298 (1980).

Wilkinson, H.A.: Percutaneous radiofrequency upper thoracic sympathectomy: a new technique. Neurosurgery *15:* 811–814 (1984).

Wilkinson, H.A.: Stereotaxic upper thoracic sympathectomy: a day surgery procedure for hyperhidrosis, Raynaud's causalgia, angina and tachyarrhythmias. J. Neurosurg. (1989) (to be published).

Willer, J.C.; Bussel, B.: Evidence for a direct spinal mechanism in morphine-induced inhibition of nociceptive reflexes in humans. Brain Res. *187:* 212–215 (1980).

Williams, N.E.; Miles, J.B.; Lipton, S.; Hipkin, L.J.; Davis, J.C.: Pain relief and pituitary function following injection of alcohol into the pituitary fossa. Ann. R. Coll. Surg. *62:* 203–207 (1980).

Willis, W.D.: Modulation of primate spinothalamic tract discharges. Adv. Pain Res. Ther. *6:* 217–240 (1984).

Willis, W.D.: The pain system (Karger, Basel 1985).

Wilson, D.H.; Chang, A.E.: Bilateral anterior cingulectomy for the relief of intractable pain. Report of 23 patients. Confinia neurol. *36:* 61–68 (1974).

Winkelmüller, W.: Experience with the control of low back pain by the dorsal column stimulation (DCS) system and by the peridural electrode system (PISCES); in Hosobuchi, Corbin, Indications for spinal cord stimulation, pp. 34–40 (Excerpta Medica, Amsterdam 1981).

Winkler, C.: L'appareil nerveux du nervus trigeminus et celui du nervus octavus; in Manuel de neurologie, vol. 1, part 2, pp. 51–59 (Bohn, Haarlem 1921).

Wirth, F.P.; Rutherford, R.B.: A civilian experience with causalgia. Archs Surg. *100:* 633–638 (1970).

Woolf, C.J.: Intrathecal high dose morphine produces hyperalgesia in the rat. Brain Res. *209:* 491–495 (1981).

Woolsey, C.N.; Erickson, T.C.; Gilson, W.E.: Localization in somatic sensory and motor areas of human cerebral cortex as determined by direct recording of evoked potentials and electrical stimulation. J. Neurosurg. *51:* 476–506 (1979).

Wycis, H.T.; Spiegel, E.A.: Long-range results in the treatment of intractable pain by stereotaxic midbrain surgery. J. Neurosurg. *19:* 101–107 (1962).

Wynn Parry, C.B.: Pain in avulsion lesions of the brachial plexus. Pain *9:* 41–53 (1980).

Wynn Parry, C.B.: Management of pain avulsion lesions of the brachial plexus. Adv. Pain Res. Ther. *5:* 751–761 (1983).

Yakovlev, P.I.; Rakic, P.: Patterns of decussation of bulbar pyramids and distribution of pyramidal tracts on two sides of the spinal cord. Trans. Am. neurol. Ass. *91:* 366–370 (1966).

Yaksh, T.L.: Spinal opiate analgesia: characteristics and principles of action. Pain *11:* 293–346 (1981).

Yaksh, T.L.: In vivo studies on spinal opiate receptor systems mediating antinociception. I. Mu and delta receptor profiles in the primate. J. Pharmac. exp. Ther. *226:* 303–316 (1983).

Yaksh, T.L.: Spinal afferent processing (Plenum Press, New York 1986).

Yaksh, T.L.: Opioid receptor systems and the endorphins: a review of their spinal organization. J. Neurosurg. *67:* 157–176 (1987a).

Yaksh, T.L.: Neurochemical mediators of analgesia in the spinal cord. Pain, suppl. *4,* p. S224 (1987b).

Yaksh, T.L.; Durant, P.A.L.; Granann, D.M.; Stevens, C.W.; Mjanger, E.: The use of receptor-selective agents as analgesics in the spinal cord: Trends and possibilities. J. Pain and Symp. Management *2:* 129–138 (1987).

Yaksh, T.L.; Jessell, T.M.; Gamse, R.; Mudge, A.W.; Leeman, S.E.: Intrathecal morphine inhibits substance P release from mammalian spinal cord in vivo. Nature *286:* 55–57 (1980).

Yaksh, T.L.; Kohl, R.L.; Rudy, T.A.: Induction of tolerance and withdrawal in rats receiving morphine in the spinal subarachnoidal space. Eur. J. Pharmacol. *42:* 275–284 (1977).

Yaksh, T.L.; Onofrio, B.M.: Retrospective consideration of the doses of morphine given intrathecally by chronic infusion in 163 patients by 19 physicians. Pain *31:* 211–223 (1987).

Yaksh, T.L.; Reddy, S.V.R.: Studies in the primate on the analgetic effects associated with intrathecal actions of opiates, α-adrenergic agonists and baclofen. Anesthesiology *54:* 451–467 (1981).

Yaksh, T.L.; Rudy, T.A.: Analgesia mediated by a direct spinal action of narcotics. Science *192:* 1357–1358 (1976).

Yaksh, T.L.; Rudy, T.A.: Narcotic analgetics; C.N.S. sites and mechanisms of action as revealed by intracerebral injection techniques. Pain *4:* 299–360 (1978).

Yamamoto, T.; Iwasaki, Y.; Konno, H.: Experimental sensory ganglionectomy by way of suicide axoplasmic transport. J. Neurosurg. *60:* 108–114 (1984).

Yao, J.S.T.; Bergan, J.J.: Predictability of vascular reactivity relative to sympathetic ablation. Archs Surg. *107:* 676–680 (1973).

Yoshii, N.; Fukuda, S.: Several clinical aspects of thalamic pulvinotomy. Appl. Neurophysiol. *39:* 162–164 (1976/77).

Yoshimasu, N.; Ishijima, B.; Sano, K.: Pain and the internal medullary lamina. 4 autopsy cases. Appl. Neurophysiol. *45:* 498–499 (1982).

Yoshioka, J.; Ueta, K.; Ohmoto, T.; Fujiwara, T.; Tabuchi, K.: Combined trigeminal and glossopharyngeal neuralgia. Surg. Neurol. *24:* 416–420 (1985).

Young, R.F.: Evaluation of dorsal column stimulation in the treatment of chronic pain. Neurosurgery *3:* 373–379 (1978a).

Young, R.F.: Unmyelinated fibers in the trigeminal motor root. J. Neurosurg. *49:* 538–543 (1978b).

Young, R.F.: Effect of trigeminal tractotomy on dental sensation in humans. J. Neurosurg. *56:* 812–818 (1982).

Young R.F.: Personal communication (1987).

Young, R.F.; Brechner, T.: Electrical stimulation of the brain for relief of intractable pain due to cancer. Cancer *57:* 1266–1272 (1986).

Young, R.F.; Chambi, V.I.: Pain relief by electrical stimulation of the periaqueductal and periventricular gray matter. Evidence for a non-opioid mechanism. J. Neurosurg. *66:* 364–371 (1987).

Young, R.F.; Feldman, R.A.; Kroening, R.; Fulton, W.; Morris, J.: Electrical stimulation of the brain in the treatment of chronic pain in man. Adv. Pain Res. Ther. *6:* 289–303 (1984).

Young, R.F.; Kroening, R.; Fulton, W.; Feldman, R.A.; Chambi, I.: Electrical stimulation of the brain in treatment of chronic pain. Experience over 5 years. J. Neurosurg. *62:* 389–396 (1985).

Young, R.F.; Perryman, K.M.: Pathways for orofacial pain sensation in the trigeminal brain-stem nuclear complex of the macaque monkey. J. Neurosurg. *61:* 563–568 (1984).

Yuen, T.G.H.; Agnew, W.R.; Bullara, L.A.; Jasques, S.; McCreery, B.: Histological evaluation of neural damage from electrical stimulation: considerations for the selection of parameters for clinical application. Neurosurgery *9:* 292–299 (1981).

Zervas, N.T.: Technique of radiofrequency hypophysectomy. Confinia neurol. *26:* 157–160 (1965).

Zervas, N.T.: Stereotaxic radiofrequency surgery of the normal and the abnormal pituitary gland. New Engl. J. Med. *280:* 429–437 (1969).

Zorman, G.; Hentall, I.D.; Adams, J.E.; Fields, H.L.: Naloxone-reversible analgesia produced by microstimulation in the rat medulla. Brain Res. *219:* 137–148 (1981).

Zorman, G.; Wilson, C.B.: Outcome following microsurgical vascular decompression or partial sensory rhizotomy in 125 cases of trigeminal neuralgia. Neurology *34:* 1362–1365 (1984).

Subject Index

Author Index